NUTRITION AND HEALTH

Adrianne Bendich, Ph.D., FASN, FACN, Series Editor

More information about this series at http://www.springer.com/series/7659

Elizabeth H. Yen • Amanda Radmer Leonard

Editors

Nutrition in Cystic Fibrosis

A Guide for Clinicians

Humana Press

Editors
Elizabeth H. Yen, M.D.
Department of Pediatrics
Division of Gastroenterology
Hepatology and Nutrition
University of California
San Francisco, CA, USA

Benioff Children's Hospital
San Francisco, CA, USA

Amanda Radmer Leonard, M.P.H., R.D., L.D., C.D.E.
The Johns Hopkins Children's Center
Department of Pediatrics
Division of Gastroenterology and Nutrition
Baltimore, MD, USA

Nutrition and Health
ISBN 978-3-319-16386-4   ISBN 978-3-319-16387-1   (eBook)
DOI 10.1007/978-3-319-16387-1

Library of Congress Control Number: 2015952012

Springer Cham Heidelberg New York Dordrecht London

Humana Press is a brand of Springer
Springer International Publishing AG Switzerland is part of Springer Science+Business Media (www.springer.com)

"We dedicate this book to all patients and families of patients with cystic fibrosis. Their dedication to their care and to the advancement of medicine and science in the field is exemplary and humbling."

Preface

Over the past half-century, advances in the treatment of cystic fibrosis have resulted in remarkable improvements in patients' quality of life and longevity. Nutritional therapies were key early interventions, and remain central to the well-being and survival of patients with cystic fibrosis. The nature of the disease causes significant alterations in a patient's ability to process and assimilate nutrients. Furthermore, many factors contribute to higher metabolic demands throughout a patient's life. In combination, maldigestion, malabsorption, and increased metabolic demands pose a high hurdle for the patient to overcome in order to maintain optimal nutritional status. Yet much data exist demonstrating the importance of good nutrition on outcomes in cystic fibrosis.

The book provides an introduction to cystic fibrosis and nutritional assessments. It also serves as a comprehensive guide to the nutritional monitoring and management of patients with cystic fibrosis, including special populations within cystic fibrosis that require additional considerations.

The book consists of 18 chapters, written by experts in their fields, and includes the most up to date scientific information. The first chapter lays the groundwork for the importance of nutritional status on outcomes. Macronucrient requirements, including how to assess for their absorption and assimilation, are the topic of the second chapter, while the third chapter goes into careful detail about specific fatty acids taking into consideration the altered fatty acid metabolism in cystic fibrosis. The important role of vitamin D in bone health and extra-skeletal co-morbidities, along with management recommendations, are presented, followed by the remainder of the micronutrient considerations in cystic fibrosis.

Cystic fibrosis patients are now living well into their adulthood. Separate chapters on infant, pediatric, and adult nutrition provide guidance for the care of cystic fibrosis patients over the lifespan, followed by a chapter dedicated to nutritional interventions. Complications of cystic fibrosis which impact nutrition are each given their own chapters, each explaining the impact of the complication on nutritional requirements, nutrition assimilation, and methods to overcome these. Nutritional requirements during pregnancy are amplified in cystic fibrosis, and this book dedicates an entire chapter to this special population, there is also a separate chapter on the treatment of patients with SEP in, a condition often neglected due to its milder impact on nutrition, but nonetheless meriting increased nutritional attention over healthy populations. The final chapters of the book address behavioral interventions for improved nutrition, and quality improvement approaches to implement in the clinic aimed at improving the nutritional status at the clinic population level.

Nutrition in Cystic Fibrosis: A Guide for Clinicians is designed as a resource for physicians, nurses, dietitians and other medical providers who deliver care for patients with cystic fibrosis. Students of medicine, nursing, nutrition, as well as professors will find value in this book.

San Francisco, CA, USA   Elizabeth H. Yen
Baltimore, MD, USA   Amanda Radmer Leonard

Series Editor Page

The great success of the Nutrition and Health Series is the result of the consistent overriding mission of providing health professionals with texts that are essential because each includes: (1) a synthesis of the state of the science, (2) timely, in-depth reviews by the leading researchers and clinicians in their respective fields, (3) extensive, up-to-date fully annotated reference lists, (4) a detailed index, (5) relevant tables and figures, (6) identification of paradigm shifts and the consequences, (7) virtually no overlap of information between chapters, but targeted, inter-chapter referrals, (8) suggestions of areas for future research and (9) balanced, data-driven answers to patient as well as health professionals questions which are based upon the totality of evidence rather than the findings of any single study.

The series volumes are not the outcome of a symposium. Rather, each editor has the potential to examine a chosen area with a broad perspective, both in subject matter and in the choice of chapter authors. The international perspective, especially with regard to public health initiatives, is emphasized where appropriate. The editors, whose trainings are both research and practice oriented, have the opportunity to develop a primary objective for their book; define the scope and focus, and then invite the leading authorities from around the world to be part of their initiative. The authors are encouraged to provide an overview of the field, discuss their own research, and relate the research findings to potential human health consequences. Because each book is developed de novo, the chapters are coordinated so that the resulting volume imparts greater knowledge than the sum of the information contained in the individual chapters.

"Nutrition in Cystic Fibrosis: A Guide for Clinicians," edited by Elizabeth H. Yen, M.D. and Amanda R. Leonard, M.P.H., R.D., C.D.E. is a welcome addition to the Nutrition and Health Series. The editors are experts in the care of cystic fibrosis (CF) patients and have significant expertise in the development of nutritional strategies to aid in the growth and development of children diagnosed with CF. They have invited the leaders in the field to develop the 18 relevant, practice-oriented chapters in this unique and clinically valuable volume. Dr. Yen is currently the Associate Director of Clinical Research in the Liver Disease Therapeutic Area at Gilead Sciences. Prior to this position, she served as Assistant Clinical Professor in Pediatric Gastroenterology at the University of California in San Francisco. Amanda R Leonard is an Advanced Nutrition Practitioner at Johns Hopkins Children's Center in Baltimore, MD, where she assesses patients with cystic fibrosis and educates staff, medical students, and the pediatric population on the topic of cystic fibrosis. She also serves as Facilitator in the CF Nutrition Mentoring Program for the Cystic Fibrosis Foundation in Bethesda, MD, where in 2008 she assisted in implementing a full-scale, national nutrition mentoring program.

"Nutrition in Cystic Fibrosis: A Guide for Clinicians" fulfills an unmet need for pediatric and adult pulmonologists and gastroenterologists, residents and fellows, internists, pediatricians, nurses, dietitians, and general practitioners who treat patients with cystic fibrosis by providing data-driven advice concerning the implementation of nutritional interventions to CF patients from infancy to adulthood. The book provides an introduction to cystic fibrosis and nutritional assessments. It serves as a comprehensive guide to the nutritional monitoring and management of patients with cystic fibrosis including special populations with both cystic fibrosis and other medical issues that require additional nutritional considerations. The chapters are written by experts in their fields and include the most up-to-date scientific and clinical information. Nutritional therapies have been key to successful care and remain central to the well-being and survival of patients with cystic fibrosis. The nature of the disease causes significant alterations in a patient's ability to process and assimilate nutrients. Electrolyte balance is a critical issue for the CF patient. Furthermore, many factors contribute to higher caloric needs throughout the patient's life. The volume provides chapters that can answer critical questions for health professionals as well as knowledgeable family members, educators and others involved in the lives of CF patients.

Chapter 1, written by the volume's co-editor, provides a comprehensive overview of cystic fibrosis from an historical perspective and reminds us that CF, although relatively rare, is the most common life-shortening inherited disease in the United States, affecting approximately 30,000 children and adults. In 1989, the gene mutation responsible for causing this recessive disorder was found to be on the gene encoding the cystic fibrosis transmembrane regulator (CFTR), which serves as an ion channel. The defect results in impaired fluid movement through the channel resulting in a dehydrated and thickened mucus layer and decreased function in the tissues and organs where the gene is active. At present, there is neonatal screening for CF and major advances have been made in the treatment of the adverse nutritional and other effects of this disease. Key effects of the disease include increased energy expenditure, small for age, loss of pancreatic enzyme production resulting in incomplete absorption of fats, and pulmonary dysfunction resulting in the inability to breathe in deeply, greater risk of infections and significantly lowered forced expiratory lung volume. Chapter 2 reviews the studies to determine the energy requirements for CF patients and also to provide guidance to healthcare providers concerning the sources of the calories (useful tables are included). This chapter also presents an historical analysis of the development of recommendations for both macro and micronutrients in addition to antioxidants. The importance of pancreatic enzyme replacement therapy (PERT) and its development are discussed. Increased caloric intake compared to age and sex-matched children is required for CF patients especially during the growth years. High fat diets that include essential fatty acids and high protein diets containing certain amino acids including taurine, essential amino acids, and fiber-rich complex carbohydrates are recommended. The next chapter, Chapter 3, follows logically and contains an extensive review of the importance of fats in the diet of CF patients. The reader is guided through the terminology used to describe dietary fats, their metabolism and the physiological effects of different fats and fatty acids. There is a detailed description of fatty acid metabolism and the importance of providing sufficient essential fatty acids especially linoleic acid in the CF patient's diet.

Chapter 4 examines the critical role of vitamin D in the bone development of CF patients. The chapter integrates clinical practice with the underlying science. CF-related bone disease, including osteoporosis, osteopenia, and/or fractures, is the second most prevalent co-morbidity in patients with CF. Adequate intake and absorption of the fat-soluble vitamin D is also important in reducing the risk of lung impairment, inflammation, diabetes, and depression that are often seen in CF. Likewise, in addition to vitamin D, other factors such as vitamin K, calcium, and physical activity are major nutrition-related contributors to bone health in CF. The author notes the importance of bone heath for the CF patients and emphasizes the importance of optimizing bone mineral density, as bone disease contributes to increased fracture risk, impaired lung function, and exclusion for lung transplant candidacy. Chapter 5 continues the discussion of the essential micronutrient requirements for CF patients. The chapter includes a review of the many reasons for low vitamin (both fat soluble and water soluble vitamins) and mineral levels in CF patients including maldigestion and malabsorption, inadequate dietary intake, inadequate adherence to therapy, incorrect use of supplements and PERT, drug–nutrient interactions, and/or medical challenges, such as bowel resection or liver disease. Sodium chloride is central both to the diagnosis and to the care of persons who have CF. Of importance is the additional requirements for women of childbearing potential with CF who are also taking oral contraceptives that are known to increase the need for folate and certain other vitamins. There are excellent tables included in the chapter that outline the nutritional content of vitamin supplements that are formulated to meet the needs of the CF patient and meet the recommendations of the International CF Foundation. Also included is a comprehensive review of each of the critical micronutrients and over 150 relevant references.

The next three chapters examine the effects of CF in the infant, in the child from age 2 to 20, and in adults. Chapter 6 describes the critical needs of the infant diagnosed with CF during the first few weeks of life and through 2 years of age. As indicated above, there is an increased requirement for calories and fats in CF infants compared to age-matched infants who do not have CF. This requirement is difficult to reach as pancreatic insufficiency is seen in up to 60 % of infants with CF diagnosed through newborn screening and increases to over 90 % of children diagnosed within the first year of life. The chapter describes the studies of dosing with PERT and its importance in helping to maintain infant growth. The importance of the trained CF Registered Dietitian is stressed as is the need for frequent weight assessments during infancy. This practice-oriented chapter provides detailed discussions of the CF Foundation Consensus Guidelines recommendations for the care of the CF infant. Chapter 7 contains a detailed description of the clinic nutrition evaluation for individuals with CF who are 2–20 years of age. Children with CF can have several complications that can adversely affect their attainment of sufficient nutrients for growth. Some of these conditions that are addressed in the chapter include maldigestion with resultant malabsorption secondary to pancreatic insufficiency; intestinal resection due to meconium ileus, poorly controlled CF-related diabetes, and impaired bile flow in cases of severe CF-related liver disease as well recurrent pulmonary infections and increased oxidative stress, fevers, and increased metabolic rates. The 11 detailed tables included in the chapter provide valuable guidelines for the assessment of the nutritional status of the CF patient during these years of growth and sexual maturation. Chapter 8 reviews the continued need to monitor the nutritional status of adults with CF to reduce the risk of malnutrition. There are discussions concerning diet, clinical assessment, pancreatic enzyme status, vitamin and mineral supplementation, gradual loss of lung function, reduced bone health, and diabetes that results from deterioration of the pancreas and gastroesophageal reflux. CF patients are living longer (average over 40 years) than ever before and are experiencing new non-respiratory illness such as diabetes, osteoporosis, overweight and obesity, and reproductive concerns. The chapter examines these relatively new issues for adult CF patients and refers to current CF Foundation and other national assessment guidelines.

The ninth chapter concentrates on the nutritional care of CF patients who experience weight loss or growth faltering. The nutrition interventions reviewed include increasing energy intake from solid food, oral supplements, and/or enteral feeding; use of appetite stimulants and parenteral nutrition are also reviewed. Behavioral strategies to increase calories without increasing food/beverage volume (boosting) that are considered to be central to optimizing energy intake in children are reviewed in detail. The use of supplemental tube feedings and the clinical studies that examined the effects on lung function are objectively evaluated. The mechanisms of action and the efficacy of several appetite stimulant drugs as well as the uses of parenteral nutrition are discussed.

Four chapters examine the effects of the major co-morbidities often seen in CF patients. Chapter 10 reviews the importance of both the exocrine and endocrine functions of the pancreas and concentrates on the development of pancreatic insufficiency, links to the genetic defect causing CF, and consequences of pancreatic insufficiency, historic development of PERT and the modern screening methods for pancreatic insufficiency that are currently available. We learn that the cystic fibrosis transmembrane regulator (CFTR) protein is expressed in the exocrine ducts of the pancreas, where it allows water and ions to enter the ducts. When there is a genetic defect in the receptor in the pancreas, duct fluid is reduced resulting in a concentration of proteins and eventual obstruction leading to pancreatic damage and fibrosis. Depending on the genetic defect, these injuries can begin in utero, and at birth the pancreas can be severely damaged. Pancreatic insufficiency (PI) is defined as greater than 85 % loss of pancreatic enzyme function, and therefore CF patients can have a greater than 50 % loss of function and still not be considered pancreatic insufficient, but would benefit from PERT. The assessment tests for pancreatic function are reviewed and compared for efficacy and the chapter contains over 100 relevant references.

In addition to the pancreas, the liver is a second organ that is adversely affected by CF. Chapter 11 reviews the disorders that occur in the liver as a result of CF nutritional deficiencies and discusses the management of cholestasis and cirrhosis, the two liver diseases in CF that directly affect nutritional status. Neonatal cholestasis results in significant decrease in bile formation with further reduction in fat absorption beyond that seen with decreased pancreatic enzyme formation. Fat soluble vitamin deficiencies, especially vitamin E deficiency, may also occur. Liver cirrhosis is discussed in detail and secondary effects are enumerated as are the nutritional consequences that may be seen in the CF patient with cirrhosis. Nutritional recommendations are included for these diseases. There is also a discussion of the nutritional role of hepatic steatosis. Both the pancreas and the liver communicate with the gastrointestinal (GI) system that is the site of nutrient absorption, formation of hormones that control eating behavior and movement of dietary components through the GI tract.

Chapter 12 examines the effects of the mutation of the CFTR in the GI tract and its adverse effects on the movement of chloride and bicarbonate across the epithelial cell membrane, altered luminal physiology with dehydrated mucus, altered pH, immune deficiency, nutrient malabsorption, and small bowel bacterial overgrowth. As a consequence of these pathological changes, diseases of the esophagus, stomach, small intestine, and colon are not uncommon in patients with CF. The chapter includes a detailed discussion of the importance of the new CFTR potentiator drug, ivacaftor and its benefit to improvements in GI functions for the CF patient. Also, there are reviews of the effects of CF on the small and large intestine. The fourth chapter that deals with comorbid conditions reviews the development of diabetes in the CF patient. Chapter 13 describes the development and consequences of Cystic Fibrosis Related Diabetes Mellitus (CFRD). CFRD is a unique form of diabetes that has both a different cause and natural history than seen with either type 1 or type 2 diabetes mellitus. CFRD requires a different approach to nutritional therapy. Patients with CFRD require insulin, yet must continue to consume high fat, high calorie diets that can be difficult as they must also be aware of their carbohydrate intakes. Lung function is directly linked to control of CFRD. The chapter includes practice-oriented details concerning insulin use, nutritional recommendations with and without acute illnesses, insulin therapy with enteral and total parenteral nutrition, pregnancy issues, and other relevant topics.

Chapter 14 provides a unique perspective on the critical importance of the nutritional status of the CF patient prior to and following lung transplant surgery. We learn that for CF patients, respiratory failure is the main cause of mortality. Lung transplantation can provide a survival advantage and improved quality of life. Optimizing nutritional status prior to transplantation can improve post-transplant outcomes; however, this is challenging. CF patients have been shown to have improvements in nutritional status after lung transplantation, however, they face multiple unique nutritional challenges that are reviewed in this chapter. Indications and contraindications for transplant and other valuable practice-related guidelines are tabulated. Chapter 15 also examines the effects of CF during the unique time of pregnancy. The chapter discusses the CF-related nutrition issues during pre-pregnancy, pregnancy, post-pregnancy, and breast-feeding. Specific areas discussed in the chapter include vitamin/mineral supplementation, GI issues affecting intake and absorption, weight gain, diabetes, and other medications. Women with CF who become pregnant are at a higher risk of gestational diabetes and screening starting at 8–10 weeks gestation is recommended. Women with CF who have diabetes prior to conception should be closely monitored to optimize blood sugar control.

The chapter includes detailed information concerning individual vitamin requirements as well as strategies for improving the intake of the added caloric needs during pregnancy.

Although the vast majority of CF patients suffer from pancreatic insufficiency that usually develops at birth through adolescence, there are CF patients who are pancreatic enzyme sufficient (PS) and Chapter 16 examines the needs of this population. Generally, PS is associated with milder CFTR phenotypes and better nutritional status. However, persons with CF PS often have gastrointestinal and/or nutritional problems including overweight and obesity. PS patients should be tested for exocrine PI annually and especially if there is evidence of pancreatic dysfunction such as diarrhea due to malabsorption, steatorrhea, abdominal pain, or weight loss. CF PS patients are at increased risk of acute pancreatitis compared to pancreatic enzyme insufficient CF patients and careful monitoring is required.

The second to last chapter of this highly informative volume includes an in-depth discussion of the role of behavioral therapy in helping clinicians respond to CF children and their parents as they attempt to reach the difficult nutritional goals associated with CF. Chapter 17 reviews the studies that have demonstrated the effectiveness of combined behavioral nutrition interventions in helping parents of children with CF manage disruptive child behaviors and promote increased energy intake and weight. Key behavioral components reviewed include monitoring energy intake, setting calorie goals and providing timely feedback, and educating and coaching parents in the use of child behavioral management strategies to promote improved behavior at mealtimes and acceptance of new foods. Inclusion of anticipatory guidance about feeding challenges and early empirically informed assessment and intervention are needed to reduce the risks of growth deficits. The authors provide examples of behavioral programs that have been shown to have efficacy with young CF children. One example is a program called Be-In-CHARGE where parents are taught several child behavioral management strategies and how to apply them at meals. Examples include how to effectively use parent attention to encourage increased energy intake and behavioral cooperation, setting specific action-oriented goals for each meal as a way to gradually increase calories over time, and tracking calories to monitor intake patterns and providing feedback toward progress with goals. Chapter 18 reviews the role of quality improvement (QI) in CF treatment strategies. The chapter reviews the value of initiating a set of quality standards for care that include patient registries, benchmarking projects, patient and family involvement and care team education in improvement methods. The chapter author, who is also the volume's co-editor, suggests that implementing nutrition quality improvement projects using a standardized approach can also potentially improve nutrition outcomes. An aspect of QI that has been of great help globally is the development of patient registries. In the USA, the CF Foundation began its registry in 1966 and tracks not only survival, but also more than 300 unique variables and can be used to identify variability and measure outcomes. Registries have been used to extract nutrition-related data and have improved patient life expectancies by increasing fat intake, as one example. The chapter includes detailed discussions of a number of successful QI programs that have resulted in improved nutritional status in CF patients.

The above description of the volume's 18 chapters attests to the depth of information provided by the 27 well-recognized and respected chapter authors. Each chapter includes complete definitions of terms with the abbreviations fully defined for the reader and consistent use of terms between chapters. The volume includes over 60 detailed tables and informative figures, an extensive, detailed index and more than 1350 up-to-date references that provide the reader with excellent sources of worthwhile information. Thus, the volume provides a broad base of knowledge concerning the physiology and pathology associated with CF and nutritionally relevant interventions that can enhance the potential for the patient's more healthful life.

In conclusion, "Nutrition in Cystic Fibrosis: A Guide for Clinicians," edited by Elizabeth H. Yen, M.D. and Amanda R. Leonard, M.P.H., R.D., C.D.E., provides health professionals in many areas of research and practice with the most up-to-date, well-referenced volume on the importance of maintaining the nutritional status of the CF patient from the day of diagnosis through the remainder of their lifetime. The volume chapters carefully document the critical value of medical nutrition evaluation by a specialized CF dietitian/nutritionist as part of the overall CF team; review the treatment support and management of CF patients who often have additional chronic diseases, such as diabetes and organ failures including the lung and/or liver. Each of the conditions is covered in depth in individual chapters. Unique chapters examine the nutritional requirements for the CF patient who undergoes lung transplant, or pregnancy, or has sufficient pancreatic enzyme capacity but is at increased risk of other nutrition-related complications. This volume will serve the reader as the benchmark in this complex area of interrelationships between diet, nutritional and enzyme supplements and the specific treatments required to optimize the GI tract, liver and pancreatic functions to help assure the nutritional status of the CF patient. Moreover, these physiological and pathological interactions are clearly delineated so that medical students, nurses, dietitians as well as practitioners can better understand the complexities of these interactions. Unique chapters that examine the importance of behavioral modification and the use of quality standards to improve patient adherence to nutritional therapies are included. These provide the health professionals involved in the treatment of CF patients with the enhanced capability of understanding the potential to improve CF patient outcomes. The editors are applauded for their efforts to develop the most authoritative resource in the field to date and this excellent text is a very welcome addition to the Nutrition and Health Series.

Morristown, NJ, USA   Adrianne Bendich, Ph.D., F.A.C.N., F.A.S.N.

About Series Editor

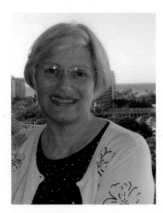

Dr. Adrianne Bendich, Ph.D., F.A.S.N., F.A.C.N. has served as the "Nutrition and Health" Series Editor for 20 years and has provided leadership and guidance to more than 200 editors who have developed the 70+ well-respected and highly recommended volumes in the Series.

In addition to *Nutrition in Cystic Fibrosis: A Guide for Clinicians*, edited by Elizabeth H. Yen, M.D. and Amanda R. Leonard, M.P.H., R.D., C.D.E., major new editions published in 2012–2016 include:

1. *Preventive Nutrition: The Comprehensive Guide For Health Professionals, Fifth Edition*, edited by Adrianne Bendich, Ph.D. and Richard J. Deckelbaum, M.D., 2016
2. *Glutamine in Clinical Nutrition*, edited by Rajkumar Rajendram, Victor R. Preedy, and Vinood B. Patel, 2015
3. *Nutrition and Bone Health, Second Edition*, edited by Michael F. Holick and Jeri W. Nieves, 2015
4. *Branched Chain Amino Acids in Clinical Nutrition, Volume 2*, edited by Rajkumar Rajendram, Victor R. Preedy, and Vinood B. Patel, 2015
5. *Branched Chain Amino Acids in Clinical Nutrition, Volume 1*, edited by Rajkumar Rajendram, Victor R. Preedy, and Vinood B. Patel, 2015
6. *Fructose, High Fructose Corn Syrup, Sucrose and Health*, edited by James M. Rippe, 2014
7. *Handbook of Clinical Nutrition and Aging, Third Edition*, edited by Connie Watkins Bales, Julie L. Locher, and Edward Saltzman, 2014
8. *Nutrition and Pediatric Pulmonary Disease*, edited by Dr. Youngran Chung and Dr. Robert Dumont, 2014
9. *Integrative Weight Management*, edited by Dr. Gerald E. Mullin, Dr. Lawrence J. Cheskin, and Dr. Laura E. Matarese, 2014

10. *Nutrition in Kidney Disease, Second Edition*, edited by Dr. Laura D. Byham-Gray, Dr. Jerrilynn D. Burrowes, and Dr. Glenn M. Chertow, 2014

11. *Handbook of Food Fortification and Health, Volume I*, edited by Dr. Victor R. Preedy, Dr. Rajaventhan Srirajaskanthan, and Dr. Vinood B. Patel, 2013

12. *Handbook of Food Fortification and Health, Volume II*, edited by Dr. Victor R. Preedy, Dr. Rajaventhan Srirajaskanthan, and Dr. Vinood B. Patel, 2013

13. *Diet Quality: An Evidence-Based Approach, Volume I*, edited by Dr. Victor R. Preedy, Dr. Lan-Ahn Hunter, and Dr. Vinood B. Patel, 2013

14. *Diet Quality: An Evidence-Based Approach, Volume II*, edited by Dr. Victor R. Preedy, Dr. Lan-Ahn Hunter, and Dr. Vinood B. Patel, 2013

15. *The Handbook of Clinical Nutrition and Stroke*, edited by Mandy L. Corrigan, M.P.H., R.D., Arlene A. Escuro, M.S., R.D., and Donald F. Kirby, M.D., F.A.C.P., F.A.C.N., F.A.C.G., 2013

16. *Nutrition in Infancy, Volume I*, edited by Dr. Ronald Ross Watson, Dr. George Grimble, Dr. Victor Preedy, and Dr. Sherma Zibadi, 2013

17. *Nutrition in Infancy, Volume II*, edited by Dr. Ronald Ross Watson, Dr. George Grimble, Dr. Victor Preedy, and Dr. Sherma Zibadi, 2013

18. *Carotenoids and Human Health*, edited by Dr. Sherry A. Tanumihardjo, 2013

19. *Bioactive Dietary Factors and Plant Extracts in Dermatology*, edited by Dr. Ronald Ross Watson and Dr. Sherma Zibadi, 2013

20. *Omega 6/3 Fatty Acids*, edited by Dr. Fabien De Meester, Dr. Ronald Ross Watson, and Dr. Sherma Zibadi, 2013

21. *Nutrition in Pediatric Pulmonary Disease*, edited by Dr. Robert Dumont and Dr. Youngran Chung, 2013

22. *Magnesium and Health*, edited by Dr. Ronald Ross Watson and Dr. Victor R. Preedy, 2012.

23. *Alcohol, Nutrition and Health Consequences*, edited by Dr. Ronald Ross Watson, Dr. Victor R. Preedy, and Dr. Sherma Zibadi, 2012

24. *Nutritional Health, Strategies for Disease Prevention, Third Edition*, edited by Norman J. Temple, Ted Wilson, and David R. Jacobs, Jr., 2012

25. *Chocolate in Health and Nutrition*, edited by Dr. Ronald Ross Watson, Dr. Victor R. Preedy, and Dr. Sherma Zibadi, 2012

26. *Iron Physiology and Pathophysiology in Humans*, edited by Dr. Gregory J. Anderson, and Dr. Gordon D. McLaren, 2012

Earlier books included *Vitamin D, Second Edition* edited by Dr. Michael Holick; *Dietary Components and Immune Function* edited by Dr. Ronald Ross Watson, Dr. Sherma Zibadi, and Dr. Victor R. Preedy; *Bioactive Compounds and Cancer* edited by Dr. John A. Milner and Dr. Donato F. Romagnolo; *Modern Dietary Fat Intakes in Disease Promotion* edited by Dr. Fabien De Meester, Dr. Sherma Zibadi, and Dr. Ronald Ross Watson; *Iron Deficiency and Overload* edited by Dr. Shlomo Yehuda and Dr. David Mostofsky; *Nutrition Guide for Physicians* edited by Dr. Edward Wilson, Dr. George A. Bray, Dr. Norman Temple, and Dr. Mary Struble; *Nutrition and Metabolism* edited by Dr. Christos Mantzoros and *Fluid and Electrolytes in Pediatrics* edited by Leonard Feld and Dr. Frederick Kaskel. Recent volumes include: *Handbook of Drug–Nutrient Interactions* edited by Dr. Joseph Boullata and Dr. Vincent Armenti; *Probiotics in Pediatric Medicine* edited by Dr. Sonia Michail and Dr. Philip Sherman; *Handbook of Nutrition and Pregnancy* edited by Dr. Carol Lammi-Keefe, Dr. Sarah Couch, and Dr. Elliot Philipson; *Nutrition and Rheumatic Disease* edited by Dr. Laura Coleman; *Nutrition and Kidney Disease* edited by Dr. Laura Byham-Grey, Dr. Jerrilynn Burrowes, and Dr. Glenn Chertow; *Nutrition and Health in Developing Countries* edited by Dr. Richard Semba and Dr. Martin Bloem; *Calcium in Human Health* edited by Dr. Robert Heaney and Dr. Connie Weaver and *Nutrition and Bone Health* edited by Dr. Michael Holick and Dr. Bess Dawson-Hughes.

Dr. Bendich is President of Consultants in Consumer Healthcare LLC, and is the editor of ten books including *Preventive Nutrition: The Comprehensive Guide for Health Professionals, Fifth Edition* co-edited with Dr. Richard Deckelbaum (www.springer.com/series/7659). Dr. Bendich serves on the Editorial Boards of the Journal of Nutrition in Gerontology and Geriatrics, and Antioxidants, and has served as Associate Editor for "Nutrition" the International Journal; served on the Editorial Board of the Journal of Women's Health and Gender-based Medicine, and served on the Board of Directors of the American College of Nutrition.

Dr. Bendich was Director of Medical Affairs at GlaxoSmithKline (GSK) Consumer Healthcare and provided medical leadership for many well-known brands including TUMS and Os-Cal. Dr. Bendich had primary responsibility for GSK's support for the Women's Health Initiative (WHI) intervention study. Prior to joining GSK, Dr. Bendich was at Roche Vitamins Inc. and was involved with the groundbreaking clinical studies showing that folic acid-containing multivitamins significantly reduced major classes of birth defects. Dr. Bendich has co-authored over 100 major clinical research studies in the area of preventive nutrition. She is recognized as a leading authority on antioxidants, nutrition and immunity and pregnancy outcomes, vitamin safety and the cost-effectiveness of vitamin/mineral supplementation.

Dr. Bendich received the Roche Research Award, is a *Tribute to Women and Industry* Awardee, and was a recipient of the Burroughs Wellcome Visiting Professorship in Basic Medical Sciences. Dr. Bendich was given the Council for Responsible Nutrition (CRN) Apple Award in recognition of her many contributions to the scientific understanding of dietary supplements. In 2012, she was recognized for her contributions to the field of clinical nutrition by the American Society for Nutrition and was elected a Fellow of ASN. Dr Bendich is Adjunct Professor at Rutgers University. She is listed in Who's Who in American Women.

About Volume Editors

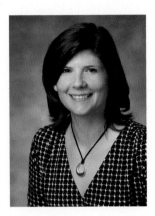

Amanda Radmer Leonard, M.P.H., R.D./L.D., C.D.E. is an Advanced Nutrition Practitioner at The Johns Hopkins Children's Center in Baltimore, M.D., where she assesses patients with cystic fibrosis and educates staff, medical students, and the pediatric population on the topic of cystic fibrosis. She has been at Hopkins since 1997. Prior to this, she worked as a pediatric dietitian at Tulane Hospital for Children in New Orleans, L.A. Ms. Leonard also serves as Facilitator in the CF Nutrition Mentoring Program for the Cystic Fibrosis Foundation in Bethesda, M.D., where in 2008 she assisted in implementing a full-scale, national nutrition mentoring program. She earned her bachelor's degree in dietetics and nutritional science from the University of Delaware in Newark and went on to get her master's of public health in nutrition from the Tulane School of Public Health and Tropical Medicine in New Orleans, L.A. She is actively involved in several professional societies including the American Dietetic Association, the ADA Pediatric Nutrition Practice group, and the Cystic Fibrosis Foundation Conference Planning Committee. Ms. Leonard has published several articles in peer-reviewed journals including the *Journal of Pediatrics*, the *Journal of Cystic Fibrosis*, and the *Journal of Pediatric Psychology*. She has given more than two dozen national and international presentations on the topic of nutrition, namely nutrition for pediatrics, diabetes, and for patients with cystic fibrosis, at conferences such as the North American Cystic Fibrosis Conference, the Brazilian Cystic Fibrosis Congress and the American Dietetic Association Food and Nutrition Expo.

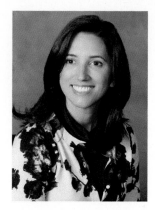

Elizabeth H. Yen, M.D. is a Board Certified Pediatric Gastroenterologist who specializes in the gastrointestinal and nutritional care of children with cystic fibrosis and University of California, San Francisco, Benioff Children's Hospital. Prior to joining UCSF, Dr. Yen worked at Boston Children's Hospital. She completed her training in Pediatric Gastroenterology at Boston Children's Hospital and Harvard Medical School. Prior to that, Dr. Yen completed her residency training in Pediatrics at the University of Washington. She received her medical degree from Weill Cornell Medical College. Her research has focused on nutrition in cystic fibrosis. Dr. Yen has authored several articles in peer reviewed journals including *Journal of Pediatrics, the Journal of Pediatric Gastroenterology and Nutrition, Journal of Cell Biology, and Molecular Biology of the Cell.* She has received grant funding from the National Institutes of Health and the Cystic Fibrosis Foundation.

Contents

Contributors

Jessica A. Alvarez, Ph.D., R.D. Division of Endocrinology, Metabolism, and Lipids Emory University School of Medicine, Atlanta, GA, USA

Molly Bozic, M.D. Pediatric Gastroenterology, Riley Hospital for Children, Indianapolis, IN, USA

Michelle Brotherwood, R.D., C.D.E. Pulmonary, Children's Hospital Los Angeles, Los Angeles, CA, USA

Kristin J. Brown, M.S., R.D., C.N.S.C. Children's Hospital Colorado, Aurora, CO, USA

Jaclyn Brownlee, R.D., C.N.S.C. Department of Nutrition and Food Service, UCSF Benioff Children's Hospital, San Francisco, San Francisco, CA, USA

Carol Brunzell, R.D., L.D., C.D.E. Diabetes Care Centers, University of Minnesota Health, Fairview, Minneapolis, MN, USA

Elissa Downs, M.D., M.P.H. Department of Pediatric Gastroenterology, Hepatology, and Nutrition, University of Minnesota Medical Center, Minneapolis, MN, USA

Stephanie S. Filigno, Ph.D. Division of Behavioral Medicine and Clinical Psychology, Cincinnati Children's Hospital Medical Center, Cincinnati, OH, USA

Judith A. Fulton, M.P.H., R.D., L.D.N. Clinical Nutrition, Children's Hospital Colorado, University of Colorado, Cystic Fibrosis Center, Aurora, CO, USA

Daniel Gelfond, M.D. WNY Pediatric Gastroenterology, Batavia, NY, USA

University of Rochester Medical Center, Rochester, NY, USA

Amanda Radmer Leonard, M.P.H., R.D., C.D.E. The Johns Hopkins Children's Center, Department of Pediatrics, Division of Gastroenterology and Nutrition, Baltimore, MD, USA

Cathy Lingard, R.D. Children's Hospital Colorado, Aurora, CO, USA

Evans Machogu, M.B.Ch.B., M.S. Section of Pediatric Pulmonology, Allergy, and Sleep Medicine, Indiana University Health, Indianapolis, IN, USA

Karen Maguiness, M.S., R.D., C.S.P. Pediatric Pulmonology, Riley Hospital for Children, Indianapolis, IN, USA

Asim Maqbool, M.D. Gastroenterology, Hepatology and Nutrition, The Children's Hospital of Philadelphia, University of Pennsylvania Perelman School of Medicine, Philadelphia, PA, USA

Maria R. Mascarenhas, M.B.B.S. Division of Gastroenterology, Hepatology and Nutrition, Children's Hospital of Philadelphia, Philadelphia, PA, USA

Perelman School of Medicine University of Pennsylvania, Philadelphia, PA, USA

Catherine M. McDonald, Ph.D., R.D.N. Division of Pediatric Gastroenterology, Department of Pediatrics, Primary Children's Hospital, University of Utah, Salt Lake City, UT, USA

Suzanne H. Michel, M.P.H., R.D., L.D.N. Pulmonary Medicine, Medical University of South Carolina, Folly Beach, SC, USA

Tami Miller, R.D., C.S.P., C.D. Cystic Fibrosis Program, Children's Hospital of Wisconsin, Milwaukee, WI, USA

Donna H. Mueller, Ph.D., R.D. F.A.D.A., L.D.N., F.C.P.P. Department of Nutrition Sciences, Drexel University, Philadelphia, Pennsylvania, USA

Michael R. Narkewicz, M.D. Children's Hospital Colorado, Aurora, CO, USA

Section of Pediatric Gastroenterology, Hepatology and Nutrition, Department of Pediatrics, University of Colorado School of Medicine, Aurora, CO, USA

Katie Larson Ode, M.D., M.S. University of Iowa Children's Hospital, Iowa City, IA, USA

John F. Pohl, M.D. Division of Pediatric Gastroenterology, Department of Pediatrics, Primary Children's Hospital, University of Utah, Salt Lake City, UT, USA

Jamie L. Ryan, Ph.D. Division of Behavioral Medicine and Clinical Psychology, Cincinnati Children's Hospital Medical Center, Center for Adherence and Self-Management, Cincinnati, OH, USA

Teresa Schindler, M.S., R.D.N. Pediatric Pulmonology, Rainbow Babies and Children's Hospital Case Medical Center, Cleveland, OH, USA

Sarah Jane Schwarzenberg, M.D. Department of Pediatric Gastroenterology, Hepatology, and Nutrition, University of Minnesota Medical Center, Minneapolis, MN, USA

Ala K. Shaikhkhalil, M.D. Division of Gastroenterology, Hepatology and Nutrition, The Ohio State University College of Medicine, Nationwide Children's Hospital, Columbus, OH, USA

Virginia A. Stallings, M.D. Division of Gastroenterology, Hepatology and Nutrition, Children's Hospital of Philadelphia, Philadelphia, PA, USA

Perelman School of Medicine University of Pennsylvania, Philadelphia, PA, USA

Lori J. Stark, Ph.D., A.B.P.P. Division of Behavioral Medicine and Clinical Psychology, Cincinnati Children's Hospital Medical Center, Cincinnati, OH, USA

Birgitta Strandvik, M.D., Ph.D. Department of Pediatrics and Department of Bioscience and Nutrition, Karolinska Institutet, Huddinge, Stockholm, Sweden

Vin Tangpricha, M.D., Ph.D. Division of Endocrinology, Metabolism, and Lipids Emory University School of Medicine, Atlanta, GA, USA

Danielle Usatin, M.D. Department of Pediatrics, Division of Gastroenterology, Hepatology and Nutrition, UCSF Benioff Children's Hospital, San Francisco, San Francisco, CA, USA

Alexandra W.M. Wilson, M.S., R.D.N., C.D.E. Food Service and Clinical Nutrition, National Jewish Health, Adult Cystic Fibrosis Program, Colorado Cystic Fibrosis Center, Denver, CO, USA

Elizabeth H. Yen, M.D. Department of Pediatrics, Division of Gastroenterology, Hepatology and Nutrition, University of California, San Francisco, CA, USA

Benioff Children's Hospital, San Francisco, CA, USA

Chapter 1
What Is Cystic Fibrosis? The Relationship Between Nutrition and Outcomes in Cystic Fibrosis

Danielle Usatin and Elizabeth H. Yen

Key Points

- Cystic fibrosis is the most common life-shortening, inherited disease in the USA
- It is known to be an autosomal recessive disorder, caused by mutations in an ion channel, affecting organs throughout the body
- Appropriate nutrition remains inexorably linked with optimized outcomes
- Optimal nutrition and growth throughout life remain the focus of the cystic fibrosis community

Keywords Cystic fibrosis • Nutrition • Outcomes • Growth • Malnutrition • Pulmonary function • Pancreatic insufficiency • PERT

Introduction

Cystic fibrosis (CF) is the most common life-shortening inherited disease in the USA, affecting approximately 30,000 children and adults. This autosomal recessive disorder is caused by mutations in the gene encoding the cystic fibrosis transmembrane regulator (CFTR) [1]. CFTR is an ion channel that is present in multiple organs throughout the body. Mutations in this gene are divided into five major categories. Class I, II, and III mutations generally result in more severe pulmonary disease and pancreatic insufficiency; CF patients with these mutations generally have symptomatic disease in infancy or childhood. Class IV and V mutations typically result in milder disease, which is often diagnosed later in life [2]. Neonatal screening catches most patients in the USA with diagnosis confirmed by sweat or genetic testing. Diagnosis in the neonatal period leads to opportunities to optimize nutrition earlier in life.

D. Usatin, M.D. (✉)
Department of Pediatrics, Division of Gastroenterology, Hepatology and Nutrition, UCSF Benioff Children's Hospital, San Francisco, Mail Code 0136, 550 16th Street, 5th Floor, San Francisco, CA 94143, USA
e-mail: danielle.usatin@ucsf.edu

E.H. Yen, M.D.
Department of Pediatrics, Division of Gastroenterology,
Hepatology and Nutrition, University of California, San Francisco, CA, USA

Benioff Children's Hospital, San Francisco, CA, USA
e-mail: Elizabeth.yen@gilead.com; Ehy2005@gmail.com

E.H. Yen, A.R. Leonard (eds.), *Nutrition in Cystic Fibrosis: A Guide for Clinicians*, Nutrition and Health, DOI 10.1007/978-3-319-16387-1_1, © Springer International Publishing Switzerland 2015

History of Cystic Fibrosis

Historically, infants with cystic fibrosis were identified by their salty sweat and failure to thrive. German literature dating back to the eighteenth century cautioned: "[w]oe to the child who tastes salty from a kiss on the brow, for he is cursed and soon must die." [3] The clinical spectrum of cystic fibrosis was not clarified until the early twentieth century. At that time, children with cystic fibrosis were often mistakenly classified as having celiac disease because of their poor growth, distended abdomen, and diarrhea (Fig. 1.1). In the 1930s, several case series reported children who carried the diagnosis of celiac disease with unusual presentations. They were born with meconium plugging and died early in life. Autopsy found them to have changes in their lung, pancreas, and liver. Dr. Dorothy Andersen first described this constellation calling it cystic fibrosis of the pancreas in 1938, differentiating these patients from those with failure to thrive and steatorrhea due to celiac disease. She linked fibrotic changes in the pancreas with bronchiectasis in the lungs [4]. Dr. Andersen's paper combined 20 of her cases with those reported by other physicians and previous publications. This seminal paper led to the recognition of cystic fibrosis as a disease of exocrine pancreatic insufficiency and recurrent pulmonary infections.

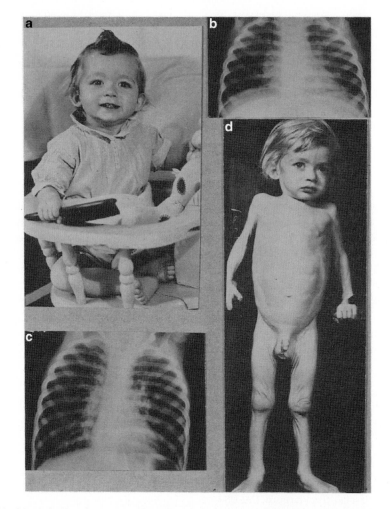

Fig. 1.1 A child with cystic fibrosis at 1 year 7 months (**a**); lungs at 1 year 2 months (**b**), lungs (**c**) and patient (**d**) at 2 years 5 months (**c**). Reprinted from The Journal of Pediatrics, Volume 34 (6), May CD and Lowe CU, "Fibrosis of the pancreas in infants and children: An illustrated review of certain clinical features with special emphasis on the pulmonary and cardiac aspects." p. 674, Copyright 1949, with permission from Elsevier

When Andersen and others described cystic fibrosis in the 1930s, malnutrition was the main cause of death. Until the mid-twentieth century, many cystic fibrosis patients died in childhood from a combination of malnutrition and lung disease. Children with cystic fibrosis were noted to be smaller in weight and stature than their healthy siblings [5].

Thanks to improvements in nutritional and pulmonary management, life expectancy has increased in this population from death in childhood to a mean survival into the fourth decade of life [6]. Despite changing therapies, malnutrition and growth retardation remain common in this patient population. In 2001, 25% of children in the Cystic Fibrosis Foundation Registry had a weight less than the 10th percentile for age according to the CDC growth curves. This has improved only slightly over the last decade, to 15% in 2011 [6].

Affects of Cystic Fibrosis on Nutrition

Cystic fibrosis affects all organ systems, causing a systemic impact on growth and nutrition. Patients suffer from increased energy expenditure, decreased caloric intake, as well as nutrient losses from malabsorption. Pulmonary exacerbations, with cough, tachypnea, infection, and post-tussive emesis lead to both increased energy expenditures and decreased appetite. Resting energy requirements in patients with cystic fibrosis are higher than their non-diseased siblings [5]. Chronic inflammation likely also results in decreased growth, although the mechanism remains poorly understood. Pancreatic insufficiency and alterations in bile salts lead to poor absorption of nutrients. Cystic fibrosis patients thus struggle to maintain adequate nutritional intake to support growth and development.

Treatment with Pancreatic Enzymes

At least 85% of patients with cystic fibrosis are born with pancreatic insufficiency. More than 25% of those remaining develop pancreatic insufficiency within 3 years of age [7–9]. Pancreatic dysfunction and destruction begins in the womb. It is caused by thickened secretions obstructing intrapancreatic ducts. Over time the pancreas undergoes autolysis and replacement of the body of the pancreas with fat [2]. When only 10% of pancreas functionality is left patients develop the symptoms of pancreatic insufficiency [9]. Pancreatic Enzyme Replacement Therapy (PERT) has long been the method of treatment for maldigestion due to pancreatic insufficiency. Porcine pancreatic enzymes were available prior to the publishing of the Federal Food, Drug and Cosmetic Act of 1938, so they were not required to undergo review by the FDA for safety and efficacy prior to marketing [10]. Early formulations of pancreatic enzyme were obtained by freeze-drying hog pancreas and then extracting and purifying the enzymes. They were recommended in children who had oily stools suggestive of fat malabsorption, but they were not well tolerated, largely due to bad taste. Many pediatricians and families felt that the enzymes adversely affected children's appetites. Thus, they were not widely used as therapy for the first 20 years.

In 1955, Harris et al. reported improvement of fat absorption from 46 to 71% of daily intake with use of pancreatin [11]. Subsequently PERT became a more standard part of therapy. In that same year, the National Cystic Fibrosis Research Foundation (later called the Cystic Fibrosis Foundation) was formed in New York. Optimizing PERT in cystic fibrosis became an active area of interest and research, largely thanks to the foundation's efforts.

In the 1970s, the formation of cystic fibrosis specialty centers in many major cities led to more consistent and aggressive treatment of malabsorption and other conditions associated with CF. As children survived through adolescence, their nutritional state and growth deteriorated progressively.

Despite the known effect of pancreatic enzymes in improving fat absorption, specialized diets high in protein and low in fat like the Allan diet [12, 13] were initially popularized and somewhat successful [14]. This was mainly due to the inconsistency and intolerability of pancreatic enzymes.

Early preparations of pancreatic enzymes were also not as effective as modern ones due to the fact that they were inactivated in the acidic environment of the stomach [10]. The co-administration of acid suppression medication with pancreatin helped alleviate this problem [15]. The Hospital for Sick Children in Toronto was one of the first centers to show improved outcomes with high fat diets and large doses of pancreatic enzymes [16]. In the 1980s, acid resistant formulations became available that were more effective and widely adopted [10]. Cystic fibrosis centers started to use dietitians as part of their integrated care approach, as evidence accumulated that early, aggressive PERT and nutritional support improved survival.

For example, a 1988 comparison of outcomes in Boston and Toronto demonstrated better survival rates in Toronto. The most significant difference between these two centers was the improved nutritional outcomes among those in Toronto. This was thought to be due to their aggressive supplementation of pancreatic enzymes and increased dietary fat and vitamin supplements [17]. This finding led to the development of more specific PERT guidelines, which were published as part of the first Cystic Fibrosis Foundation Nutritional Consensus Report in 1992 [18].

Associations with Malnutrition in Cystic Fibrosis

Poor nutritional status has long been associated with worse clinical outcomes in cystic fibrosis patients. As early as the 1970s, it was clear that vigorous attention to care with aggressive pulmonary interventions and appropriate nutrition led to longer survival [16, 19, 20]. In 1992, Kerem et al. noted that poor nutrition predicted earlier mortality [21]. Several studies followed demonstrating that nutritional rehabilitation with supplemental feedings improved lung function in patients whose Forced Expiratory Volume in 1 second (FEV_1) started at less than 40% predicted [22, 23]. Among cystic fibrosis patients with advanced lung disease, better nutritional status is associated with higher exercise tolerance [24].

Earlier diagnosis of cystic fibrosis allows for early, intensive nutritional support. This has been a major contributor to improvements in long-term survival and decreased morbidity [21, 25–31]. Multiple subsequent studies have demonstrated that early nutritional interventions and improved anthropomorphic measures have a positive impact on lung function in childhood [29, 30, 32–34].

In 2001 a randomized clinical trial compared CF diagnosis by universal neonatal screening to traditional, symptom-driven diagnostic workup. This trial reported that earlier diagnosis with neonatal screening prevented malnutrition and promoted long-term growth in the patients with CF [35]. Additional studies have repeatedly demonstrated that neonatal screening leads to fewer pulmonary exacerbations, fewer hospital days, and better growth parameters in childhood [36, 37]. Researchers hypothesize that early malnutrition affects lung growth and development. Rao et al. found in a cross sectional study that on high resolution computed tomography lung volume was very closely correlated with body length in healthy infants and toddlers [38]. Animal models also suggest that poor nutrition early in life may result in poor lung development and disease progression [39].

The links between adequate nutrition and pulmonary outcomes provided a foundation for the second Consensus Report on Nutrition commissioned by the Cystic Fibrosis Foundation in 2002. The purpose of this report was to help cystic fibrosis care centers identify undernourished patients and give guidance on interventions. This report recommended the Moore method of calculating percent Ideal Body Weight (%IBW), as well as weight-for-length percentile and BMI percentile based on the CDC 2000 growth curves. This allowed stratification of patient nutritional status as "acceptable," "at risk," or in "nutritional failure." Height was classified by genetic potential using mid parental heights.

Patients classified as having acceptable growth parameters had weight-for-length or BMI greater than the 25 percentile for age, and IBW≥90% [40]. If patients fell into the "nutritional failure" category, the guidelines recommended targeted interventions to promote growth by boosting their weight.

Subsequent to the 2002 nutritional consensus guidelines, several publications supported even more aggressive nutritional goals. Peterson et al. prospectively collected data on over 300 children followed at the Minnesota Cystic Fibrosis Center. They demonstrated that each 1 kg of weight was associated with 55 mL higher average FEV_1. During their follow-up period, children with steady weight gain had greater increases in FEV_1 than those whose weight gain was not steady [30]. Also publishing in 2003, Konstan et al. reported on the Epidemiology Study of Cystic Fibrosis (ESCF). They followed 931 patients cared for at 139 different centers in the USA and Canada from age 3 to at least age 6. They noted that weight-for-age and height-for-age were strong predictors of FEV_1 at age 6 years. Weight-for-age maintained above the 10th percentile from age 3 to 6 was associated with better lung function when compared to patients who fell below the 10th percentile at age 6 after previously being above it age 3 [29].

The implementation of %IBW as a standard for determining optimal growth parameters, as recommended in the 2002 guidelines, proved difficult and cumbersome for many centers. They found poor reproducibility of this measure between patients and in any given patient poor reducibility between examiners [41]. Furthermore, patients' nutritional status might be classified differently depending on the anthropomorphic index used [42]. Zhang and Lai compared %IBW and BMI as predictors of undernourishment and lung function in 2004. They found good agreement between the two indices in children <10 years of age with average stature. But, in older children and in children with height-for-age outside of 25–75th percentile they found that these two measures diverged significantly. Even more striking, however, was their finding that in all ranges of stature, BMI percentile more sensitively predicted improvements in lung function [43].

In 2008, the Cystic Fibrosis Foundation Subcommittee on Growth and Nutrition updated their recommendations again based on interim evidence. BMI and BMI percentile replaced %IBW for defining nutritional status. Additionally, they published a series of graphs demonstrating, in varying age categories, an association between higher BMI percentile and FEV_1 percent-predicted for age (Fig. 1.2). Furthermore, evidence suggested that among cystic fibrosis patients, reaching 50th percentile weight-for-length at age 2 years correlated significantly with higher percent-predicted FEV_1 at age 6 through 15. Higher BMI also seemed to correlate with pulmonary function in adults [44] (Fig. 1.3). BMI goals were set conservatively at ≥50th BMI percentile for all children, ≥22 kg/m^2 for adult females, and ≥23 kg/m^2 for adult males. The committee also recommended interventions to help children reach ≥50th percentile weight-for-length by 2 years of age.

More recently, Lai et al. demonstrated that children who recovered their birth weight z-score by age 2 years had overall better lung function at 6 years of age [45]. Additionally, a link between pulmonary disease severity and delayed growth velocities has been demonstrated [46]. Yen et al. demonstrated that at age 4 years, weight-for-age strongly predicted height and growth velocity. Moreover, weight-for-age percentile at age 4 predicted lung function as measured by percent-predicted FEV_1 at age 18. Weight and height-for-age percentiles at age 4 years correlated with survival, fewer pulmonary exacerbations, and fewer days in the hospital at age 18 years [47] (Fig. 1.4). Given that lung volume expands with height [48], these findings suggest that greater weight at age 4 may lead to larger lung volumes and enhanced pulmonary reserve.

Despite the strength of the literature to support the association between anthropomorphic parameters and pulmonary outcomes in cystic fibrosis there remain several areas in need of further research. Many have demonstrated that systematic implementation of PERT and enteral supplements improve weight gain [22, 23]. Clinical trials to evaluate if nutritional interventions that increase weight percentiles result in a slower rate of pulmonary functional decline are needed. Specifically, children between the 10th and 50th percentiles should be targeted to find the optimal zone for aggressive nutritional intervention. Thus far, cystic fibrosis care providers have set the goal of normal

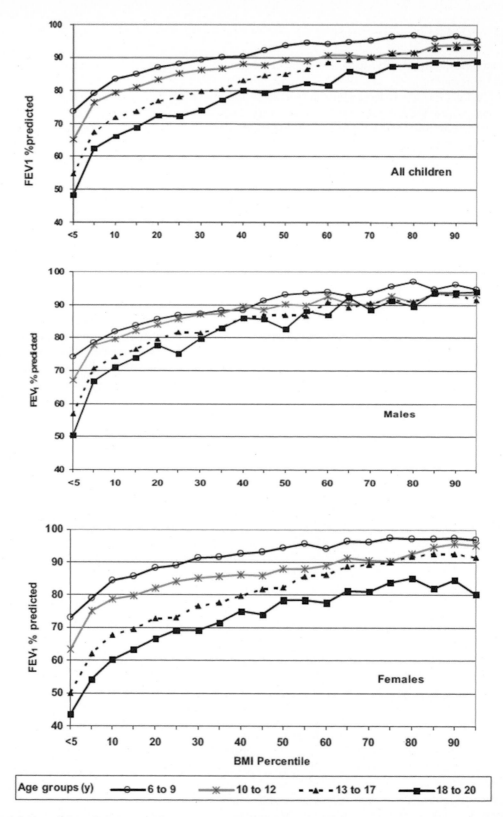

Fig. 1.2 Association of BMI percentile and percent-predicted FEV$_1$ for children with cystic fibrosis and pancreatic insufficiency by age and sex group, from the 2005 Cystic Fibrosis Patient Registry. Reprinted from Journal of the American Dietetic Association, VA Stallings, LJ Stark, KA Robinson, AP Feranchak, H Quinton, "Evidence-Based Practice Recommendations for Nutrition-Related Management of Children and Adults with Cystic Fibrosis and Pancreatic Insufficiency: Results of a Systematic Review." Pages 835, Copyright 2008, with permission from Elsevier

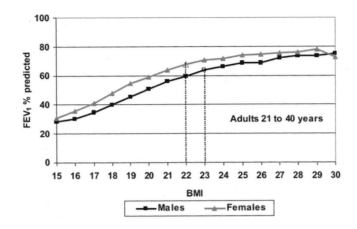

Fig. 1.3 Association of BMI and percent-predicted FEV_1 in adults aged 21 to 40 years with cystic fibrosis and pancreatic insufficiency, from the 1994 to 2003 Cystic Fibrosis Patient Registry. Reprinted from Journal of the American Dietetic Association, VA Stallings, LJ Stark, KA Robinson, AP Feranchak, H Quinton, "Evidence-Based Practice Recommendations for Nutrition-Related Management of Children and Adults with Cystic Fibrosis and Pancreatic Insufficiency: Results of a Systematic Review." Pages 836, Copyright 2008, with permission from Elsevier

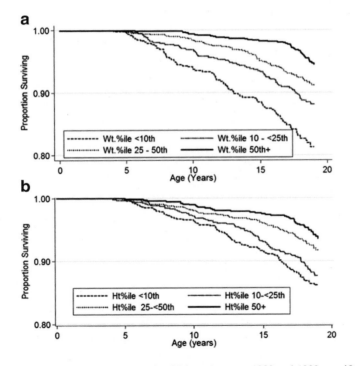

Fig. 1.4 Kaplan–Meier survival curves of patients with CF born between 1989 and 1992, stratified by A, weight and B, height categories at age 4 years. Reprinted from The Journal of Pediatrics, EH Yen, H Quinton, D Borowitz. "Better Nutritional Status in Early Childhood Is Associated with Improved Clinical Outcomes and Survival in Patients with Cystic Fibrosis." Page 533, Copyright 2013, with permission from Elsevier

anthropomorphic measures. Perhaps further consideration needs to be taken to individual inherited variance in patient size.

Prospective clinical trials to evaluate if nutritional interventions that increase weight percentiles result in a slower rate of lung function decline are needed. Significant resources and stress on the part of patients and their families go into meeting nutritional goals. It is important that a direct causal link between efforts to achieve these goals and better outcomes is made. A cluster randomization model would be an ideal method to evaluate this question and could target children with BMI ranges between the 25th and 50th percentiles with aggressive nutritional interventions versus standard of care, which already calls for increased interactions with a CF dietitian for dietary counseling. An aggressive nutritional intervention could be a combination of increased visit frequency, frequent contact with patients in between visits either via telephone calls or digital media, maximizing PERT, consultation with relevant subspecialties (e.g., Gastroenterology and Endocrinology) and introduction of high calorie nutritional supplements.

Francis and Welch identified the disease causing mutation in 1989 [1]. This breakthrough discovery marked a turning point in cystic fibrosis research and the search for a cure for the disease. At the forefront of current therapies are treatments that improve the function of the defective CFTR protein. These therapies have already shown that they can halt the progression of CF end-organ damage, and sometimes even reverse pulmonary damage. Despite the hope that these therapies hold for the health and longevity of patients with cystic fibrosis, patients will continue to require careful monitoring of their health, with special attention to their lung function and nutritional status.

References

1. Riordan JR, Rommens JM, Kerem B, Alon N, Rozmahel R, Grzelczak Z, et al. Identification of the cystic fibrosis gene: cloning and characterization of complementary DNA. Science. 1989;245(4922):1066–73.
2. O'Sullivan BP, Freedman SD. Cystic fibrosis. Lancet. 2009;373(9678):1891–904.
3. Busch R. On the history of cystic fibrosis. Acta Univ Carol Med. 1990;36(1–4):13–5.
4. Andersen DH. Cystic fibrosis of the pancreas and its relation to celiac disease: a clinical and pathologic study. Am J Dis Child. 1938;56(2):344–99.
5. Anthony H, Bines J, Phelan P, Paxton S. Relation between dietary intake and nutritional status in cystic fibrosis. Arch Dis Child. 1998;78(5):443–7.
6. Cystic Fibrosis Foundation. Patient Registry 2011: Annual Report. Bethesda, MD: Cystic Fibrosis Foundation 2011.
7. Waters DL, Dorney SF, Gaskin KJ, Gruca MA, O'Halloran M, Wilcken B. Pancreatic function in infants identified as having cystic fibrosis in a neonatal screening program. N Engl J Med. 1990;322(5):303–8.
8. Bronstein MN, Sokol RJ, Abman SH, Chatfield BA, Hammond KB, Hambidge KM, et al. Pancreatic insufficiency, growth, and nutrition in infants identified by newborn screening as having cystic fibrosis. J Pediatr. 1992;120 (4 Pt 1):533–40.
9. Couper RT, Corey M, Moore DJ, Fisher LJ, Forstner GG, Durie PR. Decline of exocrine pancreatic function in cystic fibrosis patients with pancreatic sufficiency. Pediatr Res. 1992;32(2):179–82.
10. Somaraju UR, Solis-Moya A. Pancreatic enzyme replacement therapy for people with cystic fibrosis. Cochrane Database Syst Rev. 2014;10, CD008227.
11. Harris R, Norman AP, Payne WW. The effect of pancreatin therapy on fat absorption and nitrogen retention in children with fibrocystic disease of the pancreas. Arch Dis Child. 1955;30(153):424–7.
12. Allan JD, Milner J, Moss D. Therapeutic use of an artificial diet. Lancet. 1970;1(7650):785–6.
13. Allan JD, Mason A, Moss AD. Nutritional supplementation in treatment of cystic fibrosis of the pancreas. Am J Dis Child. 1973;126(1):22–6.
14. Berry HK, Kellogg FW, Hunt MM, Ingberg RL, Richter L, Gutjahr C. Dietary supplement and nutrition in children with cystic fibrosis. Am J Dis Child. 1975;129(2):165–71.
15. Graham DY. Pancreatic enzyme replacement: the effect of antacids or cimetidine. Dig Dis Sci. 1982;27(6):485–90.
16. Crozier DN. Cystic fibrosis: a not-so-fatal disease. Pediatr Clin North Am. 1974;21(4):935–50.
17. Corey M, McLaughlin FJ, Williams M, Levison H. A comparison of survival, growth, and pulmonary function in patients with cystic fibrosis in Boston and Toronto. J Clin Epidemiol. 1988;41(6):583–91.
18. Ramsey BW, Farrell PM, Pencharz P. Nutritional assessment and management in cystic fibrosis: a consensus report. The Consensus Committee. Am J Clin Nutr. 1992;55(1):108–16.
19. Chase HP, Long MA, Lavin MH. Cystic fibrosis and malnutrition. J Pediatr. 1979;95(3):337–47.
20. Phelan PD, Allan JL, Landau LI, Barnes GL. Improved survival of patients with cystic fibrosis. Med J Aust. 1979;1(7):261–3.
21. Kerem E, Reisman J, Corey M, Canny GJ, Levison H. Prediction of mortality in patients with cystic fibrosis. N Engl J Med. 1992;326(18):1187–91.

22. Efrati O, Mei-Zahav M, Rivlin J, Kerem E, Blau H, Barak A, et al. Long term nutritional rehabilitation by gastrostomy in Israeli patients with cystic fibrosis: clinical outcome in advanced pulmonary disease. J Pediatr Gastroenterol Nutr. 2006;42(2):222–8.
23. Walker SA, Gozal D. Pulmonary function correlates in the prediction of long-term weight gain in cystic fibrosis patients with gastrostomy tube feedings. J Pediatr Gastroenterol Nutr. 1998;27(1):53–6.
24. Marcotte JE, Canny GJ, Grisdale R, Desmond K, Corey M, Zinman R, et al. Effects of nutritional status on exercise performance in advanced cystic fibrosis. Chest. 1986;90(3):375–9.
25. Augarten A, Akons H, Aviram M, Bentur L, Blau H, Picard E, et al. Prediction of mortality and timing of referral for lung transplantation in cystic fibrosis patients. Pediatr Transplant. 2001;5(5):339–42.
26. Beker LT, Russek-Cohen E, Fink RJ. Stature as a prognostic factor in cystic fibrosis survival. J Am Diet Assoc. 2001;101(4):438–42.
27. Dalzell AM, Shepherd RW, Dean B, Cleghorn GJ, Holt TL, Francis PJ. Nutritional rehabilitation in cystic fibrosis: a 5 year follow-up study. J Pediatr Gastroenterol Nutr. 1992;15(2):141–5.
28. George L, Norman AP. Life tables for cystic fibrosis. Arch Dis Child. 1971;46(246):139–43.
29. Konstan MW, Butler SM, Wohl ME, Stoddard M, Matousek R, Wagener JS, et al. Growth and nutritional indexes in early life predict pulmonary function in cystic fibrosis. J Pediatr. 2003;142(6):624–30.
30. Peterson ML, Jacobs Jr DR, Milla CE. Longitudinal changes in growth parameters are correlated with changes in pulmonary function in children with cystic fibrosis. Pediatrics. 2003;112(3 Pt 1):588–92.
31. Liou TG, Adler FR, Fitzsimmons SC, Cahill BC, Hibbs JR, Marshall BC. Predictive 5-year survivorship model of cystic fibrosis. Am J Epidemiol. 2001;153(4):345–52.
32. Zemel BS, Jawad AF, FitzSimmons S, Stallings VA. Longitudinal relationship among growth, nutritional status, and pulmonary function in children with cystic fibrosis: analysis of the Cystic Fibrosis Foundation National CF Patient Registry. J Pediatr. 2000;137(3):374–80.
33. Steinkamp G, Wiedemann B. Relationship between nutritional status and lung function in cystic fibrosis: cross sectional and longitudinal analyses from the German CF quality assurance (CFQA) project. Thorax. 2002;57(7):596–601.
34. McPhail GL, Acton JD, Fenchel MC, Amin RS, Seid M. Improvements in lung function outcomes in children with cystic fibrosis are associated with better nutrition, fewer chronic pseudomonas aeruginosa infections, and dornase alfa use. J Pediatr. 2008;153(6):752–7.
35. Farrell PM, Kosorok MR, Rock MJ, Laxova A, Zeng L, Lai HC, et al. Early diagnosis of cystic fibrosis through neonatal screening prevents severe malnutrition and improves long-term growth. Wisconsin Cystic Fibrosis Neonatal Screening Study Group. Pediatrics. 2001;107(1):1–13.
36. Siret D, Bretaudeau G, Branger B, Dabadie A, Dagorne M, David V, et al. Comparing the clinical evolution of cystic fibrosis screened neonatally to that of cystic fibrosis diagnosed from clinical symptoms: a 10-year retrospective study in a French region (Brittany). Pediatr Pulmonol. 2003;35(5):342–9.
37. Sims EJ, Clark A, McCormick J, Mehta G, Connett G, Mehta A, et al. Cystic fibrosis diagnosed after 2 months of age leads to worse outcomes and requires more therapy. Pediatrics. 2007;119(1):19–28.
38. Rao L, Tiller C, Coates C, Kimmel R, Applegate KE, Granroth-Cook J, et al. Lung growth in infants and toddlers assessed by multi-slice computed tomography. Acad Radiol. 2010;17(9):1128–35.
39. Gaultier C. Malnutrition and lung growth. Pediatr Pulmonol. 1991;10(4):278–86.
40. Borowitz D, Baker RD, Stallings V. Consensus report on nutrition for pediatric patients with cystic fibrosis. J Pediatr Gastroenterol Nutr. 2002;35(3):246–59.
41. Poustie VJ, Watling RM, Ashby D, Smyth RL. Reliability of percentage ideal weight for height. Arch Dis Child. 2000;83(2):183–4.
42. Lai HC, Kosorok MR, Sondel SA, Chen ST, FitzSimmons SC, Green CG, et al. Growth status in children with cystic fibrosis based on the National Cystic Fibrosis Patient Registry data: evaluation of various criteria used to identify malnutrition. J Pediatr. 1998;132(3 Pt 1):478–85.
43. Zhang Z, Lai HJ. Comparison of the use of body mass index percentiles and percentage of ideal body weight to screen for malnutrition in children with cystic fibrosis. Am J Clin Nutr. 2004;80(4):982–91.
44. Stallings VA, Stark LJ, Robinson KA, Feranchak AP, Quinton H, Clinical Practice Guidelines on Growth and Nutrition Subcommittee, et al. Evidence-based practice recommendations for nutrition-related management of children and adults with cystic fibrosis and pancreatic insufficiency: results of a systematic review. J Am Diet Assoc. 2008;108(5):832–9.
45. Lai HJ, Shoff SM, Farrell PM, Wisconsin Cystic Fibrosis Neonatal Screening Group. Recovery of birth weight z score within 2 years of diagnosis is positively associated with pulmonary status at 6 years of age in children with cystic fibrosis. Pediatrics. 2009;123(2):714–22.
46. Assael BM, Casazza G, Iansa P, Volpi S, Milani S. Growth and long-term lung function in cystic fibrosis: a longitudinal study of patients diagnosed by neonatal screening. Pediatr Pulmonol. 2009;44(3):209–15.
47. Yen EH, Quinton H, Borowitz D. Better nutritional status in early childhood is associated with improved clinical outcomes and survival in patients with cystic fibrosis. J Pediatr. 2013;162(3):530–535. e1.
48. Wang X, Dockery DW, Wypij D, Fay ME, Ferris Jr BG. Pulmonary function between 6 and 18 years of age. Pediatr Pulmonol. 1993;15(2):75–88.

Chapter 2
Macronutrient Requirements

Jaclyn Brownlee

Key Points

- Many individuals with cystic fibrosis will likely require higher nutrient intakes in order to overcome losses in the stool and to achieve expected growth or weight gain/maintenance. However needs are very individualized and will depend on many factors including severity of illness.
- Calorie needs will be best determined by each individual's current intake as well as their clinical and nutritional status.
- Patients, especially those with high energy needs, may benefit from a diet higher in fat (approximately 35% of total calories).
- Protein is an important nutrient to prevent catabolism; recommended intakes are 1.5–2 times greater than the recommended daily allowance or ~15% of total calories.
- There are no specific recommendations for carbohydrate provision and intake is generally adequate in people with CF.
- With adequate enzyme intake, no clear benefit of medium chain fats or hydrolyzed proteins has been found compared to long chain fats except for in patients with additional digestive and/or allergic issues.
- Due to concern about the ongoing oxidative stress it has been suggested that patients with CF may benefit from a diet rich in antioxidants to help optimize the benefits of a high fat diet.
- There is no clear consensus on the appropriate amount of fiber to provide to individuals with CF. As fiber-rich foods, in particular fruits, vegetables, legumes, and whole grains, provide the additional benefit of being rich in vitamins, minerals, and antioxidants it may be wise to recommend that patients incorporate these foods into their diets. However, it should be noted that high fiber intake may cause more problems, including calorie displacement and possible abdominal pain exacerbations.
- Personalized diet assessment and recommendations are best for patients with cystic fibrosis.
- When giving patients recommendations on recommended macronutrient intake, patients may be able to work better with the number of grams/day (as opposed to percent of diet) as this information is readily available on food labels or calorie tracker programs.

J. Brownlee, R.D., C.N.S.C. (✉)
Department of Nutrition and Food Services, UCSF Benioff Children's Hospital San Francisco,
1855 4th Street, San Francisco, CA 94143, USA
e-mail: jaclyn.brownlee@ucsf.edu; jaclyn.brownlee@ucsfmedctr.org

E.H. Yen, A.R. Leonard (eds.), *Nutrition in Cystic Fibrosis: A Guide for Clinicians*, Nutrition and Health, DOI 10.1007/978-3-319-16387-1_2, © Springer International Publishing Switzerland 2015

Keywords Calories • Energy expenditure • Estimated energy requirement • Fat • Antioxidants • Protein • Protein hydrolysate • Catabolism • Carbohydrate • Fiber

Abbreviations

BMI   Body mass index
CF   Cystic fibrosis
CFRD   Cystic fibrosis-related diabetes
DIOS   Distal intestinal obstruction syndrome
EER   Estimated energy needs
EFAD   Essential fatty acid deficiency
g   Gram
kcal   Kilocalorie
LCT   Long chain triglycerides
MCT   Medium chain triglycerides
MUFA   Monounsaturated fatty acid
PA   Physical activity
PERT   Pancreatic enzyme replacement therapy
PI   Pancreatic insufficient
PS   Pancreatic sufficient
PUFA   Polyunsaturated fatty acid
RDA   Recommended daily allowance
REE   Resting energy expenditure
RQ   Respiratory quotient
SFA   Saturated fatty acid
TEE   Total energy expenditure

Introduction

When discussing cystic fibrosis and nutrition an important topic is the question of "are all calories created equal?" This chapter will review the available literature regarding kilocalorie and macronutrient recommendations for people with cystic fibrosis (CF). The history behind and changes leading up to current nutrition standards will also be addressed. There are several recommendations about energy and nutrient requirements in CF that have been so frequently espoused that they virtually seem to be common knowledge and solid fact- when in actuality firm guidelines are difficult to find. This chapter will explore the sometimes controversial and contradictory nutrition recommendations with the goal of providing realistic calorie and macronutrient intake goals for individuals with CF based on the current state of the literature.

Calories

Given the well-defined need for people with CF to receive adequate nutrition for proper growth and to promote improved prognosis [1–7], the goal of determining just how many calories are needed has been a prominent point of many studies conducted in the CF population. Energy needs are thought to be affected by gastrointestinal symptoms [8–10] as well as pulmonary symptoms [11] in addition to the usual factors considered in the general population: gender, age, weight, height, and physical activity levels [12].

An often cited recommendation is to provide 120–150% of the recommended daily allowance (RDA) for energy to allow for the goal of normal growth for age [13–16] by compensating for malabsorption and increased calorie needs secondary to pulmonary dysfunction and any required catch up growth [13, 16]. This recommendation has historically been validated by studies which reported that individuals with CF have an increased resting energy expenditure (REE) compared to healthy controls [17–32] or to estimated values based on predictive equations [33–38]. However, controversy surrounds these findings. While many studies support increased REE and a few have observed increased total energy expenditure (TEE) [39, 40], most studies did not observe an increase in TEE when it was measured as a study outcome [30, 41–44]. A handful of studies even suggest that REE is not actually elevated in CF patients [43–45].

Energy Expenditure in Cystic Fibrosis

A multitude of studies on the measurement of energy expenditure in CF patients have resulted in conflicting findings.

Several studies have found increased REE values in CF patients based on the comparison of indirect calorimetry measurements with predictive equations and/or control subjects. This difference has appeared to be more pronounced in CF patients with more severe respiratory disease [17–19, 33, 34]. Even when the measurements were corrected for ideal weight-for-height or lean body mass, the REE measurements remained elevated in the CF subjects [17, 18]. When compared to malnourished individuals with anorexia nervosa, CF subjects had a much higher REE. The REE of the anorexic subjects was less than predicted, suggesting that the increased REE in CF was not due to malnutrition [17]. Yet other studies failed to find a relationship between REE and severity of lung disease [20–22, 35].

Pancreatic status may contribute to differences in REE, with pancreatic insufficiency associated with an elevated REE compared to pancreatic sufficiency [23, 33–35]. In fact, the pancreatic sufficient (PS) patients tended to have normal REE [33, 34]. One study observed that REE was increased in PI subjects even when compared to PS individuals with similar pulmonary function test results leading to the possible conclusion that pancreatic status contributes more to REE than respiratory status [34].

The influence of gender on REE has also been investigated. The majority of these studies have found that while CF subjects in both genders have higher REE than expected, the REE of CF females tends to be more elevated above expected values [23, 35] or more likely to increase over time [20] compared to the REE of CF males. The REE in CF females is increased compared to healthy females even when controlling for fat free mass and pubertal stage [19, 24]. In studies on the effect of puberty, REE decreased post-menarche in all subjects compared to pre-menarche but remained higher in subjects with CF [19, 24].

The effect of an acute pulmonary exacerbation on the REE of CF patients has been another area of study. While some studies have found REE measurements decrease between the early part and the end of an exacerbation, others have found no change [36, 37, 46]. REE increases during the initial days of a hospital stay may possibly be due to increased energy consumption and/or increased physical therapy and mucous clearance [37]. A trend for the patients with the highest REE at the beginning of an exacerbation to have the largest decrease by the end of the exacerbation has been observed [36, 37]. TEE has been observed to remain similar to baseline, or even lower, during the exacerbation despite increases in measured REE [46]. It is possible that the trend for a lower TEE during illness is due to decreased physical activity [46].

Studies on the energy cost of activity in CF have yielded various results. Several studies have found that CF patients required less or the same amount of additional energy on top of their REE in order to complete the same activities as controls [25, 26, 45]. A finding that TEE was not elevated above controls despite an increased REE in CF subjects led to the conclusion that CF patients are able to compensate for their increased REE [25]. Conversely, other investigations have indeed observed an elevated energy cost of activity in CF patients compared to controls [21]. Differences in the length of the measured activities and use of fat free mass to assess REE may have contributed to the contradictory findings [21].

Several researchers have suggested that the increased energy expenditure in CF patients is due to a genetically linked metabolic abnormality [18, 27–30, 47, 48]. This conclusion was reached due to noting that the increased REE or TEE was not fully explained by pulmonary function [27–29] or differences in weight [18, 39] and/or by finding differences in the energy expenditure in individuals of various CF genotypes [27–29, 48]. Mitochondrial dysfunction has been cited as a cause of increased energy expenditure [48]. However, not all studies have found evidence to support such a genetic link [20, 21], and others have suggested that at most the genetic contribution to increased energy expenditure is minimal [33]. This issue has been further explored by studying the energy expenditure of infants and young children with CF, as these patients should be without significant lung disease. Thus elevations in their energy expenditure may reflect an intrinsic energy-consuming defect. Two studies found an elevated REE in CF infants versus controls per kilogram weight and per kilogram fat free mass or total body potassium [30, 31]. Other investigators have found elevated TEE in infants older than 6 months and in toddlers [39, 40], but a lack of assessment of the effect of fat free mass on the measured energy expenditure may have contributed to this finding [39, 41]. Studies of infants under six months of age have not found a difference in TEE between CF subjects and controls [40, 42, 43], supporting the argument that disease progression, rather than an intrinsic genetic defect, is the primary cause of elevated energy needs.

Translating Energy Expenditure into Energy Needs

The vast majority of the available studies conclude that REE is generally increased in individuals with CF, from approximately 105 to 130% of expected. There is a wide variety of ages and levels of disease severity within the studied CF subjects. The methods utilized to determine the expected REE also varied between the studies. Some utilized predictive equations that have questionable accuracy in healthy groups [31] and others referred to the RDA values, which have changed over the years. Due to these factors, it is difficult to fully compare all of the studies and draw concrete conclusions for estimating energy needs in CF. Within the studies that do conclude that REE is elevated, there is still debate as to whether or not certain disease characteristics, such as pulmonary function, pancreatic status, nutritional status, and specific alleles contribute to energy expenditure. There is also not a clear finding as to whether the energy cost of activity is different in the CF population compared to the healthy population. The general consensus is that TEE is not elevated in CF compared to healthy controls. However, it is not known how CF patients may compensate for their likely high basal metabolic rate in order to yield normal TEE. It is agreed that the normalization of TEE in CF by a spontaneous decrease in physical activity should be prevented by ensuring adequate nutrition intake [25]; however it is not certain that decreased activity in CF is truly the case [25, 28].

Another factor to consider is how much of their consumed intake CF patients are able to utilize. Having similar total energy expenditure to the healthy population does not necessarily indicate that an individual with CF can consume the same amount as a healthy person and reap the same nutritional benefit. CF patients on established pancreatic enzyme replacement therapy (PERT) with controlled gastrointestinal symptoms have been found to have higher stool energy and stool fat losses than the healthy population [9, 49, 50]. This suggests that CF patients may still experience some degree of malabsorption despite receiving standard treatment for PI.

One group of investigators measured the TEE of CF children aged 6–8 years old with mild-to-moderate lung disease. Measured fecal energy loss and standardized energy required for growth were added to the TEE to better estimate the total energy requirement for each subject [51]. The results were compared to multiple predictive equations to determine which was most accurate for predicting energy needs in children with CF. The estimated energy requirement (EER) equation with an active physical activity level factor (1.26 in boys and 1.31 in girls) [12] was the most consistent with the study results at both group and individual levels. Further, it was observed that the 1989 RDA, the 1989 RDA multiplied by 1.2, and equations developed for estimating energy needs in CF all overestimated needs, with the RDA multiplied by 1.2 resulting in the largest overestimation. However, these results are not necessarily applicable to CF populations of different ages or with more progressed lung disease [51].

What Happens in Real Life?

Actual intake in CF patients has been measured many times over the years. Diet records maintained by CF individuals have been compared to control subjects and to national standards to determine if the patients actually consume the minimum goal of 120% of the recommended calorie intake for the population. Growth and nutritional status have been assessed in comparison to dietary intake. Overall, the studies from recent decades have found that individuals with CF eat considerably more than their age-matched control counterparts, but as a group they do not achieve 120% of recommended intake [52–57]. Of note, the recommended intake varied based on the country in and the time at which each study took place. Despite eating more than the control subjects, the CF subject tended to have less optimal growth and lower weight, height, weight-for-height, and/or body mass index (BMI) z-scores than expected and/or compared to controls [52–55].

When reported, approximately 11–39% of CF subjects attained the 120% recommended intake marker [52, 56, 57]. A few studies noted that in patient groups with better compliance to calorie goals and enzyme therapies, weight, growth, and pulmonary status were actually worse [52, 53]. This may indicate that compliance improves in sicker patients [52] and may also reflect higher calorie needs in sicker patients [53].

The relationship between energy intake and growth status is variable among the studies. A positive correlation between intake and growth parameters was found in some study groups [53, 54] but this correlation was not always present for each age group [53]. Some studies found that nutritional status was suboptimal in CF patients despite their consumption of 100–120% of the population recommendations for age, and 7–18% more total calories than the control subjects [54, 55]. Alternatively, other studies observed that CF patients were able to attain growth similar to control subjects while consuming less than 120% of the RDA, though calorie intakes were approximately 10–15% higher than those of the controls [56, 57]. Some of these patients were less than the tenth percentile for weight-for-height, which is of nutritional concern, particularly in CF [57].

It is not surprising to observe that in many studies comparing actual recorded intake CF patients do seem to consume and require more calories than control subjects for, at best, similar growth. It does remain important to remember that studies requiring the subjects to record diet intake may be subject to inaccurate record keeping and/or changes from baseline intake. CF patients may have consumed or been reported to consume more than usual, as that is the recommendation they often hear during clinic visits [55, 57].

Calorie Recommendations

Overall, the recommendationto provide 120–150% of the RDA for calories to all CF patients is not fully validated. The majority of data discussed above supports that as a group, CF patients require more calories than the normal population. On an individual level, this may not be the case. Healthy patients may be capable of growing and maintaining their weight with intakes similar to normal, healthy peer groups, and/or the RDA alone [43, 55, 57–60]. However, underweight or particularly sick individuals may require at least 120–150% of the RDA [52–55, 58, 60]. Recent CF Foundation guidelines promote intakes of 110–200% of the requirements established for the general population [6]. Table 2.1 presents the 2005 EER equations, which replaced the RDA for calories.

Given the wide range of clinical statuses of the CF population as well as lifestyle factors, it seems impractical to assume that there is a "one-size-fits-all" method for determining energy needs. The best practice to adopt in estimating energy needs in individuals with CF is to assess the patient's current intake and nutritional status and to then make recommendations for adjusting caloric intake as indicated for patients who are not meeting or are exceeding goals for growth or weight maintenance [5]. Adjusting intake in increments of 10% at a time is considered to be an attainable goal for

Table 2.1 2005 estimated energy requirement equations [12]

Age	Estimated energy requirement equation (kcal/day)	Physical activity (PA) factors (equivalents of miles walked)
		Sedentary = no miles walked Low active = 1.5–3 miles walked Active = 5–10 miles walked Very active = 12–22 miles walked
0–3 months	$(89 \times \text{weight} - 100) + 175$ kcal	–
4–6 months	$(89 \times \text{weight} - 100) + 56$ kcal	–
7–12 months	$(89 \times \text{weight} - 100) + 22$ kcal	–
13–36 months	$(89 \times \text{weight} - 100) + 20$ kcal	–
Boys 3–8 years	$88.5 - (61.9 \times \text{age [year]}) + \text{PA} \times (26.7 \times \text{weight [kg]} + 903 \times \text{height [m]}) + 20$ kcal	Sedentary = 1 Low active = 1.13
Boys 9–18 years	$88.5 - (61.9 \times \text{age [year]}) + \text{PA} \times (26.7 \times \text{weight [kg]} + 903 \times \text{height [m]}) + 25$ kcal	Active = 1.26 Very active = 1.42
Men >19 years	$662 - (9.53 \times \text{age [year]}) + \text{PA} \times (15.9 \times \text{weight [kg]} + 539.6 \times \text{height [m]})$	Sedentary = 1 Low active = 1.11 Active = 1.25 Very active = 1.48
Girls 3–8 years	$135.3 - (30.8 \times \text{age [year]}) + \text{PA} \times (10 \times \text{weight [kg]} + 934 \times \text{height [m]}) + 20$ kcal	Sedentary = 1 Low active = 1.16
Girls 9–18 years	$135.3 - (30.8 \times \text{age [year]}) + \text{PA} \times (10 \times \text{weight [kg]} + 934 \times \text{height [m]}) + 25$ kcal	Active = 1.31 Very active = 1.56
Women >19 years	$354 - (6.91 \times \text{age [year]}) + \text{PA} \times (9.36 \times \text{weight [kg]} + 726 \times \text{height [m]})$	Sedentary = 1 Low active = 1.12 Active = 1.27 Very active = 1.45
Pregnancy	Age appropriate + additional energy expended during pregnancy + energy deposition 1st Trimester: $\text{EER}_{\text{nonpregnant}} + 0 + 0$ 2nd Trimester: $\text{EER}_{\text{nonpregnant}} + 160$ kcal $+ 180$ kcal 3rd Trimester: $\text{EER}_{\text{nonpregnant}} + 272$ kcal $+ 180$ kcal	–
Lactation	Age appropriate EER + milk energy output − weight loss 1st 6 months: $\text{EER}_{\text{nonpregnant}} + 500 - 170$ 2nd 6 months: $\text{EER}_{\text{nonpregnant}} + 400 - 0$	–

individuals [8, 59]. Early education of families and patients on the risk of malnutrition and the potential reasons for inadequate intake soon after a patient's diagnosis is important to promote optimal growth and nutritional status [5].

Macronutrients

The recommendations for the macronutrient composition of diets of individuals with CF have shifted over the years. Given the importance of ensuring adequate caloric intake in patients who may suffer from poor appetite and unpleasant gastrointestinal symptoms [10, 15, 61], getting calories in however possible and focusing on easily digested food, such as simple sugars, were at one point more standard recommendations than ensuring a balanced diet [1]. The remainder of this chapter will explore the different macronutrients and will provide recommendations for diet composition.

Fat

Fat is a macronutrient of critical importance in CF. In the general population, fat is considered an efficient source of energy as it provides 9 cal/g. Dietary fat consists mostly of triglycerides with sterols and phospholipids making up the small remainder [62]. The majority of fat is not soluble in water; the digestion of fat requires emulsification by bile salts so that pancreatic and intestinal lipases are able to hydrolyze triglycerides and fatty acid esters to allow for absorption [62]. Digestion of fat in patients with CF is complicated by decreased availability of lipase and bile salts due to obstruction of pancreatic and gall bladder ducts with mucous [63]. This has historically affected the opinion regarding the use of fat in cystic fibrosis.

Historical Recommendations for Fat Intake in Cystic Fibrosis

Due to the difficulty digesting and thus utilizing fat, it was common practice in the 1960s and 1970s to recommend low fat diets [1, 64–66]. At that time, PERT was suboptimal and individuals with CF demonstrated only minimal improvement of fat absorption when using it [64]. It was thought that a low fat diet would help limit steatorrhea and thus improve digestion and absorption of other nutrients [64, 67, 68]. Unfortunately, this was not the case as the low fat diet was not adequate in providing the calories needed for growth and health in CF children. In fact, it was found that patients were generally only receiving 80–90% of the RDA for calories and were experiencing growth failure [64, 65].

An alternative recommendation in the 1960s and 1970s was to provide a diet high in medium chain triglycerides (MCT) [64]. This recommendation was based on a study that found that fat excretion by infants with CF drinking an MCT-based formula was normal [64]. However, it was later discovered that the method used for quantifying fat in stool was not appropriate for MCT and thus stool loss of MCT had been underestimated [64]. This recommendation also resulted in growth failure for the CF patients receiving MCT-based formulas [64].

The Shift to a High Fat Diet in Cystic Fibrosis

Despite the prevalence of the low fat diet recommendation throughout the 1960s and 1970s, the concept was questioned as early as the 1950s [67]. Dr. Crozier, of the Toronto Cystic Fibrosis Clinic, started to make the case for a higher fat diet in the early 1970s [1, 66]. Given the improved caloric density of fat compared to carbohydrate and protein, he suspected that increasing fat consumption with the simultaneous increase of PERT in patients would result in improved intake and absorption [66]. These patients consequently demonstrated improved growth despite ongoing fat malabsorption, leading to the conclusion that net energy absorption was indeed improved [66]. When Toronto clinic patients were compared to CF patients in Boston for the years 1972–1982, it was found that the patients from Toronto had much improved growth and survival compared to the Boston patients [1]. The only significant difference between the two centers was that the Toronto center encouraged a high energy, high fat diet with increased PERT and the Boston center encouraged a high energy, fat restricted diet [1].

Subsequent studies confirmed that calorie intake, absorption, and growth could be improved on a high calorie, high fat diet [64, 65, 67, 69]. Investigators were able to demonstrate that increased fat intake did not result in increased fat excretion [67]. PI was shown to be well controlled even in CF subjects who consumed diets with greater than 35% of calories from fat [70].

Defining a High Fat Diet

Initial recommendations for a high fat diet were to aim for a fat consumption of 35–45% of total calories [64, 66, 71, 72]. Recent CF nutrition consensus guidelines still promote 35–40% of dietary calories to come from fat [5]. For perspective, the acceptable macronutrient distribution range for the general healthy population is 20–35% of total energy intake from fat [62] with a normal intake considered to be approximately 30% of calories from fat [73].

It has been noted that the percentage of calories from fat may not correlate well with total calorie intake and overall nutritional status [70, 74]. Several investigators did not find an association between percent of calories provided by fat and the percentage of the recommended energy index consumed [74] or the percentage of ideal body weight [70]. Grams of fat consumed per day did positively correlate with total daily energy intake and percent ideal body weight, thus it was concluded that it would be more beneficial to set an actual daily fat gram goal for patients to achieve [70, 74]. There are several benefits to this practice, as counting grams of fat would be simpler for patients than determining percentage of dietary intake from fat and could assist with accurate dosing of PERT [70, 74].

MCT Versus LCT

As briefly mentioned above, MCT were previously recommended over long chain triglycerides (LCT) [64]. Despite the flaws of the initial study promoting the use of MCT-based formulas, MCT absorption was better than that of LCT in patients taking an older version of PERT [64]. The use of MCT in CF remains controversial. The benefits of MCT include that they are soluble in water and are absorbed directly into the intestinal enterocytes without requiring bile salts or lipase. Steatorrhea and abdominal pain were reported as being decreased in the setting of supplementation with MCT; however these patients did not gain weight during the 6-month trial [75]. MCT are also noted to cause increased diet-induced thermogenesis [76, 77], to have decreased deposition into adipose stores [76, 78], and to cause increased energy expenditure [76, 78] compared to LCT. These factors suggest that MCT would not be as beneficial of a calorie source as LCT for individuals with CF, unless the patient has additional complications that further limit absorption, such as short bowel syndrome or cholestasis [76].

Potential Benefits of a High Fat Diet in Cystic Fibrosis

A high fat diet for individuals with CF could yield other advantages in addition to caloric density. A diet high in fat could help prevent essential fatty acid deficiency (EFAD) and also may provide a more optimal fuel mix to help decrease carbon dioxide production.

Patients with CF have historically been noted to have EFAD [76, 79–84], thought to be due to the low fat diet and poor absorption of fatty acids [76, 80]. Other factors may also contribute to EFAD in CF, including defects in the metabolism of fatty acids and excessive use of fatty acids as an energy source and for production of eicosanoids [80]. Effects of a high fat diet on EFAD in CF appear to be mixed; several studies have noted that EFAD continues to exist in CF patients consuming high fat diets [80, 81] and that serum fatty acid levels do not correlate with the individual's level of fat absorption [84]. Yet, other studies have observed that serum fatty acid levels can be similar to controls in CF patients on a high fat diet with PERT [85] or can improve with consumption of high fat, particularly high linoleic acid, oral supplements [86]. While a high fat diet in CF may not completely prevent EFAD, recommendations for supplementation of specific fatty acids do not yet exist [81, 83]. Patients may benefit from increasing dietary linoleic acid and alpha-linolenic acid [81]. For further discussion and recommendations regarding the different types of dietary fat please refer to Chapter 6.

Enteral formulas high in carbohydrate can lead to an increased production of carbon dioxide, which may exacerbate the pulmonary status of patients with advanced lung disease [87, 88]. In studies comparing the use of different formulas in CF patients, the formulas which were higher in fat and lower in carbohydrate resulted in lower carbon dioxide production, lower respiratory quotient (RQ), and lower minute ventilation compared to higher carbohydrate, lower fat formulas [88, 89]. Of note, due to the increased minute ventilation on the higher carbohydrate formulas, the patients studied were able to breathe off the additional carbon dioxide to avoid increased carbon dioxide retention and hypoxia [89]. Another study verified that provision of a higher fat formula resulted in a decreased RQ compared to a higher carbohydrate formula but alternatively found that production of carbon dioxide was similar between the two formulas [90]. Overall, it remains possible that CF patients with severe lung disease who require enteral supplementation may benefit from the use of high fat formulas, especially at high levels of supplementation [87–90].

Concerns About a High Fat Diet in Cystic Fibrosis

Despite the known and potential benefits of a high fat diet, some concerns remain. In an era of increasing lifespan in CF, the co-morbidities of an aging population must be considered. A diet high in fat, particularly saturated fat, can have negative effects on cardiovascular health [91, 92]. CF patients have historically been noted to have minimal signs of atherosclerosis, very likely due to the low fat diet and poor fat absorption typical in CF patients in the past [91]. More recent studies have reported that CF patients on high fat diets have low to normal serum cholesterol levels compared to controls [85, 93–96]; although it was noted that adult patients with PS had high normal serum cholesterol levels [93, 96]. Alternatively, higher serum triglyceride levels in patients with CF compared to the standard population with several incidences of hypertriglyceridemia have been observed [94, 95]. The etiology and consequences of the elevated triglycerides are not fully known. A positive correlation between serum triglyceride level and BMI was found [96]. Otherwise, there were overall minimal significant correlations between elevated triglycerides in CF and other risk factors for cardiovascular disease, including glucose intolerance and blood pressure. Chronic inflammation, excessive carbohydrate intake or absorption and chronic high fat diets have been proposed mechanisms of elevated triglyceride levels [94–96]. Furthering the concern regarding the tolerance of a high fat diet, CF patients have recently been observed to have premature arterial damage compared to controls [97].

Table 2.2 High fat, high calorie foods and ideas for how to incorporate into diet [101, 102]

Food (serving size)	Type of fat	G fat/ serving	kcal/serving	Serving suggestions
Butter (1 tbsp)	SFA	11.5	102	• Use to cook vegetables, grains, meats
Olive oil (1 tbsp)	MUFA	13.5	119	• Serve on warm bread/grains (melts in)
Canola oil (1 tbsp)	MUFA, PUFA[a]	14	124	• Add to shakes • Add extra to served foods (vegetables, grains)
Flaxseed oil (1 tbsp)	PUFA[a]	13.6	120	
Coconut oil (1 tbsp)	SFA, MCT	13.6	117	
Avocado (½ cup cubed)	MUFA	11	120	• Make guacamole for chips, crackers, vegetables • Add to sandwiches, tacos, burritos, soups, salads • Mix into smoothies and/or shakes
Cheese, most varieties (1 oz)	SFA	6–10	85–115	• Serve with crackers, fruit • Add extra to pasta, casseroles, pizza • Add to eggs, soups, vegetables, salads • Use melted cheese as a dip for chips, vegetables, crackers, fruit
Heavy whipping cream (1 oz)	SFA	11	103	• Mix with whole milk to drink • Use in recipes that call for milk • Use to make hot cereals
Sour cream (1 tbsp)	SFA	2.4	23	• Use to make dips for chips, vegetables • Make a sweet dip for fruit • Add to soups, potatoes, casseroles
Ice cream (1/2 cup)	SFA	7.3	137	• Ice cream sundaes • Milkshakes • Soda floats
Yogurt, whole milk, plain (6 oz)	SFA	5.5	104	• Mix with granola • Use in smoothies • Make a dip for fruit (add sugar/honey)
Nuts (1 oz)	MUFA, PUFA	13–20	163–204	• Add to hot cereal, salads, baked goods • Trail mix
Peanut butter (1 tbsp)	MUFA, PUFA	8.2	96	• Serve on warm bread/grains • Add to milkshakes, smoothies • Serve with apples, bananas and celery • Peanut butter crackers, pretzels
Egg (1 large)	SFA	5.3	72	• Add extra yolk to French toast, baked goods, quiches, scrambled eggs • Add hard boiled eggs to salads, sandwiches • Add to ground meat • Use as the binder for breaded meats
Bacon (1 slice)	SFA	4	54	• Add to salads, sandwiches
Salami (1 slice)	SFA	3.2	41	• Add to sandwiches • Serve with cheese and crackers

Abbreviations: *g* gram, *kcal* kilocalorie, *SFA* saturated fatty acid, *MUFA* monounsaturated fatty acid, *PUFA* polyunsaturated fatty acid, *MCT* medium chain triglycerides
[a]Food considered to be a major source of omega-3 fatty acids

This may lead to complications in cardiovascular health, especially as the population ages [97]. Notably, myocardial infarction has been reported in CF patients [98, 99]. Due to this potential for cardiovascular disease, encouraging increased intake of monounsaturated and polyunsaturated fatty acids rather than saturated fatty acids may be wise [92, 100]. Table 2.2 presents common food sources of unsaturated and saturated fatty acids.

Table 2.3 Examples of antioxidant-rich foods [102, 104]

Food (serving size)	Calories/ serving	Grams protein/ serving	Grams fat/ serving	Grams carbohydrate/ serving
Kale (1/2 cup cooked)	18	1.24	0.26	3.66
Spinach (1/2 cup cooked)	21	2.67	0.23	3.38
Broccoli (1/2 cup cooked)	27	1.86	0.32	5.6
Carrots (1/2 cup cooked)	27	0.59	0.14	6.41
Brussels sprouts (1/2 cup cooked)	28	1.99	0.39	5.54
Red bell pepper (1/2 cup chopped raw)	23	0.74	0.22	4.49
Sweet potatoes (1/2 cup mashed)	125	2.25	0.23	29
Mango (1/2 cup chopped raw)	50	0.68	0.31	12.36
Orange (1/2 cup sections raw)	42	0.85	0.11	10.58
Strawberries (1/2 cup halves raw)	24	0.51	0.23	11.63
Blueberries (1/2 cup raw)	42	0.55	0.24	10.72
Pomegranates (1/2 cup seeds raw)	72	1.45	1.02	16.27
Millet (1/2 cup cooked)	104	3.05	0.87	20.59
Oats (1/2 cup cooked)	83	2.97	1.78	14.04
Pinto beans (1/2 cup cooked)	104	6.39	0.82	18.48
Soybeans (1/2 cup cooked)	127	11.12	5.76	9.94
Brazil nuts (1/2 cup whole)	438	9.52	44.62	7.81
Walnuts (1/2 cup halves)	387	15.04	37.08	5.99
Sunflower seeds (1/2 cup with hulls, edible portion)	134	4.78	11.84	4.6
Wild salmon (3 oz cooked)	155	21.62	6.91	–

Another concern is that a diet high in fat may be a source of increased oxidative stress in CF patients [103]. An investigation monitoring CF patients as they improved following a pulmonary exacerbation observed that as their intake of fatty foods increased so did their serum plasma fatty acids [103]. The increase in plasma fatty acids correlated with an increase in oxidative stress, which was further complicated by a lack of observed improvement in antioxidant circulation [103]. Due to concern about the ongoing oxidative stress it has been suggested that patients with CF may benefit from a diet rich in antioxidants to help optimize the benefits of a high fat diet [103]. Please refer to Table 2.3 for a review of foods high in antioxidants.

Dietary Fat Goal for Patients with Cystic Fibrosis

Individuals with CF benefit from a higher fat diet in order to more easily meet their energy needs [1, 5, 64–67, 69, 72, 73]. Consensus committees have suggested that 35–40% of calories from fat is a reasonable high fat diet goal [5]. An appropriate tactic for practitioners to use would be to determine the grams of fat necessary to achieve 35–40% of their patient's individualized calorie goal. This fat gram number could easily be provided to patients along with instructions for counting fat grams as needed. If a patient in need of additional calories is consuming significantly less fat at the time of assessment, the practitioner could start by increasing fat intake by 10%, similar to the method discussed for increasing calories. A fat gram goal could still be provided to the patient and/or the patient's family. Education on incorporating high fat foods into the diet ad libitum is another method that has shown success [69]. For high fat, high calorie foods and suggestions on how to incorporate into the diet please refer to Table 2.2.

Protein

Proteins are organic compounds made up of amino acids, nitrogen containing molecules [105]. Amino acids are necessary for building and replacing the majority of structures within the body including bones, muscles, blood, and skin [105]. They also can act as hormones, enzymes, transporters, and antibodies, work to regulate fluid balance and acid–base balance and can be utilized to provide energy and glucose if needed [105]. Protein is not as efficient of an energy source as fat; each gram of protein provides four calories. However, adequate intake of protein is critical to ensure the maintenance of bodily structures and functions and to provide the essential amino acids that the human body is unable to produce on its own [105]. In order to be absorbed in the intestine, proteins must be denatured by stomach acid and then broken down into di- and tri-peptides and free amino acids [105]. In the general population, protein intake should provide between 10 and 35% of total calorie needs, based on the recommendations for fat and carbohydrate provision [105]. Average dietary intake of protein is 10–15% of total kcal [106]. In developed countries, people are easily able to attain this goal [105].

Similar to fat, people with CF were historically noted to have difficulty with the digestion and absorption of protein with loss of nitrogen in stools [107]. Fecal loss of up to 50% of consumed protein has been recorded [61]. The recommendations for protein intake have thus also shifted over the years with improvements in PERT.

Historical Recommendations for Protein Intake in Cystic Fibrosis

As early as 1943 patients with CF were noted to have excessive loss of protein in their stool while consuming a regular diet [107]. Improvement in fecal loss of nitrogen was observed in patients placed on casein hydrolysate, despite increases in the total protein load provided to the patients [107]. Despite several early success stories use of protein hydrolysate formulas was not further considered for several decades. The concept of a low fat, high calorie diet was promoted as discussed earlier, with an emphasis on high protein intake to make up for stool protein losses [107].

Intact Versus Hydrolyzed Protein Sources

In the 1970s, a mixture of beef serum protein hydrolysate, MCT, and modified starch was found to improve growth, energy, and digestive symptoms in children with CF who consumed enough to meet greater than 80% of their total energy needs [107]. Previous attempts in using formulas with only MCT or hydrolyzed protein resulted in improved digestive symptoms but not in improved growth [107]. In trials of amino acid based supplements weight and markers of protein absorption seemed to be improved but patients did not experience any reduction in the signs and symptoms of malabsorption [108], possibly due to ongoing fat malabsorption. Further it was noted that it was difficult to continue the trial due to the high expense of the amino acid mixture [108]. In a cross-over study of nitrogen balance in CF patients on a variety of different protein sources with or without PERT, it was found that patients had similar absorption of intact protein with enzyme supplementation as they did on hydrolyzed protein without enzyme supplementation [109]. However, individual patients overall had higher nitrogen balance while on the hydrolyzed protein supplement due to decreased urinary nitrogen loss [109]. Thus throughout the 1970s and 1980s hydrolyzed protein was overall considered superior to intact protein [76].

In the late 1980s and early 1990s intact protein made a comeback. One study observed that despite intermittent issues with gastrointestinal tolerance in some patients, formulas with intact protein led to better protein deposition compared to partially hydrolyzed formulas [110]. This was attributed to the better quality protein and higher calorie content of the intact formula and resulted in the conclusion that there was no benefit of the broken down formula [110]. Additional studies found that there was no difference in the growth and growth rate of infants [111] and the weight patterns of children and young adults [112] on formulas with intact protein with enzyme replacement versus partially hydrolyzed formulas with [111] or without [112] enzyme replacement. Additional benefits include that the intact formulas are more affordable and more palatable [111, 112].

For the majority of patients with CF who require oral or enteral formula supplementation, provision of an intact formula with PERT seems to be adequate to promote growth and nutritional status [110–112]. It is important to note that a patient with an allergic or digestive issue in addition to PI, such as cow's milk protein allergy, cholestatic liver disease, or short bowel syndrome, would benefit from a protein hydrolysate formula [76]. PERT is still necessary when using broken down formulas [76].

Protein Metabolism in Cystic Fibrosis

Protein turnover and balance is an issue of significance in CF. Illness and inflammatory disease states are associated with high levels of skeletal muscle breakdown and increased synthesis of acute phase proteins [113]. Even though proteins are being synthesized, protein catabolism and loss of skeletal muscle are the main characteristics of the inflammatory response [113]. Given the importance of maintaining and improving the nutritional status of patients with CF [1–7], preventing or reversing catabolism would be a valuable outcome. There is some controversy regarding protein turnover in CF. Many studies agree that at baseline, patients with CF have higher levels of catabolism than healthy controls [114–116]. However it is thought that this may be due to malnutrition rather than an intrinsic element of CF [61]. Conversely, other investigations have not found evidence of increased protein turnover in CF compared to controls [117, 118] and conclude that observed variations in protein metabolism in CF reflect expected changes with malnutrition and infection [117]. Patients with CF do seem to be able to achieve anabolism with adequate nutrition intake of energy and protein [115, 119, 120]. Overall, it is agreed that it is imperative to promote adequate calorie and protein intake to avoid protein catabolism in CF patients [118].

Specific Amino Acids in Cystic Fibrosis

Taurine

Taurine has been suggested to be an especially important amino acid for individuals with CF by improving fat absorption [76]. Taurine and glycine are the amino acids used in the conjugation of bile salts; taurine-bound bile salts provide increased fat solubility, which could be of benefit in the PI population [76]. Due to fat malabsorption, patients with CF have been found to lose more taurine in their stools than control patients [121]. There is some evidence that supplementation with taurine normalizes bile-acid taurine levels [76, 121]. In some individuals with particularly severe fat malabsorption, 30 mg taurine per kilogram body weight per day has helped to decrease loss of fat in stools [122, 123]. More research is needed to assess for impact on nutritional status [123].

It has also been suggested that taurine may also help protect against muscular protein breakdown [119]. This theory was not substantiated by a crossover trial, as no differences in protein metabolism on and off taurine supplementation were found [119].

Leucine and Arginine

In certain situations, the amino acids leucine and arginine have helped to promote anabolism [124]. Given concern for possible excessive catabolism in CF patients [114–116] the effects of leucine enriched supplements on protein synthesis in CF have been studied; however no added benefit of leucine were observed [118]. Arginine and/or citrulline, the precursor of peripheral arginine, may yet prove to be beneficial in stimulating muscle anabolism in CF, however studies are needed to further explore this possible effect [118, 124].

Cysteine and Glutathione

Glutathione is an antioxidant comprised of three amino acids: cysteine, glutamate, and glycine, of which cysteine is a rate-limiting precursor [125]. As previously discussed, antioxidants and their possible beneficial effect on lung health is of interest in the CF population. A negative association between lymphocyte glutathione levels and lung function has been found, suggesting that there is increased utilization of glutathione in stressed lungs [125]. There is evidence that supplementation with cysteine rich foods, such as whey protein or N-acetylcysteine supplements, can help increase levels of glutathione [126, 127] and improve markers of inflammation [126]. However, changes in lung function have not been observed during the short study time frames (1–3 months) [126, 127]. It is possible that supplementation with cysteine to improve glutathione status may help stabilize lung function in the long term and may have preventative effects, especially if utilized earlier in life [126, 127]. Longer term studies in CF patients of a variety of ages are needed to better determine true effects and recommended intakes of cysteine.

Concerns About a High Protein Diet in Cystic Fibrosis

In the general population a diet exceptionally high in protein can put an individual at risk for azotemia, metabolic acidosis, and neurodevelopmental problems [113]. These effects have been observed in patients consuming 4–6 g protein per kilogram body weight [113]. Individuals with renal disease or liver disease are particularly at risk for the toxic effects of protein due to limitations metabolizing and excreting protein. There has been a report of an individual with cystic fibrosis-related liver disease becoming encephalopathic after consumption of 4.5 g protein per kilogram during a 6-h block of time [106]. This individual recovered, but the incident serves as a good reminder to be aware of total protein intake and to encourage appropriate distribution of food over the course of the day [106].

Another concern is the source of the amino acids. Protein should ideally come in the form of whole foods or regulated supplements. Patients and their providers should be wary of over-the-counter protein and amino acid supplements [105]. These supplements are often not regulated and may not be pure. They may contain an inappropriate distribution of amino acids putting individuals at risk for both deficiencies and toxicities of specific amino acids as well as unanticipated effects on metabolism [128]. Some amino acids in inappropriate quantities have been shown to affect hormonal or neurological function or may disrupt electrolyte balance [128]. Intake of protein supplements may also lead to excessive protein intake faster than intake of whole food or balanced oral supplements [105].

Dietary Protein Goal for Patients with Cystic Fibrosis

Protein requirements for individuals with CF have been expressed in different ways; however there is overall agreement that the CF diet should be high in protein. An increase of 1.5–2 times above the RDA for age has been recommended [129]. Please refer to Table 2.4 for a review of the 2005 RDA for protein. A protein intake of 15% of total calories has also been suggested [72], with others suggesting intake up to 20% of total calories [58, 65]. Some investigators have had success improving whole body protein synthesis with very high protein doses up to 5 g protein per kilogram body weight for

Table 2.4 2005 recommended daily allowance for protein [12, 105]

Age (years)	Grams protein/day	Grams protein/kilogram weight[a] per day
0–0.5	9.1	~2.2
0.5–1	13.5	1.5
1–3	13	1.1
4–8	19	0.95
9–13 male	34	0.95
14–18 male	52	0.85
≥19 male	56	0.8
9–13 female	46	0.95
14–18 female	46	0.85
≥19 female	46	0.8
Pregnancy		
1st trimester	71	1.1
2nd trimester	71	1.1
3rd trimester	71	1.1
Lactation		
1st 6 months	71	1.1
2nd 6 months	71	1.1

[a]Based on reference body weights (~50 percentile for age)

children aged 7 to 12 years old [117]; this represents 500% of the RDA for age. As just discussed, a consistent protein intake this high may have dangerous side effects.

Given the wide variety of clinical presentations and calorie needs of individuals with CF, determining protein needs based on energy needs would be helpful to promote a well-balanced diet. Approximately 12–15% of calories from protein would be consistent with the literature and recommendations to increase protein intake relative to energy intake [61, 72]. This value should be compared to the RDA times 1.5–2 to help assess appropriateness of the protein load and to avoid excessive protein intake [105]. As with fat, if recommending a protein goal to a patient, it may be best to provide the goal in total grams protein per day. It is worth noting that overall patients seem to easily achieve, at the very least, adequate intake of protein when consuming a high calorie diet [61, 119, 129–131]. For examples of protein rich foods please refer to Table 2.5.

Carbohydrate

The term carbohydrate encompasses simple carbohydrates, mono- and disaccharides, requirements. Otherwise known as sugars, and complex carbohydrates or polysaccharides, which are starches and fibers [132]. Digestible carbohydrates provide approximately 4 cal/g [132]. Fibers are not digestible and as such provide minimal calories [132]. The bacteria in the colon can convert some fiber to short chain fatty acids (SFCA) which are important fuel for colonocytes; this conversion allows fiber to contribute up to 1.5–2.5 cal/g [132]. The general population is recommended to get 45–65% of total energy from carbohydrates [132].

The digestion of carbohydrates begins in the mouth with salivary amylase and is completed with pancreatic amylases and brush border enzymes [132]. Unlike fat and protein, individuals with CF have been observed to have minimal loss of carbohydrates in their stool [133]. Carbohydrate loss has been observed to be less than 1% of consumed carbohydrate in patients on standard PERT compared to loss of approximately 40% of consumed fat and 20% of consumed protein [133].

Table 2.5 Examples of high protein foods [102]

Food (serving size)	Grams protein/serving	Calories/serving
Beef (3 oz short loin)	23	188
Pork chop (3 oz)	22	178
Chicken (3 oz breast)	28	122
Chicken (1 thigh)	23	183
Fish (tilapia fillet)	23	111
Egg (1 large)	6	72
Milk, whole (1 cup)	7.7	149
Cheese, most varieties (1 oz)	6–7	85–115
Yogurt, plain whole milk (6 oz)	5.9	104
Tofu (1/2 cup)	10	88
Tempeh (3.5 oz)	18.2	196
Nuts (1 oz)	3–7	160–200
Peanut butter (2 tbsp)	7	191
Quinoa (1/2 cup cooked)	4.1	111
Pumpkin seeds (1 oz)	5.3	126
Beans (1/2 cup)	5–8	~110

Historical Recommendations for Carbohydrate Intake in Cystic Fibrosis

Due to seemingly adequate carbohydrate absorption in CF, it was most commonly recommended for patients to achieve their high calorie needs by increasing their intake of carbohydrates [10, 66, 133]. Carbohydrates were used to replace fat in children on the historical standard low fat diet to promote improved absorption and decreased gastrointestinal side effects [10, 66]. Unfortunately, as previously discussed, patients were not able to achieve high calorie intakes on the high carbohydrate diet and growth and health suffered [1, 10, 66].

Potential Benefits of Carbohydrates in Cystic Fibrosis

Aside from being easily digested and absorbed, carbohydrates, specifically fiber, may also support colonic bacteria and result in SCFA. Several studies have observed minimal or normal loss of SCFA in the stools of CF patients, which may help to support the energy needs of colonocytes and provide additional energy to the individual [133, 134]. There is a possible downside to this mechanism as excessive production and absorption of SCFA in a person with CF may increase the systemic acid load and exacerbate the acid–base balance in someone with severe lung disease [133]. However, not all studies found reason to be concerned about excessive SFCA absorption [134].

Concerns About High Carbohydrate Intake in Cystic Fibrosis

As previously discussed, a high intake of carbohydrate has been associated with an increased production of carbon dioxide which could lead to an exacerbation of respiratory status, especially in particularly sick individuals [88–90, 135]. Some studies have found that enteral formulas with a high percentage of energy from carbohydrate increased carbon dioxide production and the RQ more than high fat formulas [88, 89], however not all corroborate this [90, 135]. All of the studies agree that patients can compensate for the increased carbohydrate load without aggravating their pulmonary status. There is still concern that at higher levels of intake or in certain situations the high carbohydrate formulas might be more detrimental than observed [88–90, 135].

With the increasing occurrence of cystic fibrosis-related diabetes (CFRD) in the aging CF population, glucose tolerance does become a concern [135]. Formulas high in carbohydrate were found to significantly increase serum glucose concentrations and thus exacerbate hyperglycemia in patients with CFRD [135]. The main goal in managing CFRD is promotion of glycemic control. This is usually accomplished with insulin and pairing carbohydrate intake with protein and/or fat to allow an unrestricted diet [136]. For patients who require enteral nutrition support, it may be of some benefit to choose a formula that is higher in fat, instead of a high carbohydrate formula, to promote improved glucose control [135]. For more information about the management of CFRD please refer to Chapter 10.

Fiber and Cystic Fibrosis

In the general population a high fiber diet, 20–35 g of fiber per day for adults, is recommended for bowel health as well as for possible cardiovascular health and cancer prevention effects [132]. In children, the typical recommendation for determining daily grams of fiber is to add five to the current years of life [137]. Due to the focus on a high calorie diet, a high fiber diet has not historically been promoted in patients with CF [138]. There have been conflicting reports about the benefit of fiber in the diets of CF patients. One study observed very low fiber intake in English CF children and noted that the patients with a higher, but still low overall, fiber intake had less abdominal pain than those with even lower fiber intakes [138]. Thus, there is some thought that a higher fiber diet may help improve appetite and intake [60]. Alternatively, a higher occurrence of distal intestinal obstruction syndrome (DIOS) was found in Belgian CF patients with fiber intakes that were adequate to meet or exceed the recommended amount of fiber for the healthy population [137]. Low dietary fiber intake was not related to gastrointestinal symptoms [137]. These conflicting findings may reflect dietary differences in the country of origin, as overall fiber intake was much lower in the English study [137, 138]. It is also possible that the Belgian children with DIOS increased their fiber intake secondary to experiencing constipation [137].

Another study also found that incidence of constipation in patients with CF was not related to fiber or fluid intake, with all patients on average consuming less than 60% of the recommended amount of fiber [139].

There is no clear consensus on the appropriate amount of fiber to provide to individuals with CF. It appears that moderate fiber intake may be helpful in limiting abdominal pain in some patients but high fiber intake may cause more problems, including calorie displacement and possible abdominal pain exacerbations. As fiber rich foods, in particular fruits, vegetables, legumes, and whole grains provide the additional benefit of being rich in vitamins, minerals, and antioxidants it may be wise to recommend that patients incorporate these foods into their diet. Patients may not benefit as much from foods with added fiber or from fiber supplements. As with the general population, individuals with CF should increase their intake of fiber slowly [132] and with close supervision by providers [138], if they increase at all. Please refer to Table 2.6 for examples of high fiber foods.

Dietary Carbohydrate Goal for Patients with Cystic Fibrosis

The contemporary recommendation is to provide a diet with a normal amount of carbohydrates [140]. Due to the recommendations for a higher fat and high protein diet, carbohydrate intake may make up a smaller proportion of the CF diet compared to the general population. Based on the recommendations of approximately 35% of calories from fat and 15% from protein, 50% remains to come from

Table 2.6 Examples of high fiber foods by food group [102, 132]

Food (serving size)	Grams fiber/ serving	Calories/ serving	Other benefits
Grains			
Barley (1/2 cup cooked)	3	97	• Good source of vitamins and minerals
Oats (1/2 cup cooked)	2	83	• Can easily add calories with butter,
Brown rice	1.8	108	oils, nut butters, cheese, whole milk
Rye bread (1 slice)	1.8	83	
Whole wheat bread (1 slice)	2.6	87	
Bran cereal (1/2 cup)	9	65	
Vegetables			
Broccoli (1/2 cup cooked)	2.6	27	• Good sources of vitamins and minerals
Zucchini (1/2 cup cooked)	0.9	14	• Rich in antioxidants
Asparagus (1/2 cup cooked)	1.8	20	• Can provide additional calories with
Cabbage (1/2 cup cooked)	1.4	17	butter, oils, bacon, cheese, sour cream,
Brussels Sprouts (1/2 cup cooked)	2	28	ranch or other salad dressings, and
Corn (1/2 cup cooked)	1.7	25	hummus
Spinach (1/2 cup cooked)	2.2	21	
Kale (1/2 cup cooked)	1.3	18	
Carrots (1/2 cup raw)	1.8	72	
Fruit			
Apple with skin (1 small-medium)	3.6	77	• Good source of vitamins A and C
Pear with skin (1 small-medium)	4.6	84	• Rich in antioxidants
Peach with skin (1 small-medium)	2	51	• Add extra calories and protein with
Orange (1 small-medium)	3.4	65	cheese, nut butters, nutella and yogurt
Banana (1 small-medium)	2.6	90	dips
Kiwi (1/2 cup raw)	2.7	55	
Strawberries (1/2 cup raw)	2.9	27	
Legumes			
Peanuts (1 oz)	2.4	166	• Good source of protein, vitamins and
Beans, most varieties (1/2 cup cooked)	5–8	~110	minerals

carbohydrate; this is on the lower end of the range suggested for the healthy population (45–65%) [132]. It is still important that patients receive, at minimum, the RDA for carbohydrate, which is based on the brain's glucose needs. The RDA is 60–95 g during the first year of life and is 130 g after that, other than during periods of pregnancy and lactation when it is 175 and 210 g, respectively [132]. This minimum goal should be easily achieved with a high calorie diet. Patients likely do not need to receive a specific carbohydrate goal, though counseling on fiber may help some.

Conclusion

This chapter opened with a question, and in conclusion, not all calories are equal in CF. While those with CF may likely have higher energy needs than is considered typical, a balanced diet with wholesome foods is still important. High fat foods will help achieve high calorie needs but encouraging intake of mono and polyunsaturated fatty acids may help prevent cardiovascular complications in a population experiencing increasing longevity. Foods that are high in protein will help limit catabolism. Carbohydrates, once the foundation of the CF diet are no longer emphasized as patients likely consume enough carbohydrate foods. Some adjustments to carbohydrate intake may be helpful as certain patients might benefit from additional fiber. Additionally, pairing carbohydrates with fat and/or protein will help promote calorie intake and glucose control.

The diet recommendations for someone with CF will be as individual and varied as their disease. Personalized assessment and recommendations are best for this population, however the recommendations provided in this chapter can serve as a guide.

References

1. Corey M, McLaughlin FJ, Williams M, Levison H. A comparison of survival, growth, and pulmonary function in patients with cystic fibrosis in Boston and Toronto. J Clin Epidemiol. 1988;41 Suppl 6:583–91.
2. Kraemer R, Ruderberg A, Hadorn B, Rossi E. Relative underweight in cystic fibrosis and its prognostic value. Acta Paediatr Scand. 1978;67:33–7.
3. Stern RD, Boat TF, Doershuk CF, Tucker AF, Primiano Jr FP, Matthews LW. Course of cystic fibrosis in 95 patients. J Pediatr. 1976;89:406–11.
4. Parsons HG, Beaudry P, Dumas A, Pencharz PB. Energy needs and growth in children with cystic fibrosis. J Pediatr Gastroenterol Nutr. 1983;2 Suppl 1:44–9.
5. Borowitz D, Baker RD, Stallings V. Consensus report on nutrition for pediatric patients with cystic fibrosis. J Pediatr Gastroenterol Nutr. 2002;35:246–59. doi:10.1097/01.MPG.0000025580.85615.14.
6. Stallings VA, Stark LJ, Robinson KA, Feranchak AP, Quinton H. Evidence-based practice recommendations for nutrition-related management of children and adults with cystic fibrosis and pancreatic insufficiency: results of a systematic review. J Am Diet Assoc. 2008;108 Suppl 5:832–9. doi:10.1016/j.jada.2008.02.020.
7. Yen EH, Quinton H, Borowitz D. Better nutritional status in early childhood is associated with improved clinical outcomes and survival in patients with cystic fibrosis. J Pediatr. 2013;162 Suppl 3:530–5. doi:10.1016/j.jpeds.2012.08.040.
8. Ramsey BW, Farrell PM, Pencharz P. Consensus Committee. Nutritional assessment and management in cystic fibrosis: a consensus report. Am J Clin Nutr. 1992;55:108–16.
9. Murphy JL, Wootton SA, Bond SA, Jackson AA. Energy content of stools in normal healthy controls and patients with cystic fibrosis. Arch Dis Child. 1991;61:495–500.
10. Chase HP, Long MA, Lavin MH. Cystic fibrosis and nutrition. J Pediatr. 1979;3 Suppl 3:337–47.
11. Schoni MH, Casaulta-Aebischer C. Nutrition and lung function in cystic fibrosis patients: review. Clin Nutr. 2000;19 Suppl 2:79–85. doi:10.1054/clnu.1999.0080.
12. Institute of Medicine. Energy. In: Dietary reference intakes for energy carbohydrate, fiber, fat, fatty acids, cholesterol, protein and amino acids. Washington: National Academy Press; 2002. p. 104–264.
13. Dodge JA. Nutritional requirements in cystic fibrosis: a review. J Pediatr Gastroenterol Nutr. 1988;7 Suppl 1:S8–11.
14. Dodge JA, Turck D. Cystic fibrosis: nutritional consequences and management. Best Pract Res Clin Gastroenterol. 2006;20 Suppl 3:531–46. doi:10.1016/j.bpg.2005.11.006.
15. Pencharz PB, Durie PR. Pathogenesis of malnutrition in cystic fibrosis, and its treatment. Clin Nutr. 2000;19 Suppl 6:387–94. doi:10.1054/clnu.1999.0079.
16. Amin R, Ratjen F. Cystic Fibrosis: a review of pulmonary and nutritional therapies. Adv Pediatr. 2008;55:99–121. doi:10.1016/j.yapd.2008.07.015.
17. Vaisman N, Pencharz PB, Corey M, Canny GJ, Hahn E. Energy expenditure of patients with cystic fibrosis. J Pediatr. 1987;111 Suppl 4:496–500.
18. Buchdahl RM, Cox M, Fulleylove C, Marchant JL, Tomkins AM, Brueton MJ, Warner JO. Increased resting energy expenditure in cystic fibrosis. J Appl Physiol. 1988;64:1810–6.
19. Stallings VA, Tomezsko JL, Schall JI, Mascarenhas MR, Stettler N, Scanlin TF, Zemel BS. Adolescent development and energy expenditure in females with cystic fibrosis. Clin Nutr. 2005;24:737–45. doi:10.1016/j.clnu.2005.02.005.
20. Zemel BS, Kawchaw DA, Cnaan A, Zhao H, Scanlin TF, Stallings VA. Prospective evaluation of resting energy expenditure, nutritional status, pulmonary function and genotype in children with cystic fibrosis. Pediatr Res. 1996;40:578–85.
21. Richards ML, Davies PSW, Bell SC. Energy cost of physical activity in cystic fibrosis. Eur J Clin Nutr. 2001;55:690–7.
22. Shepherd RW, Greer RM, McNaughton SA, Wotton M, Cleghorn GJ. Energy expenditure and the body cell mass in cystic fibrosis. Nutrition. 2001;17 Suppl 1:22–5.

23. Allen JR, McCauley JC, Selby AM, Waters DL, Gruca MA, Baur LA, Asperen PV, Gaskin KJ. Differences in resting energy expenditure between male and female children with cystic fibrosis. J Pediatr. 2003;142:15–9. doi:10.1067/mpd.2003.38.

24. Barclay A, Allen JR, Blyler E, Yap J, Gruca MA, Asperen PV, Cooper P, Gaskin KJ. Resting energy expenditure in females with cystic fibrosis: is it affected by puberty? Eur J Clin Nutr. 2007;61:1207–12. doi:10.1038/sj. ejcn.1602637.

25. Spicher V, Roulet M, Schutz Y. Assessment of total energy expenditure in free-living patients with cystic fibrosis. J Pediatr. 1991;118 Suppl 6:865–72.

26. Gunrow JE, Azcue MP, Berall G, Pencharz PB. Energy expenditure in cystic fibrosis during activities of daily living. J Pediatr. 1993;122 Suppl 2:243–6.

27. O'Rawe A, McIntosh I, Dodge JA, Brock DJ, Redmond AO, Ward R, Macpherson AJ. Increased energy expenditure in cystic fibrosis is associated with specific mutations. Clin Sci. 1992;82 Suppl 1:71–6.

28. Tomezsko JL, Stallings VA, Kawchak DA, Goin JE, Diamond G, Scanlin TF. Energy expenditure and genotype of children with cystic fibrosis. Pediatr Res. 1994;35 Suppl 4:451–60.

29. Thomson MA, Wilmott RW, Wainwright C, Masters B, Francis PJ, Shepherd RW. Resting energy expenditure, pulmonary inflammation, and genotype in the early course of cystic fibrosis. J Pediatr. 1996;129 Suppl 3:367–73.

30. Girardet JP, Tounian P, Sardet A, Veinberg F, Grimfeld A, Tournier G, Fontaine JL. Resting energy expenditure in infants with cystic fibrosis. J Pediatr Gastroenterol Nutr. 1994;18 Suppl 2:214–9.

31. Thomson MA, Bucolo S, Quirk P, Shepherd RW. Measured versus predicted energy expenditure in infants: a need for reappraisal. J Pediatr. 1995;126 Suppl 1:21–7.

32. Bell SC, Saunders MJ, Elborn JS, Shale DJ. Resting energy expenditure and oxygen cost of breathing in patients with cystic fibrosis. Thorax. 1996;51:126–31.

33. Fried MD, Durie PR, Tsui LC, Corey M, Levison H, Pencharz PB. The cystic fibrosis gene and resting energy expenditure. J Pediatr. 1991;119 Suppl 6:913–6.

34. Moudiou T, Galli-Tsinopoulou A, Vamvakoudis E, Nousia-Arvanitakis S. Resting energy expenditure in cystic fibrosis as an indicator of disease severity. J Cyst Fibros. 2007;6:131–6. doi:10.1016/j.jcf.2006.06.001.

35. Magoffin A, Allen JR, McCauley J, Gruca MA, Peat J, Asperen PV, Gaskin K. Longitudinal analysis of resting energy expenditure in patients with cystic fibrosis. J Pediatr. 2008;152:703–8. doi:10.1016/j.jpeds.2007.10.021.

36. Steinkamp G, Drommer A, von der Hardt H. Resting energy expenditure before and after treatment for *Pseudomonas aeroginosa* in patients with cystic fibrosis. Am J Clin Nutr. 1993;57:685–9.

37. Stallings VA, Fung EB, Hofley PM, Scanlin TF. Acute pulmonary exacerbation is not associated with increased energy expenditure in children with cystic fibrosis. J Pediatr. 1998;132 Suppl 3:493–9.

38. Groleau V, Schall JI, Dougherty KA, Latham NE, Maqbool A, Mascarenhas MR, Stallings VA. Effect of dietary intervention on growth and energy expenditure in children with cystic fibrosis. J Cyst Fibros. 2014. doi:10.1016/j. jcf.2014.01.009.

39. Shepherd RW, Vasques-Velasquez L, Prentice A, Holt TL, Coward WA, Lucas A. Increased energy expenditure in young children with cystic fibrosis. Lancet. 1988;2:1300–3.

40. Davies PSW, Erskine JM, Hambridge KM, Accurso FJ. Longitudinal investigation of energy expenditure in infants with cystic fibrosis. Eur J Clin Nutr. 2002;56:940–6.

41. Pencharz PB, Berall G, Vaisman N, Corey M, Canny G. Energy expenditure in children with cystic fibrosis. Lancet. 1988;2:513–4.

42. Bronstein MN, Davies PS, Hambidge KM, Accurso FJ. Normal energy expenditure in the infant with presymptomatic cystic fibrosis. J Pediatr. 1995;126 Suppl 1:28–33.

43. Bines JE, Truby HD, Armstrong DA, Phelan PD, Grimwood K. Energy metabolism in infants with cystic fibrosis. J Pediatr. 2002;140 Suppl 5:527–33. doi:10.1067/mpd.2002.123284.

44. Marin VB, Velandia S, Hunter B, Gattas V, Fielbaum O, Herrera O, Diaz E. Energy expenditure, nutrition status and body composition in children with cystic fibrosis. Nutrition. 2004;20 Suppl 2:181–6. doi:10.1016/j. nutr.2003.10.010.

45. Johnson MR, Ferkol TW, Shepherd RW. Energy cost of activity and exercise in children and adolescents with cystic fibrosis. J Cyst Fibros. 2006;5:53–8. doi:10.1016/j.jcf.2005.10.001.

46. McCloskey M, Redmond AOB, McCabe C, Pyper S, Westerterp KR, Elborn SJ. Energy balance in cystic fibrosis when stable and during a respiratory exacerbation. Clin Nutr. 2004;23:1405–12. doi:10.1016/j.clnu.2004.06.010.

47. Shapiro BL. Mitochondrial dysfunction, energy expenditure and cystic fibrosis. Lancet. 1988;2:289.

48. O'Rawe A, Dodge JA, Redmond AOB, McIntosh I, Brock DJH. Gene/energy interaction in cystic fibrosis. Lancet. 1990;2:552–3.

49. Kuhn RD, Gelrud A, Munck A, Caras S. CREON (pancrelipase delayed release capsules) for the treatment of exocrine pancreatic insufficiency. Adv Ther. 2010;27 Suppl 12:895–916. doi:10.1007/s12325-010-0085-7.

50. Walkowiak J, Nousia-Arvanitakis S, Henker J, Stern M, Sinaasappel M, Dodge JA. Indirect pancreatic function tests in children. J Pediatr Gastroenterol Nutr. 2005;40 Suppl 2:107–14.

51. Trabulsi J, Ittenbach RF, Schall JI, Olsen IE, Yudkoff M, Daikhin Y, Zemel BS, Stallings VA. Evaluation of formulas for calculating total energy requirements of preadolescent children with cystic fibrosis. Am J Clin Nutr. 2007;85:144–51.

52. Schall JI, Bentley T, Stallings VA. Meal patterns, dietary fat intake and pancreatic enzyme use in preadolescent children with cystic fibrosis. J Pediatr Gastroenterol Nutr. 2006;43 Suppl 5:651–9.

53. White H, Wolfe SP, Foy J, Morton A, Conway SP, Brownlee KB. Nutritional intake and status in children with cystic fibrosis: does age matter? J Pediatr Gastroenterol Nutr. 2007;44 Suppl 1:116–23.

54. Kawchak DA, Zhao H, Scanlin TF, Tomezsko JL, Cnaan A, Stallings VA. Longitudinal, prospective analysis of dietary intake in children with cystic fibrosis. J Pediatr. 1996;129 Suppl 1:119–29.

55. Woestenenk JW, Castelijns SJAM, van der Ent CK, Houwen RHJ. Dietary intake in children and adolescents with cystic fibrosis. Clin Nutr. 2014;33:528–32. doi:10.1016/j.clnu.2013.07.011.

56. Tomezsko JL, Stallings VA, Scanlin TF. Dietary intake of healthy children with cystic fibrosis compared with normal control children. J Pediatr. 1992;90:547–53.

57. Powers SW, Patton SR, Byars KC, Mitchell MJ, Jelalian E, Mulvihill MM, Hovell MF, Stark LJ. Caloric intake and eating behavior in infants and toddlers with cystic fibrosis. J Pediatr. 2002. doi:10.1542/peds.109.5.e75.

58. Macdonald A, Holden C, Harris G. Nutritional strategies in cystic fibrosis: current issues. J R Soc Med. 1991;84 Suppl 18:28–35.

59. Pencharz PB, Berall G, Corey M, Durie P, Vaisman N. Energy intake in cystic fibrosis. Nutr Rev. 1989;47:31–2.

60. Sinaasappel M, Stern M, Littlewood J, Wolfe S, Steinkamp G, Heijerman HGM, Robberecht E, Doring G. Nutrition in patients with cystic fibrosis: a European consensus. J Cyst Fibros. 2002;1:51–75.

61. Turck D, Michaud L. Cystic fibrosis: nutritional consequences and management. Baillieres Clin Gastroenterol. 1998;12 Suppl 4:805–22.

62. Hise ME, Brown JC. Lipids. In: Gottschlich MM, DeLegge MH, Mattox T, Mueller C, Worthington P, editors. The A.S.P.E.N. nutrition support core curriculum: a case based approach – the adult patient. USA: American Society for Parenteral and Enteral Nutrition; 2007. p. 48–70.

63. Green MR, Buchanan E, Weaver LT. Nutritional management of the infant with cystic fibrosis. Arch Dis Child. 1995;72:452–6.

64. Gaskin KJ. Nutritional care in children with cystic fibrosis: are our patients becoming better? Eur J Clin Nutr. 2013;67:558–64. doi: 10.1038/ejcn.2013.20.

65. Luder E, Kattan M, Thornton JC, Koehler KM, Bonforte RJ. Efficacy of a nonrestricted fat diet in patients with cystic fibrosis. Am J Dis Child. 1989;143:458–64.

66. Pencharz PB. Energy intakes and low-fat diets in children with cystic fibrosis. J Pediatr Gastroenterol Nutr. 1983;2:400–2.

67. Daniels L, Davidson GP, Martin JA. Comparison of the macronutrient intake of healthy controls and children with cystic fibrosis on low fat or nonrestricted fat diets. J Pediatr Gastroenterol Nutr. 1987;6 Suppl 3:381–6.

68. Marlotta RB, Floch MH. Dietary therapy of steatorrhea. Gastroenterol Clin North Am. 1989;18:485–512.

69. Walkowiak J, Przyslawski J. Five-year prospective analysis of dietary intake and clinical status in malnourished cystic fibrosis patients. J Hum Nutr Diet. 2003;16:225–31.

70. Anthony H, Bines J, Phelan P, Paxton S. Relation between dietary intake and nutritional status in cystic fibrosis. Arch Dis Child. 1998;78:443–7.

71. Landon C, Kerner JA, Castillo R, Adams L, Whalen R, Lewiston NJ. Oral correction of essential fatty acid deficiency in cystic fibrosis. J Parenter Enteral Nutr. 1981;5:501–4. doi:10.1177/0148607181005006501.

72. Macdonald A. Nutritional management of cystic fibrosis. Arch Dis Child. 1996;74:81–7.

73. Robinson P. Nutritional status and requirements in cystic fibrosis. Clin Nutr. 2001;20 Suppl 1:81–6. doi:10.1054/clnu.2001.0408.

74. Collins CE, O'Loughlin EV, Henry RL. Fat gram target to achieve high energy intake in cystic fibrosis. J Paediatr Child Health. 1997;31:142–7.

75. Widhalm K, Gotz M. Long-term use of medium chain triglycerides in cystic fibrosis (author's translation). Wien Klin Wochenschr. 1976;88 Suppl 17:557–61.

76. Koletzko S, Reinhardt D. Nutritional challenges of infants with cystic fibrosis. Early Hum Dev. 2001;65:S53–61.

77. Kasai M, Nosaka N, Maki H, Suzuki Y, Takeuchi H, Aoyama T, Ohra A, Harada Y, Okazaki M, Kondo K. Comparison of diet-induced thermogenesis of foods containing medium- versus long-chain triacylglycerols. J Nutr Sci Vitaminol. 2002;48:536–40.

78. Clegg ME. Medium-chain triglycerides are advantageous in promoting weight loss although not beneficial to exercise performance. Int J Food Sci Nutr. 2010;61 Suppl 7:653–79. doi:10.3109/09637481003702114.

79. Maqbool A, Schall JI, Garcia-Espana JF, Zemel BS, Strandvik B, Stallings VA. Serum linoleic acid status as a clinical indicator of essential fatty acid status in children with cystic fibrosis. J Pediatr Gastroenterol Nutr. 2008;47:635–44.

80. Roulet M, Frascarolo P, Rappaz I, Pilet M. Essential fatty acid deficiency in well nourished young cystic fibrosis patients. Eur J Pediatr. 1997;156:952–6.

81. Maqbool A, Schall JI, Gallagher PR, Zemel BS, Strandvik B, Stallings VA. Relation between dietary fat intake type and serum fatty acid status in children with cystic fibrosis. J Pediatr Gastroenterol Nutr. 2012;5:605–11. doi:10.1097/MPG.0b013e3182618f33.

82. Al-Turkmani RM, Freedman SD, Laposata M. Fatty acid alterations and n-3 fatty acid supplementation in cystic fibrosis. Prostaglandins Leukot Essent Fatty Acids. 2007;77:309–18. doi:10.1016/j.plefa.2007.10.009.

83. Coste TC, Armand M, Lebacq J, Lebecque P, Wallemacq P, Leal T. An overview of monitoring and supplementation of omega 3 fatty acids in cystic fibrosis. Clin Biochem. 2007;40:511–20. doi:10.1016/j.clinbiochem.2007.01.002.

84. Thompson GN. Relationships between essential fatty acid levels, pulmonary function and fat absorption in pre-adolescent cystic fibrosis children with good clinical scores. Eur J Pediatr. 1989;148:327–9.

85. Burdge GC, Goodale AJ, Hill CM, Halford PH, Lambert EJ, Postle AD, Rolles CJ. Plasma lipid concentrations in children with cystic fibrosis: the value of a high fat diet and pancreatic supplementation. Br J Nutr. 1994;71:959–64.

86. Rettammel AL, Marcus MS, Farrell PM, Sondel SA, Koscik RE, Mischler EH. Oral supplementation with a high-fat, high-energy product improves nutritional status and alters serum lipids in patients with cystic fibrosis. J Am Diet Assoc. 1995;95 Suppl 4:454–9.

87. Heymsfield SB, Casper K, Funfar J. Physiologic response and clinical implications of nutrition support. Am J Cardiol. 1987;60:75G–81.

88. Kane RE, Hobbs P. Energy and respiratory metabolism in cystic fibrosis: the influence of carbohydrate content of nutritional supplements. J Pediatr Gastroenterol Nutr. 1991;12 Suppl 2:217–23.

89. Kane RE, Hobbs PH, Black PG. Comparison on low, medium, and high carbohydrate formulas for nighttime enteral feedings in cystic fibrosis patients. J Parenter Enteral Nutr. 1990;14 Suppl 1:47–52. doi:10.1177/014860719001400147.

90. Gottrand F, Hankard R, Michaud L, Ategbo S, Dabadie A, Druon D, Turck D. Effect of glucose to fat ratio on energy substrate disposal in children with cystic fibrosis fed enterally. Clin Nutr. 1999;18 Suppl 5:297–300.

91. Moss TJ, Austin GE, Moss AJ. Preatherosclerotic aortic lesions in cystic fibrosis. J Pediatr. 1979;1:32–7.

92. Smith C, Winn A, Seddon P, Ranganathan S. A fat log of good: balance and trends in fat intake in children with cystic fibrosis. J Cyst Fibros. 2012;11:154–7. doi:10.1016/j.jcf.2011.10.007.

93. Slesinski MJ, Gloninger MF, Costantino JP, Orenstein DM. Lipid levels in adults with cystic fibrosis. J Am Diet Assoc. 1994;94 Suppl 4:402–8. doi:10.1016/0002-8223(94).

94. Figueroa V, Milla C, Parks EJ, Schwarzenberg SJ, Moran A. Abnormal lipid concentrations in cystic fibrosis. Am J Clin Nutr. 2002;75:1005–11.

95. Georgiopoulou VV, Denker A, Bishop KL, Brown JM, Hirsh B, Wolfenden L, Sperling L. Metabolic abnormalities in adults with cystic fibrosis. Respirology. 2010;15:823–9. doi:10.1111/j.1440-1843.2010.01771.x.

96. Rhodes B, Nash EF, Tullis E, Pencharz PB, Brotherwood M, Dupuis A, Stephenson A. Prevalence of dyslipidemia in adults with cystic fibrosis. J Cyst Fibros. 2010;9:24–8. doi:10.1016/j.jcf.2009.09.002.

97. Hull JH, Garrod R, Ho TB, Knight RK, Cockcroft JR, Shale DJ, Bolton CE. Increased augmentation index in patients with cystic fibrosis. Eur Respir J. 2009;34 Suppl 6:1322–8.

98. O'Nady GM, Farinet CL. An adult cystic fibrosis patient presenting with persistent dyspnea: case report. BMC Pulm Med. 2006;6:9–12. doi:10.1186/1471-2466-6-9.

99. Aratari MT, Venuta F, De Giacoma T, Rendina EA, Anile M, Diso D, Francioni F, Quattrucci S, Rolla M, Pugliese F, Liparulo V, Di Stasio M, Ricella C, Tsagkaropoulos S, Ferretti G, Coloni CF. Lung transplantation for cystic fibrosis: ten years of experience. Transplant Proc. 2008;40:2001–2. doi:10.1016/j.transproceed.2008.05.029.

100. De Aragao Dantas Alves C, Seabra Lima D. Cystic fibrosis-related dyslipidemia. J Bras Pneumol. 2008;34 Suppl 10:829–39.

101. Whitney E, Rolfes SR. The lipids: triglycerides, phospholipids and sterols. In: Understanding nutrition. 10th ed. USA: Thomson Wadsworth; 2005. p. 140–79.

102. USDA National Nutrient Database for Standard Reference. USDA National Agricultural Library. Beltsville MD. 2011. http://ndb.nal.usda.gov. Accessed 30 Sept 2014, 3 Oct 2014, 4 Oct 2014.

103. Wood LG, Fitzgerald DA, Gibson PG, Cooper DM, Garg ML. Increased plasma fatty acid concentration after respiratory exacerbations are associated with elevated oxidative stress in cystic fibrosis patients. Am J Clin Nutr. 2002;75:668–75.

104. Whitney E, Rolfes SR. Antioxidant nutrients in disease prevention. In: Understanding nutrition. 10th ed. USA: Thomson Wadsworth; 2005. p. 389–93.

105. Whitney E, Rolfes SR. Protein: amino Acids. In: Understanding nutrition. 10th ed. USA: Thomson Wadsworth; 2005. p. 180–206.

106. Pandit C, Graham C, Selvadurai H, Gaskin K, Cooper P, van Asperan P. Festival food coma in cystic fibrosis. Pediatr Pulmonol. 2013;48:725–7. doi:10.1002/ppul.22702.

107. Berry HK, Kellogg FW, Hunt MM, Ingberg RL, Richter L, Guthar C. Dietary supplement and nutrition in children with cystic fibrosis. Am J Dis Child. 1975;129:165–71.

108. Darby C, Seakins JWT. Trial of amino acid supplements in cystic fibrosis of the pancreas. Arch Dis Child. 1971;46 Suppl 250:866–7.
109. Clegg KM. Nitrogen balance trials in cystic fibrosis patients. Nutr Metab. 1977;21 Suppl 1:77–9.
110. Pelekanos JT, Holt TL, Ward LC, Cleghorn GJ, Shepherd RW. Protein turnover in malnourished patients with cystic fibrosis: effects of elemental and nonelemental nutritional supplements. J Pediatr Gastroenterol Nutr. 1990;10 Suppl 3:339–43.
111. Ellis L, Kalnins D, Corey M, Brennan J, Pencharz P, Durie P. Do infants with cystic fibrosis need a protein hydrolysate formula? A prospective, randomized comparative study. J Pediatr. 1998;132 Suppl 2:270–6.
112. Erskine JM, Lingard CD, Sontag MK, Accurso FJ. Enteral nutrition for patients with cystic fibrosis: comparison of a semi-elemental and nonelemental formula. J Pediatr. 1998;132 Suppl 2:265–9.
113. Mehta NM, Compher C, ASPEN Board of Directors. A.S.P.E.N. clinical guidelines: nutrition support or the critically ill child. J Parenter Enteral Nutr. 2009;33:260–77. doi:10.1177/0148607109333114.
114. Holt TL, Ward LC, Francis PJ, Isles A, Cooksley WGE, Shepherd RW. Whole body protein turnover in malnourished cystic fibrosis patients and its relationship to pulmonary disease. Am J Clin Nutr. 1985;41:1061–6.
115. Shepherd RW, Holt TL, Thomas BJ, Kay L, Ilsles A, Francis MD, Ward LC. Nutritional rehabilitation in cystic fibrosis: controlled studies of effects on nutritional growth retardation, body protein turnover and course of pulmonary disease. J Pediatr. 1986;109 Suppl 5:788–94.
116. Hardin DS, Ellis KJ, Dyson M, Rice J, McConnell R, Seilheimer DK. Growth hormone decreases protein catabolism in children with cystic fibrosis. J Clin Endocrinol Metab. 2001;86 Suppl 9:4424–8.
117. Thompson GN, Tomas FM. Protein metabolism in cystic fibrosis: responses to malnutrition and taurine supplementation. Am J Clin Nutr. 1987;46:606–13.
118. Vaisman N, Clarke R, Rossi M, Goldberg E, Zello GA, Pencharz PB. Protein turnover and resting energy expenditure in patients with under nutrition and chronic lung disease. Am J Clin Nutr. 1992;55:63–9.
119. Geukers VGM, Oudshoorn JH, Taminiau JAJM, van der Ent CK, Schilte P, Ruiter AFC, Ackermans MT, Endert E, Jonkers-Schuitema CF, Heymans HAS, Sauerwein HP. Short-term protein intake and stimulation of protein synthesis in stunted children with cystic fibrosis. Am J Clin Nutr. 2005;81:605–10.
120. Engelen MPKJ, Com G, Wolfe RR, Deutz NEP. Dietary essential amino acids are highly anabolic in pediatric patients with cystic fibrosis. J Cyst Fibros. 2013;12:445–53. doi:10.1016/j.jcf.2012.12.011.
121. Thompson GN. Excessive fecal taurine loss predisposes to taurine deficiency in cystic fibrosis. J Pediatr Gastroenterol Nutr. 1988;7:214–9.
122. Belli DC, Levy E, Darling P, Leroy C, Lepage G, Giguere R, Roy CC. Taurine improves the absorption of a fat meal in patients with cystic fibrosis. Pediatrics. 1987;80:517–23.
123. Smith LJ, Lacaille F, Lepage G, Ronco N, Lamarre A, Roy CC. Taurine decreases fecal fatty acid and sterol excretion in cystic fibrosis. Am J Dis Child. 1991;145:1401–4.
124. Jonker R, Engelen MPKJ, Deutz NEP. Role of specific dietary amino acids in clinical conditions. Br J Nutr. 2012;108:S139–48. doi:10.1017/S0007114512002358.
125. Lands LC, Grey V, Smountas AA, Kramer VG, McKenna D. Lymphocyte glutathione levels in children with cystic fibrosis. Chest. 1999;116 Suppl 1:201–5.
126. Tirouvanziam R, Conrad CK, Bottiglieri T, Herzenberg LA, Moss RB, Herzenberg LA. High-dose oral N-acetylcysteine, a glutathione prodrug, modulates inflammation in cystic fibrosis. Proc Natl Acad Sci U S A. 2006;103 Suppl 12:4628–33.
127. Grey V, Mohammed SR, Smountas AA, Bahlool R, Lands LC. Improved glutathione status in young adult patients with cystic fibrosis supplemented with whey protein. J Cyst Fibros. 2003;2:195–8. doi:10.1016/S1569-1993(03)00097-3.
128. Garlick PJ. Assessment of the safety of glutamin and other amino acids. J Nutr. 2001;131:2556S–61.
129. Leonard A, Schindler T. Cystic fibrosis nutrition 101: getting started 6th edition. 2014. https://portcf2dev.cff.org/RegistryLaunch/Documents/CFNutrition101version20140722.pdf. Accessed 20 Sept 2014.
130. Hanning RM, Blimkie CJR, Bar-Or O, Lands LC, Moss LA, Wilson WM. Relationships among nutritional status and skeletal and respiratory muscle function in cystic fibrosis: does early dietary supplementation make a difference? Am J Clin Nutr. 1993;57:580–7.
131. Michel SH, Maqbool A, Hanna MD, Mascarenhas M. Nutrition management of pediatric patients who have cystic fibrosis. Pediatr Clin North Am. 2009;56:1123–41. doi:10.1016/j.pcl.2009.06.008.
132. Whitney E, Rolfes SR. The carbohydrates: sugars, starches, and fibers. In: Understanding nutrition. 10th ed. USA: Thomson Wadsworth; 2005. p. 102–131.
133. Hoffman RD, Isenberg N, Powell GK. Carbohydrate malabsorption in minimal in school-age cystic fibrosis children. Dig Dis Sci. 1987;32 Suppl 10:1071–4.
134. Vaisman N, Tabachnik E, Sklan D. Short-chain fatty acid absorption in patients with cystic fibrosis. J Pediatr Gastroenterol Nutr. 1992;15 Suppl 2:146–9.

135. Milla C, Doherty L, Raatz S, Schwarzenberg SJ, Regelmann W, Moran A. Glycemic response to dietary supplements in cystic fibrosis is dependent on the carbohydrate content of the formula. J Parenter Enteral Nutr. 1996;20:182–6. doi:10.1177/0148607196020003182.

136. Wilson DC, Kalnin C, Stewart C, Hamilton N, Hanna AK, Durie PR, Tullis E, Pencharz PB. Challenges in the dietary treatment of cystic fibrosis related diabetes mellitus. Clin Nutr. 2000;19 Suppl 2:87–93.

137. Proesmans M, De Boeck K. Evaluation of dietary fiber intake in Belgian children with cystic fibrosis: is there a link with gastrointestinal complaints. J Pediatr Gastroenterol Nutr. 2002;35:610–4.

138. Gavin J, Ellis J, Dewar AL, Rolles CJ, Connett GJ. Dietary fibre and the occurrence of gut symptoms in cystic fibrosis. Arch Dis Child. 1997;76:35–7.

139. Van der Doef HPJ, Kokke FTM, Beek FJA, Woestenenk JW, Froeling SP, Houwen RHJ. Constipation in pediatric cystic fibrosis patients: an underestimated medical condition. J Cyst Fibros. 2010;9:59–63. doi:10.1016/j.jcf.2009.11.003.

140. Anton DT, Moraru D, Cirdei E, Bozomitu L. Malnutrition and complex nutritional therapy in cystic fibrosis. Rev Med Chir Soc Med Nat Iasi. 2006;110 Suppl 4:801–6.

Chapter 3
Dietary Fat and Fat Metabolism in CF

Asim Maqbool and Birgitta Strandvik

Key Points

- Patients with cystic fibrosis are at risk for essential fatty acid deficiency and for fatty acid abnormalities, which may be multifactorial in etiology.
- While the debate over whether to restrict fat or to promote fat in the diet has been decided in favor of the latter, there still remains controversy about what fats to recommend.
- Linoleic acid deficiency is well documented, as well as its association with growth impairment and clinical outcomes in patients with CF.
- Improving linoleic acid status is a goal, as status is associated with many important clinical outcomes of interest, including growth, anthropometric measures, and lung function (FEV_1).
- There is concern that providing linoleic acid in the diet may drive inflammation, as demonstrated by in vitro and animal models, mostly.
- In contrast, clinical pediatric studies have shown that LA and energy supplementation have been associated with improved growth and other clinical outcomes of interest.
- Energy intake remains an important factor and variable in this discussion and fat remains an important source of energy intake.
- Docosahexaenoic acid (DHA) is also frequently low in patients with CF, and supplementation with DHA is thought to be safe, improves DHA levels, but has improved clinical status in only one human study.
- Rather than focus on normalization of fatty acid status as a function of what is observed in the general population, the goal of energy and fat quality in patients with CF shown be directed towards interventions that help improve growth, improve or preserve FEV_1, and other clinical outcomes of interest.
- An approach to modify dietary fat based on the medical literature helps forge a direction and a path forward. Additional prospective studies are required to more precisely determine specific dietary fat needs by age and life stage in patients with CF.

A. Maqbool, M.D. (✉)
Gastroenterology, Hepatology and Nutrition, The Children's Hospital of Philadelphia, University of Pennsylvania Perelman School of Medicine, 34 and Civic Center Boulevard, Room 8C09H, Philadelphia, PA 19104, USA
e-mail: maqbool@email.chop.edu

B. Strandvik, M.D., Ph.D.
Department of Biosciences and Nutrition, Karolinska Institutet,
NOVUM, Halsovagen 7-9, 14183 Huddinge, Stockholm, Sweden
e-mail: birgitta.strandvik@ki.se

E.H. Yen, A.R. Leonard (eds.), *Nutrition in Cystic Fibrosis: A Guide for Clinicians*, Nutrition and Health, DOI 10.1007/978-3-319-16387-1_3, © Springer International Publishing Switzerland 2015

Keywords Essential fatty acid deficiency • Linoleic acid • Docosahexaenoic acid • DHA • Metabolism • Inflammation • Eicosanoid • Dietary and outcome goals

Introduction

Individuals with cystic fibrosis (CF) and in particular those with pancreatic insufficiency (PI) are prone to fatty acid abnormalities, especially essential fatty acid (EFA) deficiency, which may be multifactorial in origin. While the debate of whether or not to restrict fat in the diet has been settled with respect to clinical outcomes favoring fat supplementation, the amount and quality of fat in the diet required for improving health outcomes by life stage groups has yet to be defined. Furthermore, while there have been advancements in our understanding of the importance of specific types of fats in the diet, there is discordance between the clinical data and basic science data regarding the essential fats. Moving beyond these existing controversies, consensus may be forming about a paradigm shift in how we think about these dietary fats and fatty acids—less maybe to "normalize them"—than to modify their status towards one associated with improving clinical outcomes.

Dietary Fat Requirements

Dietary fat intake is required to provide EFAs and fat soluble vitamins. Dietary fat is also important to provide energy substrate to meet needs for normal growth, development, and energy expenditure. We require approximately 1–2% of our dietary intake to be from EFAs to meet our needs [1, 2], but actual daily intake is about 10% in the form of linoleic acid [2]. The current Acceptable Macronutrient Distribution Range for fat intake as a function of energy intake is between 30 and 40% for children one to three years of age and 20–35% for children greater than four years of age and for adults [1]. Fat constitutes 50% of the energy intake from breast milk [3].

A Primer on Fatty Acid Metabolism

Fat Tissue Compartments and Reporting Modalities

Fatty acid status is determined in different tissue compartments, including cholesterol esters, triglycerides, erythrocyte and total phospholipids in plasma and cell membranes. Fatty acid status can be presented as a relative measure, weight/weight (mol%), or in absolute units [umol/L] [4]. Fat obtained from the diet is predominantly as triglycerides. However, when discussing fat tissue compartments from a metabolic perspective, the phospholipid compartment is perhaps the most relevant, as it represents the environment of cell metabolism. When total lipids in plasma (or serum) are presented, all the classes of fat compartments are included. It is noteworthy that the most labile of these tissue compartments with respect to fatty acid composition in circulation is that of triglycerides. Triglyceride fatty acid profiles undergo dramatic shifts in the post-prandial period.

Essential Fatty Acids and Their Metabolism

Humans are unable to synthesize fatty acids with a double bond proximal to the ω6 position, and therefore are dependent on dietary fat sources to meet their EFA requirements, i.e. the fatty acids of the ω6 and ω3 series. Linoleic acid (LA; 18:2ω6) is the essential ω6 polyunsaturated fatty acid (PUFA), and it has important structural and functional roles, and is an important constituent of the lipid bilayer membrane. Alpha linolenic acid (ALA; 18:3ω3) is the essential ω3 PUFA. These EFAs are enzymatically sequentially desaturated and elongated to long-chain polyunsaturated fatty acids (LCPUFA), which have important structural and functional roles in human health and disease states (Fig. 3.1). ALA is desaturated and elongated to eicosapentaenoic acid (EPA; 20:5ω3) and docosahexaenoic acid (DHA; 22:6ω3), whereas LA is desaturated and elongated to di-homo-gamma-linolenic acid (DHGLA; 20:3 ω6) and arachidonic acid (ARA; 20:4ω6).These LCPUFA exert negative feedback on the desaturases. EFA deficiency, conversely, is associated with increased elongation of precursor fatty acids to their respective longer chain counterparts, to effect or maintain membrane fluidity and preserve function. The metabolic pathways for these fatty acids are parallel and inter-related, and there is substrate competition between these fatty acid series for the desaturases and elongases. The rate limiting step is at the level of the delta 6 desaturase, which is the first enzyme in this cascade. Certain dietary factors may inhibit or facilitate the respective enzymes in these transformations. Humans can synthesize fatty acids of the ω9 and ω7 series, which are desaturated and

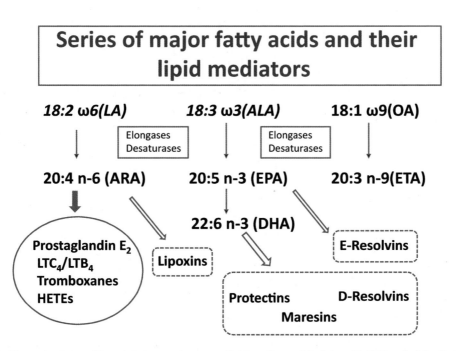

Fig. 3.1 The major fatty acids and their most important lipid mediators. Linoleic acid (LA) and alpha-linolenic acid (ALA) are the essential fatty acids, and humans are dependant on dietary intake provide these and meet our needs. LA and ALA are transformed by desaturation (see text) to highly unsaturated fatty acids and by elongases to longer fatty acids (more carbons). The most important long-chain fatty acids are arachidonic acid (ARA), eicosapentaenoic acid (EPA) and docosahexaenoic acid (DHA). ARA is mainly transformed to pro-inflammatory mediators (indicated by *filled arrow*) and EPA and DHA mainly to anti-inflammatory mediators (indicated by *open arrows*). The transformation steps compete about the same enzymes. In the setting of essential fatty acid deficiency, oleic acid (OA), which can be synthesized in the body, is transformed to eicosatrienoic acid (Mead acid). For further explanations, see text

elongated to compensate for longer chain ω6 and ω3 LCPUFA in the setting of decreased LA or ALA availability. Transformation of the ω9 series of fatty acids results in increased concentrations of Mead Acid (eicosatrienoic acid, 20:3ω9). Biochemically, EFA deficiency is primarily characterized by decreased levels of LA as well as by an increased triene: tetraene (20:3ω9/20:4ω6; T: T) ratio (Fig. 3.1). The T:T ratio was initially described by Holman et al. in the 1960s as abnormal if >0.04, and was later revised in the 1990s to abnormal if greater than >0.02 by the same investigators, reflecting changes in dietary intake in the general population, in which EFA deficiency is rare [5, 6]. Refinement in analytical techniques led to a revision of the cutoffs to one decimal place (0.4 or 0.2) [7]. The clinical consequences of EFA deficiency include impaired growth, seborrhea, platelet dysfunction, and poor wound healing [8, 9].

Membrane function follows membrane structure, and PUFA confer fluidity to the membrane. The LCPUFA have several important structural and functional roles. ARA has been suggested as important for growth and development. DHA is the most important structural component of the retina and of the central nervous system. Both ARA and DHA are actively transported across the placenta (most actively in the third trimester). They are also enriched in early breast milk and are frequently supplemented in infant formulae [10, 11]. ARA is the precursor to eicosanoids (prostaglandins, thromboxanes and leukotrienes) which are pro-inflammatory; however, ARA is also the precursor for lipoxin A, which has anti-inflammatory function. DHGLA and EPA are precursors to different prostaglandins, thromboxanes, and leukotrienes, which have other functions. The most important products of EPA and DHA are the anti-inflammatory lipid mediators named resolvins, protectins, and maresins (Fig. 3.1). These mediators function to resolve acute inflammation, and are necessary to prevent a chronic inflammatory state [12]. The balance of ω6 and ω3 fatty acids in the diet is thought to have changed at a population level over time, in transitioning from traditional and historical diets to the modern Western diet [13], and is postulated to be associated with the increase in the incidence and prevalence of several non-communicable diseases characterized by inflammatory states. The ratio of ARA to DHA serves as a surrogate marker for inflammation, and may differ by tissue type based on respective disease processes. For example, in patients with CF, this ratio is abnormal in serum [14] and in nasal epithelium [15].

Fatty Acid Abnormalities and Cystic Fibrosis: Concepts and Controversies

Fat malabsorption and steatorrhea are common in individuals with CF and PI. Steatorrhea has historically posed a challenge for quality of life for subjects with CF, more pronounced prior to the recent development of more efficient pancreatic enzyme replacement therapy (PERT). Restricting fat in the diet for individuals with CF versus not restricting fat has been associated with comparatively worse clinical outcomes [16]. Currently, fat intake is encouraged and recommended for individuals with CF, and in infants, the CF Foundation has suggested that ~35–40% of calories in the diet be from fat [17]. EFA deficiency has been described in subjects with CF and PI for more than 50 years [18], and is present in neonates with CF [19, 20] and in apparently well-nourished children with CF [14, 21]. There is evidence that the etiology of EFA deficiency in subjects with CF is multifactorial, and in addition to pancreatic insufficiency and fat malabsorption [22, 23], may relate to increased oxidative stress [24], increased membrane turnover [25], abnormal release of ARA from the cell membrane [26], increased expression and activity of desaturases as a primary event [27], to defects that may relate to genotype [14, 28], and to increased energy expenditure and imbalance, as reviewed elsewhere [29].

LA deficiency was the first fatty acid abnormality described in patients with CF in 1962 [18]. DHA deficiency was subsequently described a decade later [30]. LA and DHA are the most frequently described FA abnormalities in CF. ARA levels are not reported consequently to be abnormal in patients with CF; according to some reports, ARA levels may be increased, the same/similar to, or less than those observed in control subjects [14, 31].

EFA and PUFA abnormalities in CF may be multifactorial. PUFA abnormalities may relate to fat malabsorption [23], which conversely may be related to EFA deficiency and fatty acid abnormalities influencing the intestinal phospholipids [32], which may explain in part malabsorption that persists despite PERT [22]. Bile acid deficiency does not seem to contribute significantly to PUFA malabsorption in CF [33, 34]. Abnormal release of ARA from the lipid membrane bilayer has been previously described, mediated by phospholipase A_2, and may contribute to LA deficiency, as LA may be elongated to compensate for low membrane ARA levels [26, 28]. DHA deficiency may also relate to dietary intake, (since ω3 consumption is relatively much less relative to LA consumption [13, 35] or to an increased turnover of phosphatidylcholine in the membranes) [25, 29]. Less than 0.5% of ALA is converted to DHA in healthy subjects [36]. In CF models, the conversion of ALA to DHA may be impaired, further contributing to DHA deficiency [37].

While there is agreement that individuals with CF are prone to EFA deficiency, the approach to management remains controversial. Given the potential health consequences of EFA deficiency in patients with CF and PI, and the similarities in symptoms between animal models with EFA deficiency and patients with CF [38–40], several investigators have studied approaches to correct EFA deficiency; these warrant some discussion.

Nutritional Interventions

There are many short-term studies with supplementation in order to improve LA status, and, more recently, with ω3 fatty acids to improve DHA status. Supplementation studies with high energy foods or supplements rich in LA have yielded similar results as giving LA enterally [41–44] or parentally [45, 46] (see relevant reviews[29, 47]). These studies highlight the observation that adequate energy intake is required (but not always sufficient in itself) to preserve EFA to act as a membrane constituent and precursor to long chain counterparts, respectively, and to prevent these fats from being oxidized for energy. Energy intake has been described as an important factor in infants as much as supplementation with LA, and has been the source of a confounding variable in subsequent studies examining the relationship between type of dietary fat intake and serum FA status in children and adults with CF [48, 49]. Subsequent clinical pediatric studies in subjects with CF which controlled for energy as a confounding variable did find an association between type of dietary fat intake and serum fatty acid status [31, 50, 51]. Long-term LA supplementation studies have been demonstrated to influence the pathophysiology of the disease [46, 52, 53]. LA supplementation in the diet improves serum LA status. More importantly, dietary LA intake has been shown to be associated with improvements in growth in children with CF [31, 41, 42, 50, 54]. Following these landmark fatty acid supplementation studies demonstrating improvements in the pathophysiology of disease in CF in Sweden [46, 52, 53], the Swedish model of CF care has subsequently included both parenteral and oral supplementation to all patients as part of clinical standard of care practices [55]. These interventions are thought to have contributed to the improved clinical status and outcomes of CF patients with respect to pulmonary status, bone status, and anthropometry into adulthood [55–58].

As started above, LA status and LA intake have been associated with important clinical outcomes with CF. Improving LA status is clearly a goal and is not controversial. However, the manner in which we approach improving LA status has generated some debate. Specifically, there is concern that LA supplementation to improve LA status may increase transformation to ARA and to pro-inflammatory eicosanoids [59, 60]. However, high LA has an inhibitory effect on ARA in human cells [61], and similar results have been demonstrated in human subjects with CF[62]; in these studies, dietary intake of ARA only (not LA) was associated with high serum levels of ARA [63], as shown in healthy individuals [64].

DHA supplementation studies in subjects with CF have had multiple aims: to improve DHA status, to increase the anti-inflammatory DHA lipid mediators, and to influence the elongases and desaturases by exerting competitive inhibition of the elongation of LA to ARA. DHA also may have antibacterial properties towards Burkholderia cenocepacia, which may be desirable in individuals with CF [65]. Mouse model studies in CF have suggested that LA supplementation increases ARA, and DHA supplementation (in some studies) improves LA status and does not contribute to increased ARA production, but, via pathway interactions, may decrease ileal inflammation, and may reverse some of the CF related morphological pancreatic changes observed [60, 66–69]. The case for supplementation of DHA has been made on the basis of these studies and other studies reviewed elsewhere [47, 70].

DHA supplementation is thought to be safe, and oral supplementation of DHA may increase DHA concentrations in erythrocyte membranes [71], in serum phospholipids [72] and in plasma [73]. Enteral supplementation of ω3 fatty acids has also been demonstrated to increase EPA levels in neutrophils [74]. DHA supplementation in adult subjects was associated with improving DHA in plasma, erythrocyte, and duodenal tissue [75]. Intravenous supplementation of fish oil (which is rich in ω3 fatty acids) likewise increased DHA and EPA levels. DHA supplementation has been associated with decreasing the AA:DHA ratio [73], and in decreasing the ratio of pro-inflammatory to anti-inflammatory leukotrienes as well [74]. Perhaps the strongest case for EPA and DHA supplementation for patients with CF comes from an eight-month EPA and DHA supplementation trial in pediatric subjects with CF, which demonstrated increased levels of DHA and EPA in erythrocyte membranes, and decreased levels of ARA. The same study showed increases in LA alongside decreases in inflammatory markers, and is the only study that demonstrated an improvement in FEV_1 [76]. Other DHA supplementation studies in human subjects with CF varied from 6 weeks to 1 year in duration, and while improvements in DHA status were noted, did not demonstrate an effect on clinical outcomes of interest, including FEV_1 [71–73]. Interestingly, weekly intravenous ω3 supplementation over a 12-week period improved DHA status, but did not improve oxidation markers, and was actually associated deleterious effects of decreased glutathione levels and weight loss [77]. Contrary to most studies in patients with CF [71, 72, 74], some animal studies have shown benefit of DHA supplementation without a decrease or increase of ARA [66, 67, 78]. The primary beneficial effects of DHA on pancreas and ileum in a small study [69] have to date not been replicated in subsequently performed longer term studies [79]. However, liver histopathological/pathophysiological abnormalities appear to have been prevented in a longer term supplementation study [79]. Patients with CF related liver disease have been shown to have lower serum concentration of DHA than patients without that specific complication [80]. A Cochrane report, while stating that there may be some benefits to the use of ω3 fatty acids, did not currently support DHA or ω3 FA supplementation in CF [81].

How then to account for the discordance between DHA supplementation versus LA supplementation studies? Some of these observed differences may relate to the animal models versus human studies, since murine CFTR has only 70% homology to human CFTR. There are also different study populations across these studies, specifically, pediatric versus adult studies; growth is an important variable in the former, for which the intake requirements for LA may be greater as compared to needs for fully grown or adult subjects, in which deterioration of lung status might be most prominent. The type of supplement used may also affect study results. The duration of these respective supplementation studies may also be a factor; the duration of supplementation may need to be several months or longer prior to observing not only changes in concentrations of these respective fatty acids, but also changes in inflammatory markers and eventually outcomes of clinical interest [52].

Fatty Acid Status in CF: Normalization or Modification?

EFA deficiency is rare in the general population. The revision of the definition what constitutes a "normal" T:T ratio was based on trends in the general population and likely reflected changes in dietary fat intake patterns. The ratio of ω6:ω3 fatty acids has risen following the industrial revolution, and across populations globally, following departure from traditional diets to the modern Western diet. Parallel to these shifts, the incidence and prevalence of non-communicable diseases and inflammatory diseases has also increased [2, 13, 82]. These observations as well as EFA deficiency lead to the question: what should our goals be for fatty acid supplementation in CF?

"Normalization" is a natural goal, but is not always readily achievable [20, 83]. Christophe et al. [84] have proposed targeted modification of FA status associated with clinical outcomes, as opposed to correction of status as a function of levels seen in the general population. This line of reasoning would suggest that we have to examine the various fatty acid status markers routinely used and clinically available in relation to outcomes as a starting point. We then need to review not only how EFA status is defined currently, but also which of the markers are more clinically relevant. EFA status is defined by LA status, ALA status, or by an abnormal T:T ratio. Maqbool et al. [54] studied these markers of EFA status in relationship to clinically relevant outcomes (growth and pulmonary function) in pre-adolescent children with CF and PI, and reported that LA status predicted these outcomes of interest; LA cut points between 18 and 26 mol% were evaluated in this study, with a threshold effect noted in LA > 21 mol%. Of note, neither the 0.2 nor 0.4 T:T cut points were associated with clinically relevant outcomes. It is important to recognize that the T:T ratio may be influenced by other PUFAs in addition to LA [85]. Furthermore, EFA status as reported by LA or T:T reported similar biochemical information [54]. Shoff et al. also reported better growth status for infants and young children with CF to be associated with LA status [50]. These studies suggest that LA status may be more clinically relevant biomarker than the T:T ratio.

Therefore, our thinking regarding EFA status is undergoing a paradigm shift, from defining status as function of the healthy population to that associated with pulmonary and growth outcomes. Modification of the diet to provide sufficient energy, LA as well as ALA and longer chain ω3 PUFAS may be a reasonable approach. Olveira et al. [86] recently demonstrated that supplementation of a combination of EPA, DHA, LA, and gamma-linolenic acid in 17 adult subjects with CF for 1 year resulted in increased DHA, total ω3 PUFA, and LA levels, decreased the AA:DHA ratio, and decreased serum TNF-alpha, IgG, and IgM levels. Additionally, supplementation was associated with improvements in spirometry, and decreased number of days of respiratory exacerbations and antibiotic use. These results were similar to those reported from Sweden [55]. Fat free mass and handgrip dynamometry also improved, and were reportedly satisfactory in the Swedish population giving regular supplementation [87, 88]. This dietary fat modification study by Olveira and colleagues [86] and the more than 30 years of practical experience in Sweden reinforces the need for both LA and DHA, and suggests a path forward.

Other nutritional considerations for correcting the fatty acid abnormalities observed in individuals with CF relate to membrane phospholipids and their metabolic interfaces. Choline is the major component of phosphatidylcholine as the major phospholipid in the outer layer of the bilayer membrane, and is also at risk for deficiency in subjects with CF [89, 90]. Choline is required for methyl metabolism, cholinergic neurotransmission, transmembrane signaling, lipid cholesterol transport, and metabolism [91]. Choline supplementation studies have demonstrated improvement in choline status in CF [92]. Supplementation with LYM-X-SORB™, a novel organized lipid matrix containing choline and fatty acids, was shown to improve fatty acid and fat soluble vitamin status in pediatric subjects with CF [93]. Choline phospholipid metabolism intersects with 1-methyl metabolism, and supplementation with vitamin 5-tetrahydrofolate (a co-factor for these pathways) may improve choline status in subjects with CF as well [94]. There may be increased choline and membrane turnover in patients with CF [25], which may also explain the low DHA [29] and account for some of the phospholipid and fatty acid abnormalities observed in CF.

Abnormalities in ceramide metabolism have also been reported in CF, but the reports are divergent, which might refer to differences in species of ceramides [95–97]. Fenretinide blocks IL1-β formation and influences ceramide transformation, normalizing the fatty acid profile in an animal model of CF [95]. The implications of ceramide supplementation for patients with CF-particularly in limiting ARA production are intriguing, if these animal study results can be replicated in human subjects with CF.

There are indications that oxidative stress may contribute to EFA deficiency [24, 98, 99]. Fatty acids contain a number of double bonds, and are prone to oxidative damage. The high levels of markers of oxidative products frequently reported support this hypothesis; however, some studies also support these findings to be more indicative of the inflammatory and infectious status of these study subjects [100]. The relation between glutathione and CFTR in particular might suggest a link to defective oxidation defense. Of note, while intravenous ω3 fatty acid supplementation improved DHA status in patients with CF, it was also associated with a decrease in glutathione [101]; DHA has six double bonds, and may be more prone to oxidative stress. The role of lung transplantation in correcting FA abnormalities in CF may have to do with decreasing inflammation by restoring CFTR function to that specific tissue [102]. However, although the absolute fatty acid levels normalize, the pathological relation between the fatty acid concentrations persisted [102]. Lastly, basic science and animal models suggest that CFTR dysfunction may lead the PUFA abnormalities observed in CF [29, 103, 104], which might indicate that future treatment regulating CFTR expression might also compensate for the fatty acid abnormality by modulating the binding to the bilayer of the membranes [105] and/or could relate to additional or different mechanisms [29]. This association between CFTR and the lipid abnormalities described may also explain in part the relationship to genotype [14], and the difficulty in "normalizing" or improving LA concentrations by supplementation [44, 84].

Dietary Requirements: What We Know, and What We Don't Know

It is clear that individuals with CF have better outcomes by not restricting fat in their diets. Energy intake with energy dense nutrients such as fat is an important factor in thinking about fatty acids. Providing sufficient fat in the diet to reduce utilization of essential fats as a source of energy is an important goal, as essential fats are needed to contribute to cell membrane structure and function. The 2002 CF nutrition consensus statement may have suggested fat intake to comprise 35–40% of total caloric intake [17]. The work of Shoff et al. has suggested that greater than 120% of the estimated energy requirement may be indicated for young children with CF [50]. The relationship between LA energy intake and growth has also shown that regular supplementation with LA-rich supplements was associated with normal growth in pediatric subjects with CF, and did not require energy intake in excess of that recommended for normal individuals [106]. Energy intake requirements for pre-adolescent children with CF has been determined to be in "active" physical activity range of the estimated energy requirement (EER) of the Dietary Reference Intakes using doubly labelled water experiments [107, 108].

Until recently the type of dietary fat intake to improve serum FA status has not been defined. The data by Shoff et al. suggested that both energy intake and LA intake predict LA status [50]. Walkowiak et al. [31] and subsequently Maqbool et al. [54] showed that type of dietary fat intake does in fact predict serum fatty acid status. Similar to recommendations for the general population, limiting saturated fats, eliminating trans fats, and increasing monounsaturated fatty acids and PUFA are desirable. The high ω6 PUFA intake currently observed in the general population may be beneficial for patients with CF- but is questionable for the general population itself [109]. This area of dietary recommendation divergence can be navigated with some careful consideration. As an example of making sensible food choices, tuna has many health benefits, including provision of important ω3 PUFA. Balancing health benefits and risks, light canned tuna in water may be the better product for the general population, as it is a good source of ω3 LCPUFA, has a desirable low ω6:ω3 ratio, and is relatively lower in mercury content than albacore tuna; the canned tuna in oil (which is actually packaged in vegetable oil and is rich in LA) could be a better choice for individuals with CF [110]. LA intake and interventions associated with improving LA status are associated with improved clinical and growth outcomes. DHA intake and improved DHA status is associated with decrease in inflammatory markers. The clinical data supports LA supplementation, and the DHA data supports DHA supplementation. The data published by Olveira et al. demonstrated that a DHA, EPA, LA, and gamma linolenic acid supplementation improved FA status, markers of inflammation, and also important clinical outcomes, and provides insights for future studies to help forge a path forward [86]. Fat and energy intake requirements may change by life stage group, physical activity, and other factors which need to be determined by means of prospective studies. Early identification of CF and early nutritional interventions are required, as these may improve survival and clinical outcomes [19, 111].

Conclusion

Cystic fibrosis is a condition frequently associated with steatorrhea, and with fatty acid abnormalities. Adequate energy intake to meet needs is key to improve clinical outcomes. Fat intake is important in patients with CF. There are indications that fat intake for people with CF should be similar to those recommended for the general population, in choosing less saturated fat and more MUFA and PUFA. Intake of LA in excess of that recommended for the general population may be of benefit for patients with CF. Fat intake goals should be oriented towards improving growth in pediatric patients in particular, as well as clinical outcomes in patients with CF of all ages. Further studies are required to determine amount and type of fat intake required by life stage group, and what blend of dietary fats and dietary fat supplements are required to reach these goals. Interventions that improve CFTR function may improve fatty acid status as well as clinical outcomes of interest in CF.

References

1. Institute of Medicine. Dietary reference intakes for energy, carbohydrate, fiber, fat, fatty acids, cholesterol, protein and amino acids. Washington: National Academy Press; 2002.
2. Lands B. Historical perspectives on the impact of n-3 and n-6 nutrients on health. Prog Lipid Res. 2014;55:17–29.
3. Innis SM. Human milk and formula fatty acids. J Pediatr. 1992;120(4 Pt 2):S56–61.
4. Lagerstedt SA, Hinrichs DR, Batt SM, Magera MJ, Rinaldo P, McConnell JP. Quantitative determination of plasma c8-c26 total fatty acids for the biochemical diagnosis of nutritional and metabolic disorders. Mol Genet Metab. 2001;73(1):38–45.
5. Holman RT. The ratio of trienoic: tetraenoic acids in tissue lipids as a measure of essential fatty acid requirement. J Nutr. 1960;70:405–10.
6. Holman RT, Johnson SB, Ogburn PL. Deficiency of essential fatty acids and membrane fluidity during pregnancy and lactation. Proc Natl Acad Sci U S A. 1991;88(11):4835–9.
7. Siguel EN, Chee KM, Gong JX, Schaefer EJ. Criteria for essential fatty acid deficiency in plasma as assessed by capillary column gas–liquid chromatography. Clin Chem. 1987;33(10):1869–73.
8. Hansen RC, Lemen R, Revsin B. Cystic-fibrosis manifesting with acrodermatitis enteropathica-like eruption – association with essential fatty-acid and zinc deficiencies. Arch Dermatol. 1983;119(1):51–5.
9. Hansen AE, Haggard ME, Boelsche AN, Adam DJ, Wiese HF. Essential fatty acids in infant nutrition. III. Clinical manifestations of linoleic acid deficiency. J Nutr. 1958;66(4):565–76.

10. Hanebutt FL, Demmelmair H, Schiessl B, Larque E, Koletzko B. Long-chain polyunsaturated fatty acid (LC-PUFA) transfer across the placenta. Clin Nutr. 2008;27(5):685–93.
11. Koletzko B, Lien E, Agostoni C, Bohles H, Campoy C, Cetin I, et al. The roles of long-chain polyunsaturated fatty acids in pregnancy, lactation and infancy: review of current knowledge and consensus recommendations. J Perinat Med. 2008;36(1):5–14.
12. Levy BD, Serhan CN. Resolution of acute inflammation in the lung. Annu Rev Physiol. 2014;76:467–92.
13. Simopoulos AP. Importance of the ratio of omega-6/omega-3 essential fatty acids: evolutionary aspects. World Rev Nutr Diet. 2003;92:1–22.
14. Strandvik B, Gronowitz E, Enlund F, Martinsson T, Wahlstrom J. Essential fatty acid deficiency in relation to genotype in patients with cystic fibrosis. J Pediatr. 2001;139(5):650–5.
15. Freedman SD, Blanco PG, Zaman MM, Shea JC, Ollero M, Hopper IK, et al. Association of cystic fibrosis with abnormalities in fatty acid metabolism. N Engl J Med. 2004;350(6):560–9.
16. Corey M, McLaughlin FJ, Williams M, Levison H. A comparison of survival, growth, and pulmonary function in patients with cystic fibrosis in Boston and Toronto. J Clin Epidemiol. 1988;41(6):583–91.
17. Borowitz D, Baker RD, Stallings V. Consensus report on nutrition for pediatric patients with cystic fibrosis. J Pediatr Gastroenterol Nutr. 2002;35(3):246–59.
18. Kuo PT, Huang NN, Bassett R. The fatty acid composition of the serum chylomicrons and adipose tissue of children with cystic fibrosis of the pancreas. J Pediatr. 1962;60:394–403.
19. Marcus MS, Sondel SA, Farrell PM, Laxova A, Carey PM, Langhough R, et al. Nutritional status of infants with cystic fibrosis associated with early diagnosis and intervention. Am J Clin Nutr. 1991;54(3):578–85.
20. Lai HC, Kosorok MR, Laxova A, Davis LA, FitzSimmon SC, Farrell PM. Nutritional status of patients with cystic fibrosis with meconium ileus: a comparison with patients without meconium ileus and diagnosed early through neonatal screening. Pediatrics. 2000;105(1 Pt 1):53–61.
21. Roulet M, Frascarolo P, Rappaz I, Pilet M. Essential fatty acid deficiency in well nourished young cystic fibrosis patients. Eur J Pediatr. 1997;156(12):952–6.
22. Kalivianakis M, Minich DM, Bijleveld CM, van Aalderen WM, Stellaard F, Laseur M, et al. Fat malabsorption in cystic fibrosis patients receiving enzyme replacement therapy is due to impaired intestinal uptake of long-chain fatty acids. Am J Clin Nutr. 1999;69(1):127–34.
23. Kalivianakis M, Verkade HJ. The mechanisms of fat malabsorption in cystic fibrosis patients. Nutrition. 1999;15(2):167–9.
24. Wood LG, Fitzgerald DA, Lee AK, Garg ML. Improved antioxidant and fatty acid status of patients with cystic fibrosis after antioxidant supplementation is linked to improved lung function. Am J Clin Nutr. 2003;77(1): 150–9.
25. Ulane MM, Butler JD, Peri A, Miele L, Ulane RE, Hubbard VS. Cystic fibrosis and phosphatidylcholine biosynthesis. Clin Chim Acta. 1994;230(2):109–16.
26. Carlstedt-Duke J, Bronnegard M, Strandvik B. Pathological regulation of arachidonic acid release in cystic fibrosis: the putative basic defect. Proc Natl Acad Sci U S A. 1986;83(23):9202–6.
27. Seegmiller AC. Abnormal unsaturated fatty acid metabolism in cystic fibrosis: biochemical mechanisms and clinical implications. Int J Mol Sci. 2014;15(9):16083–99.
28. Bhura-Bandali FN, Suh M, Man SFP, Clandinin MT. The Delta F508 mutation in the cystic fibrosis transmembrane conductance regulator alters control of essential fatty acid utilization in epithelial cells. J Nutr. 2000;130(12):2870–5.
29. Strandvik B. Fatty acid metabolism in cystic fibrosis. Prostaglandins Leukot Essent Fatty Acids. 2010; 83(3):121–9.
30. Underwood BA, Denning CR, Navab M. Polyunsaturated fatty acids and tocopherol levels in patients with cystic fibrosis. Ann N Y Acad Sci. 1972;203:237–47.
31. Walkowiak J, Lisowska A, Blaszczynski M, Przyslawski J, Walczak M. Polyunsaturated fatty acids in cystic fibrosis are related to nutrition and clinical expression of the disease. J Pediatr Gastroenterol Nutr. 2007;45(4): 488–9. author reply 9.
32. Korotkova M, Strandvik B. Essential fatty acid deficiency affects the fatty acid composition of the rat small intestinal and colonic mucosa differently. Biochim Biophys Acta. 2000;1487(2–3):319–25.
33. Strandvik B, Einarsson K, Lindblad A, Angelin B. Bile acid kinetics and biliary lipid composition in cystic fibrosis. J Hepatol. 1996;25(1):43–8.
34. Werner A, Minich DM, Havinga R, Bloks V, Van Goor H, Kuipers F, et al. Fat malabsorption in essential fatty acid-deficient mice is not due to impaired bile formation. Am J Physiol Gastrointest Liver Physiol. 2002;283(4):G900–8.
35. Simopoulos AP. Overview of evolutionary aspects of omega 3 fatty acids in the diet. World Rev Nutr Diet. 1998;83:1–11.
36. Vermunt SH, Mensink RP, Simonis MM, Hornstra G. Effects of dietary alpha-linolenic acid on the conversion and oxidation of 13C-alpha-linolenic acid. Lipids. 2000;35(2):137–42.

37. Njoroge SW, Seegmiller AC, Katrangi W, Laposata M. Increased Delta5- and Delta6-desaturase, cyclooxygenase-2, and lipoxygenase-5 expression and activity are associated with fatty acid and eicosanoid changes in cystic fibrosis. Biochim Biophys Acta. 2011;1811(7–8):431–40.

38. Aaes-Jorgensen E, Leppik EE, Hayes HW, Holman RT. Essential fatty acid deficiency. II. In adult rats. J Nutr. 1958;66(2):245–59.

39. Hjelte L, Larsson M, Alvestrand A, Malmborg AS, Strandvik B. Renal function in rats with essential fatty acid deficiency. Clin Sci (Lond). 1990;79(4):299–305.

40. Hjelte L, Ahren B, Andren-Sandberg A, Bottcher G, Strandvik B. Pancreatic function in the essential fatty acid deficient rat. Metabolism. 1990;39(8):871–5.

41. Steinkamp G, Demmelmair H, Ruhl-Bagheri I, von der Hardt H, Koletzko B. Energy supplements rich in linoleic acid improve body weight and essential fatty acid status of cystic fibrosis patients. J Pediatr Gastroenterol Nutr. 2000;31(4):418–23.

42. Rettammel AL, Marcus MS, Farrell PM, Sondel SA, Koscik RE, Mischler EH. Oral supplementation with a high-fat, high-energy product improves nutritional-status and alters serum-lipids in patients with cystic-fibrosis. J Am Diet Assoc. 1995;95(4):454–9.

43. Parsons HG, Oloughlin EV, Forbes D, Cooper D, Gall DG. Supplemental calories improve essential fatty-acid deficiency in cystic-fibrosis patients. Pediatr Res. 1988;24(3):353–6.

44. Lloyd-Still JD, Johnson SB, Holman RT. Essential fatty acid status in cystic fibrosis and the effects of safflower oil supplementation. Am J Clin Nutr. 1981;34(1):1–7.

45. Chase HP, Cotton EK, Elliott RB. Intravenous linoleic acid supplementation in children with cystic fibrosis. Pediatrics. 1979;64(2):207–13.

46. Kusoffsky E, Strandvik B, Troell S. Prospective study of fatty acid supplementation over 3 years in patients with cystic fibrosis. J Pediatr Gastroenterol Nutr. 1983;2(3):434–8.

47. Coste TC, Armand M, Lebacq J, Lebecque P, Wallemacq P, Leal T. An overview of monitoring and supplementation of omega 3 fatty acids in cystic fibrosis. Clin Biochem. 2007;40(8):511–20.

48. Colombo C, Bennato V, Costantini D, Valmarana L, Dacco V, Zazzeron L, et al. Dietary and circulating polyunsaturated fatty acids in cystic fibrosis: are they related to clinical outcomes? J Pediatr Gastroenterol Nutr. 2006;43(5):660–5.

49. Olveira G, Dorado A, Olveira C, Padilla A, Rojo-Martinez G, Garcia-Escobar E, et al. Serum phospholipid fatty acid profile and dietary intake in an adult Mediterranean population with cystic fibrosis. Br J Nutr. 2006;96(2):343–9.

50. Shoff SM, Ahn HY, Davis L, Lai H. Temporal associations among energy intake, plasma linoleic acid, and growth improvement in response to treatment initiation after diagnosis of cystic fibrosis. Pediatrics. 2006;117(2): 391–400.

51. Maqbool A, Schall JI, Gallagher PR, Zemel BS, Strandvik B, Stallings VA. Relation between dietary fat intake type and serum fatty acid status in children with cystic fibrosis. J Pediatr Gastroenterol Nutr. 2012;55(5):605–11.

52. Strandvik B, Berg U, Kallner A, Kusoffsky E. Effect on renal function of essential fatty acid supplementation in cystic fibrosis. J Pediatr. 1989;115(2):242–50.

53. Strandvik B, Hultcrantz R. Liver function and morphology during long-term fatty acid supplementation in cystic fibrosis. Liver. 1994;14(1):32–6.

54. Maqbool A, Schall JI, Garcia-Espana JF, Zemel BS, Strandvik B, Stallings VA. Serum linoleic acid status as a clinical indicator of essential fatty acid status in children with cystic fibrosis. J Pediatr Gastroenterol Nutr. 2008;47(5):635–44.

55. Strandvik B. Care of patients with cystic fibrosis: treatment, screening, and clinical outcome. Annales Nestle' Birgitta. 2006;2006(64):131–40.

56. Sahlberg M, Eriksson BO, Sixt R, Strandvik B. Cardiopulmonary data in response to 6 months of training in physically active adult patients with classic cystic fibrosis. Respiration. 2008;76(4):413–20.

57. Gronowitz E, Garemo M, Lindblad A, Mellstrom D, Strandvik B. Decreased bone mineral density in normal-growing patients with cystic fibrosis. Acta Paediatr. 2003;92(6):688–93.

58. Gronowitz E, Mellstrom D, Strandvik B. Normal annual increase of bone mineral density during two years in patients with cystic fibrosis. Pediatrics. 2004;114(2):435–42.

59. Zaman MM, Martin CR, Andersson C, Bhutta AQ, Cluette-Brown JE, Laposata M, et al. Linoleic acid supplementation results in increased arachidonic acid and eicosanoid production in CF airway cells and in cftr −/− transgenic mice. Am J Physiol Lung Cell Mol Physiol. 2010;299(5):L599–606.

60. Katrangi W, Lawrenz J, Seegmiller AC, Laposata M. Interactions of linoleic and alpha-linolenic acids in the development of fatty acid alterations in cystic fibrosis. Lipids. 2013;48(4):333–42.

61. Spector AA, Kaduce TL, Hoak JC, Fry GL. Utilization of arachidonic and linoleic acids by cultured human endothelial cells. J Clin Invest. 1981;68(4):1003–11.

62. Strandvik B, Holmberg B. Plasma phospholipid arachidonic acid is inversely correlated to the linoleic acid concentration also in patients with cystic fibrosis. J Cyst Fibros. 2011;10 Suppl 1:S73.

63. Keen C, Olin AC, Eriksson S, Ekman A, Lindblad A, Basu S, et al. Supplementation with fatty acids influences the airway nitric oxide and inflammatory markers in patients with cystic fibrosis. J Pediatr Gastroenterol Nutr. 2010;50(5):537–44.
64. Strandvik B, Chen Y, Dangardt F, Eriksson S, Friberg P, Garemo M, et al. From the Swedish to the Mediterranean diet and the omega-6/omega-3 balance. World Rev Nutr Diet. 2011;102:73–80.
65. Mil-Homens D, Bernardes N, Fialho AM. The antibacterial properties of docosahexaenoic omega-3 fatty acid against the cystic fibrosis multiresistant pathogen Burkholderia cenocepacia. FEMS Microbiol Lett. 2012; 328(1):61–9.
66. Al-Turkmani MR, Andersson C, Alturkmani R, Katrangi W, Cluette-Brown JE, Freedman SD, et al. A mechanism accounting for the low cellular level of linoleic acid in cystic fibrosis and its reversal by DHA. J Lipid Res. 2008;49(9):1946–54.
67. Mimoun M, Coste TC, Lebacq J, Lebecque P, Wallemacq P, Leal T, et al. Increased tissue arachidonic acid and reduced linoleic acid in a mouse model of cystic fibrosis are reversed by supplemental glycerophospholipids enriched in docosahexaenoic acid. J Nutr. 2009;139(12):2358–64.
68. Njoroge SW, Laposata M, Boyd KL, Seegmiller AC. Polyunsaturated fatty acid supplementation reverses cystic fibrosis-related fatty acid abnormalities in CFTR −/− mice by suppressing fatty acid desaturases. J Nutr Biochem. 2015;26(1):36–43.
69. Freedman SD, Katz MH, Parker EM, Laposata M, Urman MY, Alvarez JG. A membrane lipid imbalance plays a role in the phenotypic expression of cystic fibrosis in cftr −/− mice. Proc Natl Acad Sci. 1999;96(24): 13995–4000.
70. Cawood AL, Carroll MP, Wootton SA, Calder PC. Is there a case for n-3 fatty acid supplementation in cystic fibrosis? Curr Opin Clin Nutr Metab Care. 2005;8(2):153–9.
71. Lloyd-Still JD, Powers CA, Hoffman DR, Boyd-Trull K, Lester LA, Benisek DC, et al. Bioavailability and safety of a high dose of docosahexaenoic acid triacylglycerol of algal origin in cystic fibrosis patients: a randomized, controlled study. Nutrition. 2006;22(1):36–46.
72. Van Biervliet S, Devos M, Delhaye T, Van Biervliet JP, Robberecht E, Christophe A. Oral DHA supplementation in DeltaF508 homozygous cystic fibrosis patients. Prostaglandins Leukot Essent Fatty Acids. 2008;78(2): 109–15.
73. Alicandro G, Faelli N, Gagliardini R, Santini B, Magazzu G, Biffi A, et al. A randomized placebo-controlled study on high-dose oral algal docosahexaenoic acid supplementation in children with cystic fibrosis. Prostaglandins Leukot Essent Fatty Acids. 2013;88(2):163–9.
74. Panchaud A, Sauty A, Kernen Y, Decosterd LA, Buclin T, Boulat O, et al. Biological effects of a dietary omega-3 polyunsaturated fatty acids supplementation in cystic fibrosis patients: a randomized, crossover placebo-controlled trial. Clin Nutr. 2006;25(3):418–27.
75. Jumpsen JA, Brown NE, Thomson AB, Paul Man SF, Goh YK, Ma D, et al. Fatty acids in blood and intestine following docosahexaenoic acid supplementation in adults with cystic fibrosis. J Cyst Fibros. 2006;5(2):77–84.
76. De Vizia B, Raia V, Spano C, Pavlidis C, Coruzzo A, Allesio M. Effect of an 8-month treatment with omega-3 fatty acids (eicosapentaenoic and docosahexaenoic) in patients with cystic fibrosis. J Parenter Enteral Nutr. 2003;27(1):52–7.
77. Durieu I, Vericel E, Guichardant D, Roth H, Steghens JP, Drai J, et al. Fatty acids platelets and oxidative markers following intravenous n-3 fatty acids administration in cystic fibrosis: an open pilot observational study. J Cyst Fibros. 2007;6(5):320–6.
78. Njoroge SW, Laposata M, Katrangi W, Seegmiller AC. DHA and EPA reverse cystic fibrosis-related FA abnormalities by suppressing FA desaturase expression and activity. J Lipid Res. 2012;53(2):257–65.
79. Beharry S, Ackerley C, Corey M, Kent G, Heng YM, Christensen H, et al. Long-term docosahexaenoic acid therapy in a congenic murine model of cystic fibrosis. Am J Physiol Gastrointest Liver Physiol. 2007;292(3): G839–48.
80. Van Biervliet S, Van Biervliet JP, Robberecht E, Christophe A. Fatty acid composition of serum phospholipids in cystic fibrosis (CF) patients with or without CF related liver disease. Clin Chem Lab Med. 2010;48(12):1751–5.
81. Oliver C, Watson H. Omega-3 fatty acids for cystic fibrosis. Cochrane Database Syst Rev. 2013;11, CD002201.
82. Shoda R, Matsueda K, Yamato S, Umeda N. Epidemiologic analysis of Crohn disease in Japan: increased dietary intake of n-6 polyunsaturated fatty acids and animal protein relates to the increased incidence of Crohn disease in Japan. Am J Clin Nutr. 1996;63(5):741–5.
83. Aldamiz-Echevarria L, Prieto JA, Andrade F, Elorz J, Sojo A, Lage S, et al. Persistence of essential fatty acid deficiency in cystic fibrosis despite nutritional therapy. Pediatr Res. 2009;66(5):585–9.
84. Christophe A, Robberecht E. Directed modification instead of normalization of fatty acid patterns in cystic fibrosis: an emerging concept. Curr Opin Clin Nutr Metab Care. 2001;4(2):111–3.
85. Sabel KG, Lundqvist-Persson C, Bona E, Petzold M, Strandvik B. Fatty acid patterns early after premature birth, simultaneously analysed in mothers' food, breast milk and serum phospholipids of mothers and infants. Lipids Health Dis. 2009;8:20.

86. Olveira G, Olveira C, Acosta E, Espildora F, Garrido-Sanchez L, Garcia-Escobar E, et al. Fatty acid supplements improve respiratory, inflammatory and nutritional parameters in adults with cystic fibrosis. Arch Bronconeumol. 2010;46(2):70–7.
87. Gronowitz E, Lorentzon M, Ohlsson C, Mellstrom D, Strandvik B. Docosahexaenoic acid is associated with endosteal circumference in long bones in young males with cystic fibrosis. Br J Nutr. 2008;99(1):160–7.
88. Sahlberg ME, Svantesson U, Thomas EM, Strandvik B. Muscular strength and function in patients with cystic fibrosis. Chest. 2005;127(5):1587–92.
89. Innis SM, Davidson AG, Chen A, Dyer R, Melnyk S, James SJ. Increased plasma homocysteine and S-adenosylhomocysteine and decreased methionine is associated with altered phosphatidylcholine and phosphatidylethanolamine in cystic fibrosis. J Pediatr. 2003;143(3):351–6.
90. Innis SM, Davidson A, Chen A, Dyer RA. Malabsorption of phosphatidylcholine and lysophosphatidylcholine occur concurrently with altered phospholipid and thiol metabolism in children with cystic fibrosis. Pediatr Pulmonol. 2003;Suppl 25.
91. Zeisel SH. Choline: an essential nutrient for humans. Nutrition. 2000;16(7–8):669–71.
92. Innis SM, Davidson A, James S, Hasman D, Melnyk S. Choline-related supplements improve abnormal methyl metabolism and glutathione balance in children with cystic fibrosis. Pediatr Pulmonol. 2006;Suppl 29:383.
93. Lepage G, Yesair DW, Ronco N, Champagne J, Bureau N, Chemtob S, et al. Effect of an organized lipid matrix on lipid absorption and clinical outcomes in patients with cystic fibrosis. J Pediatr. 2002;141(2):178–85.
94. Scambi C, De Franceschi L, Guarini P, Poli F, Siciliano A, Pattini P, et al. Preliminary evidence for cell membrane amelioration in children with cystic fibrosis by 5-MTHF and vitamin B12 supplementation: a single arm trial. PLoS One. 2009;4(3), e4782.
95. Guilbault C, De Sanctis JB, Wojewodka G, Saeed Z, Lachance C, Skinner TAA, et al. Fenretinide corrects newly found ceramide deficiency in cystic fibrosis. Am J Respir Cell Mol Biol. 2008;38(1):47–56.
96. Guilbault C, Wojewodka G, Saeed Z, Hajduch M, Matouk E, De Sanctis JB, et al. Cystic fibrosis fatty acid imbalance is linked to ceramide deficiency and corrected by fenretinide. Am J Respir Cell Mol Biol. 2009;41(1):100–6.
97. Teichgraber V, Ulrich M, Endlich N, Riethmuller J, Wilker B, De Oliveira-Munding CC, et al. Ceramide accumulation mediates inflammation, cell death and infection susceptibility in cystic fibrosis. Nat Med. 2008;14(4):382–91.
98. Wood LG, Fitzgerald DA, Garg ML. Hypothesis: vitamin E complements polyunsaturated fatty acids in essential fatty acid deficiency in cystic fibrosis. J Am Coll Nutr. 2003;22(4):253–7.
99. Brown RK, Kelly FJ. Role of free-radicals in the pathogenesis of cystic-fibrosis. Thorax. 1994;49(8):738–42.
100. McKeon DJ, Cadwallader KA, Idris S, Cowburn AS, Pasteur MC, Barker H, et al. Cystic fibrosis neutrophils have normal intrinsic reactive oxygen species generation. Eur Respir J. 2010;35(6):1264–72.
101. de Lima Marson FA, Bertuzzo CS, Secolin R, Ribeiro AF, Ribeiro JD. Genetic interaction of GSH metabolic pathway genes in cystic fibrosis. BMC Med Genet. 2013;14:60.
102. Witters P, Dupont L, Vermeulen F, Proesmans M, Cassiman D, Wallemacq P, et al. Lung transplantation in cystic fibrosis normalizes essential fatty acid profiles. J Cyst Fibros. 2013;12(3):222–8.
103. Andersson C, Al-Turkmani MR, Savaille JE, Alturkmani R, Katrangi W, Cluette-Brown JE, et al. Cell culture models demonstrate that CFTR dysfunction leads to defective fatty acid composition and metabolism. J Lipid Res. 2008;49(8):1692–700.
104. Strandvik B, Bronnegard M, Gilljam H, Carlstedt-Duke J. Relation between defective regulation of arachidonic acid release and symptoms in cystic fibrosis. Scand J Gastroenterol Suppl. 1988;143:1–4.
105. Artigas P, Al'aref SJ, Hobart EA, Diaz LF, Sakaguchi M, Straw S, et al. 2,3-butanedione monoxime affects cystic fibrosis transmembrane conductance regulator channel function through phosphorylation-dependent and phosphorylation-independent mechanisms: the role of bilayer material properties. Mol Pharmacol. 2006;70(6):2015–26.
106. Kindstedt-Arfwidson K, Strandvik B. Food intake in patients with cystic fibrosis on an ordinary diet. Scand J Gastroenterol Suppl. 1988;143:160–2.
107. Trabulsi J, Schall JI, Ittenbach RF, Olsen IE, Yudkoff M, Daikhin Y, et al. Energy balance and the accuracy of reported energy intake in preadolescent children with cystic fibrosis. Am J Clin Nutr. 2006;84(3):523–30.
108. Trabulsi J, Ittenbach RF, Schall JI, Olsen IE, Yudkoff M, Daikhin Y, et al. Evaluation of formulas for calculating total energy requirements of preadolescent children with cystic fibrosis. Am J Clin Nutr. 2007;85(1):144–51.
109. Baum SJ, Kris-Etherton PM, Willett WC, Lichtenstein AH, Rudel LL, Maki KC, et al. Fatty acids in cardiovascular health and disease: a comprehensive update. J Clin Lipidol. 2012;6(3):216–34.
110. Maqbool A, Strandvik B, Stallings VA. The skinny on tuna fat: health implications. Public Health Nutr. 2011;14(11):2049–54.
111. Yen EH, Quinton H, Borowitz D. Better nutritional status in early childhood is associated with improved clinical outcomes and survival in patients with cystic fibrosis. J Pediatr. 2013;162(3):530–5. 3.

Chapter 4
Vitamin D and Bone Health

Jessica A. Alvarez and Vin Tangpricha

Key Points

- Both vitamin D insufficiency and bone disease are widespread in cystic fibrosis.
- Vitamin D deficiency is linked to bone health and additional extra-skeletal outcomes in CF such as lung impairment and inflammation.
- Bone mineral density screening should be performed regularly with dual energy X-ray absorptiometry.
- Nutritional prevention and management of CF-related bone disease includes optimization of vitamin D, vitamin K, and calcium status and intake as well as other bone-related nutrients.
- Physical activity and maintenance of lean body mass are important factors in bone health.
- Guidelines exist for the prevention and management of both vitamin D deficiency and bone disease in CF.

Keywords Vitamin D • Cholecalciferol • 25-hydroxyvitamin D • Bone • Dual energy X-ray absorptiometry • Cystic fibrosis • Nutrition

Abbreviations

$1,25(OH)_2D$	1,25-dihydroxyvitamin D or calcitriol
25(OH)D	25-hydroxyvitamin D
BMD	Bone mineral density
BMI	Body mass index
CF	Cystic fibrosis
CFTR	Cystic fibrosis transmembrane conductance regulator
DEXA	Dual energy X-ray absorptiometry
HPLC	High-performance liquid chromatography
IGF-1	Insulin-like growth factor
IL-6	Interleukin-6

J.A. Alvarez, Ph.D., R.D. (✉) • V. Tangpricha, M.D., Ph.D.
Division of Endocrinology, Metabolism, and Lipids Emory University School of Medicine,
101 Woodruff Memorial Research Cr, WMRB 1313, Atlanta, GA 30322, USA
e-mail: jessica.alvarez@emory.edu; vin.tangpricha@emory.edu

E.H. Yen, A.R. Leonard (eds.), *Nutrition in Cystic Fibrosis: A Guide for Clinicians*, Nutrition and Health,
DOI 10.1007/978-3-319-16387-1_4, © Springer International Publishing Switzerland 2015

LC-MS/MS	Liquid chromatography tandem mass spectroscopy
LL-37	Cathelicidin
PICP	Carboxy-terminal propeptide of type I procollagen
PINP	Amino-terminal propeptide of type I procollagen
PIVKA-II	Prothrombin induced by vitamin K absence or antagonism
PTH	Parathyroid hormone
RANKL	Receptor activator of nuclear factor kappa-B ligand
TNF-α	Tumor necrosis factor-α
ucOC	Undercarboxylated osteocalcin
VDBP	Vitamin D binding protein
VDR	Vitamin D receptor
VDRE	Vitamin D response element

Introduction

There has been a global increased awareness of the importance of vitamin D in health and disease. Whereas the role of vitamin D in bone outcomes is well characterized, investigations within the past several decades have shifted focus to understand the role of vitamin D in extra-skeletal health outcomes. Both vitamin D insufficiency and bone disease are common manifestations in individuals with cystic fibrosis (CF). Although the two conditions are linked, vitamin D deficiency/insufficiency has been connected to additional extra-skeletal CF health outcomes such as lung function and inflammation, and bone disease is influenced by additional nutritional and endocrine factors. This chapter provides background and nutritional guidance on the prevention and maintenance of optimal vitamin D and bone health status in CF.

Vitamin D

A basic understanding of vitamin D nomenclature and physiology is essential for managing vitamin D status in CF, other diseases, and health in general. Vitamin D as a nutrient is available in two forms, vitamin D_2 (ergocalciferol) or vitamin D_3 (cholecalciferol) [1]. Ergocalciferol is derived from UVB irradiation of the plant sterol, ergosterol, and is typically obtained through vitamin D-fortified foods and supplements and irradiated mushrooms. Cholecalciferol can be produced endogenously upon exposure to UVB radiation or can be acquired through fortified foods (such as dairy products, cereal, and orange juice) and supplements, as well as a limited number of foods naturally containing cholecalciferol (such as fatty fish). Common foods and CF supplements containing vitamin D are listed in Table 4.1. Endogenous production involves the conversion of 7-dehydrocholesterol in the skin to pre-vitamin D_3 which undergoes a thermally induced isomerization to form the nutrient, cholecalciferol. Factors influencing endogenous production of vitamin D include sunscreen and clothing practices, angle of the sun (latitude, time of year), skin pigmentation (melanin competition with 7-dehydrocholesterol for UVB radiation), and age-related decreases in 7-dehydrocholesterol. Vitamin D (either as cholecalciferol or ergocalciferol) has a circulating half-life of approximately 24 h [2] and is quickly converted by the enzyme, 25-hydroxylase, to 25-hydroxyvitamin D [25(OH)D] in the liver or is distributed into adipose tissue. Blood 25(OH)D is the primary circulating vitamin D metabolite and has a half-life of approximately 2–3 weeks. Both vitamin D and 25(OH)D are generally considered to be relatively inactive forms. They are transported throughout circulation bound to vitamin D binding protein (VDBP). A second hydroxylation step occurs, catalyzed by the enzyme 1α-hydroxylase (also known as CYP27B1), to convert 25(OH)D to 1,25-dihydroxyvitamin D [1,25(OH)$_2$D or calcitriol], the

Table 4.1 Potential sources of vitamin D in individuals with cystic fibrosis

	Estimated amount of vitamin D	Type of vitamin D
Dietary sources		
Salmon, fresh	Wild-caught: ~600–1000 IU per 3.5 oz	Vitamin D_3
	Farmed: ~100–250 IU per 3.5 oz	
Canned fish (sardines, tuna)	~236–300 IU per 3.5 oz	Vitamin D_3
Shiitake mushrooms	Sun-dried: ~1600 IU per 3.5 oz	Vitamin D_2
	Fresh: ~100 IU per 3.5 oz	
Fortified milk or orange juice	100 IU per 8 fl oz	Vitamin D_3
Infant formula	100 IU per 8 fl oz	Vitamin D_3
Fortified yogurt	100 IU per 8 fl oz	Vitamin D_3
Fortified breakfast cereals	~100–200 IU per serving	Vitamin D_3
Supplemental sources		
General multivitamin	400–1000 IU per serving	Vitamin D_3
Over-the-counter vitamin D	400–50,000 IU per serving	Vitamin D_3 or D_2
Prescription vitamin D	50,000 IU per serving	Vitamin D_3 or D_2
AquADEKs®, CF fat-soluble vitamins	Liquid: 600 IU per mL	Vitamin D_3
	Chewable: 600 IU per chewable	
	Softgel: 1200 IU per softgel	
Libertas ABDEKs, CF fat-soluble vitamins	Liquid: 500 IU per mL	Vitamin D_3
	Chewable: 1000 IU per chewable	
	Softgel: 1000 IU per softgel	
Vitamax®, CF fat-soluble vitamins	Liquid: 400 IU per mL	Vitamin D_3
	Chewable: 400 IU per chewable	
MVW Complete Formulation™, CF fat-soluble vitamins	Liquid: 1500 IU per mL	Vitamin D_3
	Chewable: 1500 IU per chewable	
	Softgel: 1500 IU per softgel	
MVW Complete Formulation™ D3000, CF fat-soluble vitamins	3000 IU per softgel	Vitamin D_3
ChoiceFul, CF fat-soluble vitamins	Chewable: 800 IU per chewable	Vitamin D_3
	Softgel: 1000 IU per softgel	

Sources: (1) Holick MF. Vitamin D deficiency. N Engl J Med. 2007;357:266–81. (2) Michel, S. MVW Nutritionals Vitamin Comparison Chart 2014, available at: http://mvwnutritionals.com/wp-content/uploads/2014/12/VitaminTable-12_1_14.pdf

biologically active vitamin D metabolite with an estimated half-life of 4–6 h [3]. The production of $1,25(OH)_2D$ primarily occurs in the kidneys for the regulation of calcium and phosphorus metabolism in bone homeostasis, although numerous other tissues are recognized as being capable of producing $1,25(OH)_2D$ via the 1α-hydroxylase enzyme [4–8]. The biological action of $1,25(OH)_2D$ is initiated by its binding to a nuclear vitamin D receptor (VDR) and its heterodimerization with a retinoic X receptor [1, 9]. This complex subsequently binds to a vitamin D response element (VDRE) in the promoter region of target genes to modulate gene transcription. A non-genomic mechanism of action of $1,25(OH)_2D$ has also been described in which $1,25(OH)_2D$ binds to a membrane VDR and activates second messenger systems, including calcium mobilization and signaling.

The clinical determinant of vitamin D status is measurement of circulating total 25(OH)D concentrations, given its longer half-life and reflection of both endogenous and exogenous vitamin D production/intake. Several assays are available for measurement of circulating 25(OH)D levels, including radioimmunoassays, enzyme-immunoassays, high-performance liquid chromatography (HPLC), and liquid chromatography tandem mass spectroscopy (LC-MS/MS) [10]. An advantage of HPLC and LC-MS/MS is the ability to distinguish 25(OH)D derived from ergocalciferol ($25(OH)D_2$) and cholecalciferol ($25(OH)D_3$). Because analytic variability exists between assays, practitioners should choose laboratories that participate in external vitamin D standardization testing programs, such as the Vitamin D External Quality Assurance Survey, the Centers for Disease Control

Hormone Standardization program, or the National Institutes of Health Vitamin D Metabolites Quality Assurance Program. Also, to avoid misinterpretation, care should be taken to use proper nomenclature when ordering laboratory assays for assessing vitamin D status.

Vitamin D Pathophysiology in CF

Prevalence estimates of suboptimal vitamin D status in CF have varied widely, with reports of up to 90% prevalence [11, 12]. Numerous factors preclude inadequate vitamin D status in CF [13, 14]. Exocrine pancreas insufficiency induces intestinal malabsorption of fat and fat-soluble vitamins, including vitamin D. Vitamin D malabsorption may also occur independently of pancreatic function in CF, as suggested in a vitamin D_2 absorption study [15]. Overall dietary intake may be low secondary to illness and reduced appetite. Sun exposure may be limited due to frequent illness and use of antibiotic-induced photosensitivity [16]. Low body fat may reduce the storage capability of fat-soluble vitamins. Adherence to prescribed supplements might also be considered [17]. Additional hypotheses have been proposed based on indirect evidence: Circulating VDBP is reduced in CF [18, 19], potentially reducing the transport and availability of vitamin D metabolites [12]. Enhanced 25(OH)D degradation may be present secondary to elevated cytochrome P450 enzyme activity in CF [20]. Altered membrane phospholipid composition in CF [21] or cystic fibrosis transmembrane conductance regulator (CFTR) in the epidermis [22] may potentially influence photobiosynthesis of cholecalciferol [12]. Elevated urinary excretion of low-molecular weight proteins in CF [23] may influence excretion of VDBP-bound 25(OH)D [12]. Finally, frequent corticosteroid use in CF may promote degradation of vitamin D metabolites through enhanced 24-hydroxylase expression [24, 25]. Further research will be needed to directly address causes of low vitamin D status in CF.

Role of Vitamin D in CF Health

The biologically active form of vitamin D, $1,25(OH)_2D$, plays a critical role in maintaining optimal circulating calcium and phosphorus concentrations. For normal physiological function, blood calcium concentrations require tight regulation within a narrow range. Decreases in blood calcium will stimulate $1,25(OH)_2D$ production (via parathyroid hormone, PTH) which enables normalization of blood calcium levels by (1) binding to nuclear VDR in the intestine and stimulating absorption of dietary calcium and phosphorus, and (2) if dietary calcium is insufficient, promoting the formation and activation of bone resorbing osteoclasts for release of calcium in conjunction with PTH [26, 27]. This latter action may lead to loss of skeletal calcium and promote risk of osteoporosis. Another function of the vitamin D system is to suppress hyperplasia of the parathyroid gland and secretion of PTH [27]. Vitamin D deficiency can therefore lead to secondary hyperparathyroidism, thus further promoting calcium mobilization from bone. In individuals with CF, vitamin D deficiency is associated lower bone mineral density (BMD) [28–33] and is a risk factor for CF-related bone disease (discussed below).

The vitamin D system is becoming increasingly recognized for its role in innate and adaptive immunity [34]. Cells involved in immune function, such as macrophages, monocytes, and respiratory epithelial cells contain the machinery needed to convert 25(OH)D to $1,25(OH)_2D$ [35–38]. When activated, this pathway promotes the upregulation of the antimicrobial peptide cathelicidin (LL-37) and other host defenses and reduces pro-inflammatory cytokine production [38, 39]. Given the large microbial and inflammatory burden in individuals with CF, this immunomodulatory action of the vitamin D system may be critical in management of the disease. Human studies in CF, although relatively few in number, provide some evidence. Grossmann et al. [40] reported a decrease in the pro-inflammatory cytokines, tumor necrosis factor-α (TNF-α), and interleukin-6 (IL-6) (but no change in LL-37) in a pilot randomized, placebo-controlled trial of a bolus oral dose of 250,000 IU cholecalciferol in hospitalized adults with CF. Vitamin D allocation also improved one-year survival in this pilot study [41]. Some cross-sectional studies in CF have also linked vitamin D status to lung function [42, 43], inflammation [44], rates of pulmonary exacerbation [43], hospitalization [45], and history of Pseudomonas colonization [46].

Additional health outcomes in CF may be linked to vitamin D status. In a large CF cohort, vitamin D deficiency was associated with the presence of CF-related diabetes and elevated glycosylated hemoglobin concentrations [47]. The vitamin D system has been suggested to influence both insulin resistance and insulin secretion, potentially through direct effects on insulin signaling or through its anti-inflammatory effects [48]. Vitamin D has also been hypothesized to influence brain function [49]. Two small cross-sectional studies in patients with CF have indicated a relationship between vitamin D status and depression [50, 51]. A 2014 Cochrane Review of vitamin D supplementation was unable to establish a clear benefit or harm in vitamin D supplementation for CF, given the limited number of studies (3 full studies, 3 abstracts) and unclear risk of bias [52]. Further prospective studies will need to confirm the role vitamin D plays in extra-skeletal CF health.

Vitamin D Management in CF

The North American Cystic Fibrosis Foundation (CFF) developed guidelines in 2012 specifically for the screening, diagnosis, and management of vitamin D deficiency in CF [14] (see Table 4.2 for summary). Vitamin D status should be assessed with total circulating 25(OH)D concentrations, and a minimum target goal level is 30 ng/mL (75 nmol/L). Total 25(OH)D levels should be measured annually, at the end of winter when 25(OH)D levels are at their lowest. Routine measurement of other markers (i.e., PTH, calcitriol, alkaline phosphatase, osteocalcin) is not recommended for assessment of vitamin D status. This latter guideline differs from the 2011 European Bone Mineralization Guidelines for CF [53]; however, the CF Foundation considered the increased cost and lack of evidence that other markers reflect vitamin D status [14].

The CF Foundation developed an age-specific stepwise approach to improving vitamin D status (described in Table 4.2) [14]. The use of cholecalciferol (vitamin D_3), as opposed to ergocalciferol (vitamin D_2), is recommended. Cholecalciferol has been suggested to more effectively increase blood 25(OH)D concentrations compared to ergocalciferol [54]. Indeed, in a head-to-head study in CF comparing cholecalciferol to ergocalciferol (50,000 IU vitamin D for 12 weeks), cholecalciferol achieved a better total 25(OH)D response [55]. Both vitamin D_3 and vitamin D_2 are available by prescription (or over the counter in smaller doses). Clinicians should be aware of the vitamin D formulation prescribed and being taken as supplements by patients. Absorption of fat-soluble vitamins may be improved when taken with food, and in CF, supplements should be taken with pancreatic enzymes, if applicable [14]. The question of oil-based vs. powder-based vitamin D supplements remains a topic of investigation in CF. The CF Foundation does not give specific recommendations for the frequency of supplementation (i.e., daily, weekly, monthly); the dosing schedule may be individualized and should be sufficient to maintain a minimum serum 25(OH)D level of 30 ng/mL. The use of ultraviolet lamps to improve vitamin D status has been considered [55, 56]; however, insufficient evidence is available to make recommendations and the potential for increased photosensitivity and/or burns is a concern [14]. A specialist with expertise in vitamin D therapy should be consulted in difficult-to-treat vitamin D deficiency. Supplementation with hydroxylated vitamin D compounds (oral 25(OH)D supplement) may be considered if vitamin D therapy does not work, although there are insufficient studies available to affirm their safety or efficacy [14]. Likewise, calcitriol or other vitamin D analogs (doxercalciferol or paricalcitol) may be considered in cases of difficult-to-treat vitamin D deficiency, but only in consultation with a vitamin D specialist.

Table 4.2 Summary of cystic fibrosis foundation guidelines for the screening, diagnosis, management, and treatment of vitamin D deficiency

Assessment of vitamin D status
- Vitamin D status should be assessed with serum 25(OH)D at least annually at the end of winter.
- The goal serum 25(OH)D concentrations should be at least 30 ng/mL (75 nmol/L).
- Adherence to vitamin D prescriptions should be assessed in individuals with serum 25(OH)D < 30 ng/mL.

Treatment and management of vitamin D deficiency
- Cholecalciferol (vitamin D_3) should be used as a once-daily therapy or its weekly equivalent to achieve and maintain goal serum 25(OH)D concentrations.
- For infants <12 months of age, an initial dose of daily 400–500 IU vitamin D_3 is recommended with an increase to 800–1000 IU per day if serum 25(OH)D concentrations are between 20 and 30 ng/mL (50 and 75 nmol/L) or to a maximum of 2000 IU per day if serum 25(OH)D levels are less than 20 ng/mL (50 nmol/L) or persist at a range of 20–30 ng/mL (50–75 nmol/L).
- Infants 12 months of age with a serum 25(OH)D concentration <10 ng/mL (<25 nmol/L) should be assessed for rickets and urgently managed in consultation with a specialist.
- For children between 1 and 10 years of age, an initial dose of daily 800–1000 IU vitamin D_3 is recommended with an increase to 1600–3000 IU per day if serum 25(OH)D concentrations are between 20 and 30 ng/mL (50–75 nmol/L) or to a maximum of 4000 IU per day if serum 25(OH)D levels are less than 20 ng/mL (50 nmol/L) or persist at a range of 20–30 ng/mL (50–75 nmol/L).
- For all individuals greater than 10 years of age, an initial dose of daily 800–2000 IU vitamin D_3 is recommended with an increase to 1600–6000 IU per day if serum 25(OH)D concentrations are between 20 and 30 ng/mL (50–75 nmol/L) or to a maximum of 10,000 IU per day if serum 25(OH)D levels are less than 20 ng/mL (50 nmol/L) or persist at a range of 20–30 ng/mL (50–75 nmol/L).
- For individuals unable to meet goal 25(OH)D concentrations after maximum recommended intake, and confirmed adherence to prescribed therapy, vitamin D treatment should be managed in consultation with a specialist.
- Vitamin D deficiency that is difficult to treat should be managed with calcitriol or other vitamin D analogs only in consultation with a specialist.
- Serum 25(OH)D concentrations should be re-checked 3 months after a change in vitamin D dosing.

Adapted from Tangpricha et al. *J Clin Endocrinol Metab* 2011;97:1082–1093.
Abbreviations: *25(OH)D*; 25-hydroxyvitamin D

Vitamin D toxicity is rare and manifests as hypercalcemia (blood calcium concentration >10.5 mg/dL). The CF Foundation recommends that blood 25(OH)D concentrations not exceed 100 ng/mL (250 nmol/L) [14]. This is the level at which the risk for hypercalcemia increases [4]. Symptoms of hypercalcemia are nonspecific and include fatigue, anorexia, polydipsia, polyuria, nausea, constipation, diarrhea, vomiting, abdominal pain, muscle weakness or pain, memory loss, confusion, and/or nephrocalcinosis [57]. A diagnosis of vitamin D intoxication is based on the presence of elevated blood 25(OH)D concentrations with hypercalcemia or hypercalciuria and hyperphosphatemia. Treatment for vitamin D toxicity includes removal of vitamin D source and intravenous hydration with or without loop diuretics to increase calcium excretion. Thiazides promote calcium resorption and, therefore, should be avoided. Persistent hypercalcemia may be treated with glucocorticoids. Additional treatment options for vitamin D toxicity include intravenous hydration, calcitonin, bisphosphonates, and as a last resort, hemodialysis [57].

Cystic Fibrosis-Related Bone Disease

CF-related bone disease, manifesting as osteoporosis, osteopenia, and/or fractures, is the second most prevalent co-morbidity in patients with CF. In 2012, the CF Patient registry report indicated that 14.8% of all patients with CF had bone disease [58]. The prevalence among adults aged 35 and older is greater than 36% [58]. This prevalence is expected to increase as the CF population ages. The pathophysiology of CF-related bone disease remains a topic of scientific investigation, although it is a multifactorial disease, as described below.

CF-related bone disease can contribute to existing lung impairment in this population. Specifically, manifestations of bone disease in CF that influence lung function include rib and vertebral fractures, kyphosis (curving of the spine), and chest wall deformities, which may result in reduced lung volumes and ineffective cough and airway clearance [59–64]. Severe bone disease may also be an exclusion factor for lung transplant candidacy. Thus, management of bone disease is critical for optimizing health in CF. Maintenance of adequate nutritional status plays an integral role in preventing and treating CF-related bone disease. A summary of recommendations for prevention and nutritional management of bone disease is provided in Table 4.3.

Pathophysiology of Bone Disease in CF

The pathophysiology of CF-related bone disease is a multifactorial process resulting in insufficient bone accrual during puberty and accelerated bone loss during adulthood [64]. Direct nutritional factors, discussed below, include general malnutrition, inadequate intake of nutrients important for bone health, vitamin D and vitamin K malabsorption secondary to pancreatic insufficiency, and physical inactivity. Endocrine factors contributing to bone disease include delayed puberty, hypogonadism, and insulin deficiency. Puberty is a critical developmental period for bone mineral accrual, which is largely influenced by sex steroids and the growth hormone-insulin-like growth factor-1 (IGF-1) axis [65]. Individuals with CF are at risk for delayed puberty during childhood, potentially impeding normal bone mineral accretion, and for hypogonadism as adults, potentially accelerating bone loss [66]. Circulating IGF-1 levels are known to be lower in CF compared to healthy controls [67] and are positively associated with BMD and bone mineral content in CF [68, 69]. Insulin is an anabolic hormone that stimulates osteoblast activity [70]. Thus CF-related diabetes, characterized by both impaired insulin secretion and sensitivity, may contribute to bone disease [64]. Additional factors relate to CF care and the disease progression, including glucocorticoid therapy and chronic inflammation, respectively. Glucocorticoids reduce intestinal calcium absorption, increase urinary calcium excretion, and directly affect bone cells [62, 71]. Oral steroid use increases the risk of osteoporosis in CF [72]. Pro-inflammatory cytokines promote bone-resorptive pathways [73] and circulating levels are inversely associated with bone mass in CF [68]. The defective CFTR protein may also directly contribute to bone pathophysiology. CFTR protein is expressed in human osteoclasts and osteoblasts [74] and has been shown to regulate osteoprotegerin and prostaglandin E_2, which are involved in inhibiting and inducing osteoclast differentiation, respectively [75]. Together, these multiple factors result in a combination of reduced osteoblast and increased osteoclast activity, leading to an imbalance between bone formation and resorption, and ultimately, to CF-related bone disease [62, 76].

Assessment of Bone Health

BMD measured with dual energy X-ray absorptiometry (DEXA) is the gold standard method to assess bone health [11, 53, 64]. DEXA is widely available, emits a minimal radiation dose, and has good reproducibility [53]. Per CF Foundation guidelines, a DEXA scan is recommended for all individuals with CF by 18 years of age, with repeat testing every 5 years if BMD is normal (Table 4.3) [64]. An initial DEXA screen is also recommended for children greater than 8 years of age with the following risk factors: ideal body weight <90%, FEV1 <50% predicted, long-term glucocorticoid treatment

Table 4.3 Summary of nutrition-related recommendations for bone health in cystic fibrosis

Assessment of bone health[a]

- Bone mineral density should be assessed with dual energy X-ray absorptiometry (DEXA).
- DEXA screens should be performed in all adults ≥18 years.
- DEXA screens should be performed in children if:
  - ideal body weight is <90%
  - FEV1 <50% predicted
  - glucocorticoid intake is ≥5 mg/day for ≥90 days/year
  - puberty is delayed
  - there is a history of fractures
- Z-score should be used to assess BMD in children <18 years of age. Z- or T-score can be used in adults aged 18–30 years. T-score should be used in adults ≥30 years of age.
- Repeat DEXA scan every 5 years if BMD Z- or T-score is ≥ −1.0, every 2–4 years if BMD Z- or T-score is between −1.0 and −2.0, and annually if BMD Z- or T-score is ≤ −2.0 or there is a history of fragility fracture or a significant reduction in BMD (>3% in the lumbar spine or >5–6% in the proximal femur).

Nutritional assessment and recommendations for bone health[b]

- Maintain an optimal BMI through adequate energy and macronutrient intake, with emphasis on lean body mass:
  - ≥50th percentile on BMI growth chart for children and adolescents ≤ 20 years[c]
  - ≥23 kg/m^2 for men, ≥22 kg/m^2 for women > 20 years[c]
- Assess dietary intake (energy, protein, calcium, etc.) at least annually, and more frequently in cases of abnormal growth or weight loss, by a registered dietitian.
- Ensure daily calcium intake meets the age-specific Institute of Medicine Dietary Reference Intakes: 0–6 months, 200 mg; 7–12 months, 260 mg; 1–3 years, 700 mg; 4–8 years, 1000 mg; 9–18 years, 1300 mg; 19–50 years, 1000 mg; >50 years, 1200 mg (females) and 1000 mg (males).[d]
- Increase dietary sources of calcium when indicated with calcium supplements if necessary.
- Minimize intake of substances that may inhibit calcium absorption and/or inhibit bone formation when consumed in excess: phosphorus (found in colas), caffeine, aluminum-containing antacids, alcohol, or supplementary retinol.
- For optimal vitamin D status, achieve or maintain a blood 25-hydroxyvitamin D (25(OH)D) level ≥30 ng/mL. Refer to the 2012 CF Foundation Guidelines for vitamin D recommendations.
- Vitamin D status and calcium intake and vitamin D status should be corrected before prescribing bisphosphonates or other medical treatments.
- Vitamin K status should be assessed with circulating PIVKA-II, vitamin K$_1$, and undercarboxylated osteocalcin concentrations.
- All pancreatic insufficient patients should take a vitamin K supplement.
- Daily vitamin K intake should be at least 0.3–0.5 mg/day.
- For vitamin K deficiency, starting doses of vitamin K should be: 0.5–2.0 mg/day in infants <1 year of age, 1–10 mg/day in children and adults ≥1 year of age.
- Encourage weight-bearing exercise for all (20–30 min three times per week for children and adolescents; regular weight bearing and resistance activities for adults).

[a]From Aris RM, et al. Guide to bone health and disease in cystic fibrosis. J Clin Endocrinol Metab. 2005 Mar;90(3):1888–96

[b]From Aris RM, et al. Guide to bone health and disease in cystic fibrosis. J Clin Endocrinol Metab. 2005 Mar;90(3): 1888–96 and Sermet-Gaudelus I, et al. European cystic fibrosis bone mineralisation guidelines. J Cyst Fibros. 2011 Jun;10 Suppl 2:S16-23

[c]From Stallings VA et al. Evidence-based practice recommendations for nutrition-related management of children and adults with cystic fibrosis and pancreatic insufficiency: results of a systematic review. J Am Diet Assoc. 2008 May;108:832–9

[d]From Food and Nutrition Board, Institute of Medicine. Dietary Reference Intakes for Calcium and Vitamin D. National Academy Press, Washington, D.C., 2010

(≥5 mg/day for ≥90 days/year), delayed puberty, or a history of fractures. The European CF Society guidelines recommend that DXA screens should begin in all CF children at 8 years of age [53].

BMD should be expressed in terms of Z-scores or T-scores [53, 64]. A BMD Z-score is the difference in standard deviations between an individual's BMD value and the mean BMD value of an age- and gender-matched healthy reference group. Z-scores should be used to interpret BMD in children <18 years of age. A BMD T-score is the difference in standard deviations between an individual's BMD value and the mean BMD value of a sex-matched, healthy young adult (30 years of age) reference population. T-score should be used in adults ≥30 years of age. Z- or T-score can be used in adults aged 18–30 years, as they are generally equivalent [64]. According to CF Foundation Guidelines, DEXA scans should be repeated every 5 years if BMD Z- or T-score is ≥−1.0, every 2–4 years if BMD Z- or T-score is between −1.0 and −2.0, and annually if BMD Z- or T-score is ≤−2.0 or there is a history of fragility fracture or a significant reduction in BMD (>3% in the lumbar spine or >5–6% in the proximal femur).

Nutritional Management of Bone Health

Assessment of anthropometric changes (height, weight, BMI) in individuals with CF is a clinically useful method of monitoring nutritional status and, subsequently, risk for bone disease. A goal of clinical management of CF should be to achieve and maintain an optimal weight-for-height status. In children and adolescents, growth should be assessed using appropriate percentile charts (weight-for-length, BMI-for-age) at every clinic and in-patient visit [53]. Infants should meet or exceed a weight-for-length in the 50th percentile by the age of 2 years [77]. Children and adolescents aged 2–20 years should meet or exceed a BMI in the 50th percentile. In adults, BMI should be assessed at every clinic and in-patient visit [53]. Women should maintain a BMI ≥22 kg/m^2; men should maintain a BMI ≥23 kg/m^2 at minimum [77] (Table 4.3). Dietary intake of energy, protein, and key micronutrients involved in bone health should be assessed at least annually by a registered dietitian, and more frequently in cases of weight loss or abnormal growth velocity [53].

Calcium

Bone, which is comprised of 39.9% calcium, is the storage reservoir of more than 99% of body calcium [78]. Optimization of calcium intake is therefore critical for bone health. Schulze et al. [79–81] have conducted calcium balance studies in pancreatic sufficient girls with CF and indicated that intestinal calcium absorption is normal, yet the rate of bone calcium deposition during pre- and late puberty is lower than healthy controls. This is possibly related to the observed excess endogenous fecal calcium losses in CF [80]. There is little data available from supplemental calcium studies in CF. Hillman et al. [82] did not find changes in serum calcium concentrations, calcium absorption, or bone mineralization with 1 g calcium supplementation (±cholecalciferol) for 6 months in children with CF. Given the absence of CF-specific data, consensus statements from both the North American and European CF Foundations recommend adherence to the Institute of Medicine Dietary Reference Intakes for calcium [53, 64] (Table 4.3).

Several dietary factors inhibit calcium absorption and/or bioavailability and may be particularly detrimental to bone in the absence of adequate dietary calcium intake. Excess phosphorus can form complexes with calcium leading to interference with calcium absorption and increasing PTH secretion and subsequent bone resorption [83–85]. Cola sodas are a major source of excess phosphorus (in the form of phosphoric acid) [85]. Epidemiological studies in relatively healthy populations have indicated that cola consumption is associated with lower BMD [86] and fracture risk [87]. Caffeine increases urinary calcium excretion and is associated with reduced BMD and increased fracture risk in epidemiological studies [85, 88, 89], although these findings are typically in the setting of inadequate calcium intake [90–93]. Aluminum-containing antacids increase fecal and urinary calcium excretion

[94, 95], and their use should be limited in CF. Sodium, which is typically supplemented in CF to offset skin losses [96], also promotes renal calcium excretion [85, 97]. To offset any potential interfering dietary factors, it is imperative that calcium intake is optimized in individuals with CF.

Vitamin K

Despite routine supplementation, the prevalence of suboptimal vitamin K status is high in CF populations [17, 32, 98, 99]. In addition to fat-soluble vitamins malabsorption and inadequate intake as a cause for low vitamin D status, long-term use of antibiotics may limit gut-derived vitamin K production by normal intestinal flora [100]. Low vitamin K status is associated with an increased risk for bone disease in the general population [101]. Vitamin K is an enzyme cofactor for γ-glutamyl carboxylase, which is required for proper function of the bone protein, osteocalcin that is involved in the regulation of bone mineralization, maturation, and remodeling.

Vitamin K status can be assessed with circulating levels of undercarboxylated prothrombin (PIVKA-II, prothrombin induced by vitamin K absence or antagonism), undercarboxylated osteocalcin (ucOC), vitamin K_1 concentrations, and prothrombin time [53], although the latter two assays (vitamin K_1 and prothrombin time) should be interpreted with caution. Serum vitamin K_1 may be influenced by recent dietary intake [102], and prothrombin time is an indicator of advanced vitamin K deficiency [100]. Because bone is more susceptible to vitamin K deficiency than the liver, ucOC is a highly sensitive indicator of vitamin K status [100], although the assay is not widely available and reference values have not been established. The link between ucOC and bone mineral outcomes has only been investigated in two published studies in CF, with one reporting a positive association [103] and the other reporting no statistically significant association [99]. Vitamin K_1 supplementation should be considered in individuals with low serum vitamin K_1 levels (reference range=0.29–2.64 nmol/L) or increased serum PIVKA-II (reference range <2 nmol/L [102]), or prothrombin time (reference range 11.1–13.1 s) [53, 102, 104].

An optimal vitamin K intake range for bone health in CF has not yet been defined [64]. Randomized, controlled vitamin K supplementation studies in CF have been limited, and none have included BMD as an outcome [105]. In an open, non-randomized clinical trial, Nicolaidou et al. [106] reported improved serum markers of bone formation [increased total osteocalcin, increased amino-terminal propeptide of type I procollagen (PINP), increased carboxy-terminal propeptide of type I procollagen (PICP), and decreased ucOC] and reduced serum PTH with 10 mg/week vitamin K supplementation for 1 year in children and adolescents with CF, although BMD did not change. The CF Foundation recommends a daily vitamin K intake of 0.3–0.5 mg/day [64, 96]. For vitamin K deficiency, the European bone guidelines recommend a starting vitamin K dose of 1–10 mg/day [53].

Additional Nutrients for Bone Health

Numerous other nutrients are involved in bone homeostasis, and optimal intake should be ensured. Bone matrix contains additional nutrients such as protein, magnesium, and phosphorus [85]. Dietary protein is the source of amino acids required for building the bone matrix [107]. Magnesium plays a role in the crystallization of hydroxyapatite and directly affects osteoblasts and osteoclasts [108]. Although excess phosphorus is a more likely scenario, phosphorus deficiency leads to reduced bone mineralization [109]. Potassium enhances renal calcium retention [85] and has been shown to increase serum osteocalcin and decrease urinary hydroxyproline [110]. Iron, copper, and vitamin C are cofactors in the formation and maintenance of collagen, the protein providing the structural framework of bone [85]. The antioxidant effects of vitamin E may protect against bone resorptive factors, although potential detrimental effects of high-dose supplementation have also been proposed [111, 112]. Vitamins B_{12}, B_6, and folate may influence bone by regulating homocysteine, which has been suggested to impair collagen cross-linking, alter osteoclast and osteoblast activity, and decrease bone blood flow [85, 113, 114]. Carotenoids may stimulate bone formation and inhibit resorption [115]. The relationships between these nutrients and bone health are supported by some epidemiological studies and interventions in non-CF populations, although their relationships with bone health have not been investigated in CF populations.

Additional dietary factors may inhibit bone formation or promote bone resorption. Heavy alcohol intake increases risk for multiple nutrient deficiencies, but also may have direct effects on osteocyte apoptosis and other bone resorptive pathways [85, 116]. Higher retinol (vitamin A) intake and blood levels are associated with fracture risk in some epidemiological studies [117–119], possibly via competition with vitamin D at the retinoic X receptor or by direct action on bone cells [120]. Serum retinol levels should be monitored in CF, given the current vitamin A supplementation practices [121].

Physical Activity and Body Composition

Impaired lung function and repeated illness may reduce or limit physical activity in CF. Increased physical activity and fitness, however, is strongly associated with greater BMD both in CF and general populations [72, 122–124]. Increased mechanical load (strain) from exercise induces a mechanotransduction pathway, whereby osteocytes detect the load and respond by signaling the bone remodeling process in an effort to strengthen the area under strain [125, 126]. Physical activity, particularly weight-bearing exercises such as jogging, jumping, and dancing, should therefore be promoted in individuals with CF. The European CF Bone Mineralization Guidelines provide detailed physical activity recommendations: in addition to usual activities, children and adolescents should perform weight-bearing activities at least three times per week for 20–30 min, and adults should perform weight bearing and resistance exercises regularly [53].

A normal BMI with an emphasis on lean body mass (i.e., muscle) should be maintained [53]. Total body weight is positively associated with BMD, likely through the effect of mechanical loading induced by gravity [127]. Weight-loss studies in generally healthy subjects have shown that a 10% loss in body weight is associated with a 1–2% loss in BMD [85, 128]. Independent of body weight, muscle contractions induce the largest physiological strain on bones [129, 130], thus reinforcing the need to maintain lean body mass. In CF, lean body mass depletion is associated with bone loss [131, 132].

Medical Treatment of Bone Disease

Medical treatment of CF-related bone disease should include management of CF-related diabetes and sex steroid deficiency or pubertal delay, if applicable, as well as correction of vitamin D insufficiency or suboptimal calcium intake [53, 64]. Per CF Foundation consensus guidelines, bisphosphonate therapy should be considered as treatment for individuals with a T- or Z-score ≤-2 or those with a T- or Z-score between −1 and −2 with fragility fractures, a BMD loss of >3–5% per year, and/or awaiting organ transplantation [64]. Bisphosphonates effectively increase BMD in adults with CF; although their effect on fracture reduction has not yet been confirmed CF and side effects include severe bone pain and flu-like symptoms [133]. Additional therapeutic options may include teriparatide (a recombinant human PTH analog), growth hormone, IGF-1 therapy, or denosumab [an inhibitor of receptor activator of nuclear factor kappa-B ligand (RANKL)], although clinical trials in CF are needed [62, 69, 134].

Conclusion

The underlying pathophysiology of CF places individuals with the disease at risk for vitamin D deficiency and bone disease. Vitamin D deficiency is a known risk factor for bone disease but it has also been linked to impaired pulmonary function, inflammation, and other extra-skeletal outcomes in CF. In addition to vitamin D, nutritional prevention and management of bone disease includes ensuring adequate calcium intake and absorption, maintaining proper vitamin K status and that of other bone-related nutrients, and encouraging physical activity. Consensus guidelines for vitamin D deficiency and bone health in CF should be followed, although there is a general lack of randomized, controlled trials available to specifically address the role of nutrition in CF bone health and other related outcomes. The registered dietitian is a vital member of the CF care team and is key in optimizing nutrition status for the prevention and management of vitamin D deficiency and bone disease in CF.

References

1. Lips P. Vitamin D physiology. Prog Biophys Mol Biol. 2006;92:4–8.
2. Holick MF. The use and interpretation of assays for vitamin D and its metabolites. J Nutr. 1990;120 Suppl 11:1464–9.
3. Holick MF. Vitamin D status: measurement, interpretation, and clinical application. Ann Epidemiol. 2009;19:73–8.
4. Holick MF. Vitamin D deficiency. N Engl J Med. 2007;357:266–81.
5. Somjen D, Weisman Y, Kohen F, Gayer B, Limor R, Sharon O, et al. 25-hydroxyvitamin d3-1alpha-hydroxylase is expressed in human vascular smooth muscle cells and is upregulated by parathyroid hormone and estrogenic compounds. Circulation. 2005;111:1666–71.
6. Jablonski KL, Chonchol M, Pierce GL, Walker AE, Seals DR. 25-hydroxyvitamin D deficiency is associated with inflammation-linked vascular endothelial dysfunction in middle-aged and older adults. Hypertension. 2011;57:63–9.
7. Zehnder D, Bland R, Chana RS, Wheeler DC, Howie AJ, Williams MC, et al. Synthesis of 1,25-dihydroxyvitamin D(3) by human endothelial cells is regulated by inflammatory cytokines: a novel autocrine determinant of vascular cell adhesion. J Am Soc Nephrol. 2002;13:621–9.
8. Bland R, Markovic D, Hills CE, Hughes SV, Chan SL, Squires PE, et al. Expression of 25-hydroxyvitamin d3-1alpha-hydroxylase in pancreatic islets. J Steroid Biochem Mol Biol. 2004;89–90:121–5.
9. Mizwicki MT, Norman AW. The vitamin D sterol-vitamin D receptor ensemble model offers unique insights into both genomic and rapid-response signaling. Sci Signal. 2009;2:re4.
10. Granado Lorencio F, Blanco-Navarro I, Perez-Sacristan B. Critical evaluation of assays for vitamin D status. Curr Opin Clin Nutr Metab Care. 2013;16:734–40.
11. Siwamogsatham O, Alvarez JA, Tangpricha V. Diagnosis and treatment of endocrine comorbidities in patients with cystic fibrosis. Curr Opin Endocrinol Diabetes Obes. 2014;21:422–9.
12. Mailhot G. Vitamin D bioavailability in cystic fibrosis: a cause for concern? Nutr Rev. 2012;70:280–93.
13. Hall WB, Sparks AA, Aris RM. Vitamin D deficiency in cystic fibrosis. Int J Endocrinol. 2010;2010:218691.
14. Tangpricha V, Kelly A, Stephenson A, Maguiness K, Enders J, Robinson KA, et al. An update on the screening, diagnosis, management, and treatment of vitamin D deficiency in individuals with cystic fibrosis: evidence-based recommendations from the cystic fibrosis foundation. J Clin Endocrinol Metab. 2012;97:1082–93.
15. Lark RK, Lester GE, Ontjes DA, Blackwood AD, Hollis BW, Hensler MM, et al. Diminished and erratic absorption of ergocalciferol in adult cystic fibrosis patients. Am J Clin Nutr. 2001;73:602–6.
16. Burdge DR, Nakielna EM, Rabin HR. Photosensitivity associated with ciprofloxacin use in adult patients with cystic fibrosis. Antimicrob Agents Chemother. 1995;39:793.
17. Siwamogsatham O, Dong W, Binongo JN, Chowdhury R, Alvarez JA, Feinman SJ, et al. Relationship between fat-soluble vitamin supplementation and blood concentrations in adolescent and adult patients with cystic fibrosis. Nutr Clin Pract. 2014;29:491–7.
18. Coppenhaver D, Kueppers F, Schidlow D, Bee D, Isenburg JN, Barnett D, et al. Serum concentrations of vitamin D-binding protein (group-specific component) in cystic fibrosis. Hum Genet. 1981;57:399–403.
19. Speeckaert MM, Wehlou C, Vandewalle S, Taes YE, Robberecht E, Delanghe JR. Vitamin D binding protein, a new nutritional marker in cystic fibrosis patients. Clin Chem Lab Med. 2008;46:365–70.

20. Rey E, Tréluyer JM, Pons G. Drug disposition in cystic fibrosis. Clin Pharmacokinet. 1998;35:313–29.
21. Rogiers V, Crokaert R, Vis H-L. Altered phospholipid composition and changed fatty acid pattern of the various phospholipid fractions of red cell membranes of cystic fibrosis children with pancreatic insufficiency. Clin Chim Acta. 1980;105:105–15.
22. Sato F, Soos G, Link C, Sato K. Cystic fibrosis transport regulator and its mRNA are expressed in human epidermis. J Invest Dermatol. 2002;119:1224–30.
23. Jouret F, Bernard A, Hermans C, Dom G, Terryn S, Leal T, et al. Cystic fibrosis is associated with a defect in apical receptor–mediated endocytosis in mouse and human kidney. J Am Soc Nephrol. 2007;18:707–18.
24. Kurahashi I, Matsunuma A, Kawane T, Abe M, Horiuchi N. Dexamethasone enhances vitamin d-24-hydroxylase expression in osteoblastic (UMR-106) and renal (LLC-PK1) cells treated with 1α,25-dihydroxyvitamin d3. Endocrine. 2002;17:109–18.
25. Herscovitch K, Dauletbaev N, Lands LC. Vitamin D as an anti-microbial and anti-inflammatory therapy for cystic fibrosis. Paediatr Respir Rev. 2014;15:154–62.
26. Holick MF. Vitamin D and bone health. J Nutr. 1996;126:1159S–64.
27. DeLuca HF. Overview of general physiologic features and functions of vitamin D. Am J Clin Nutr. 2004;80: 1689S–96.
28. Donovan DS, Papadopoulos A, Staron RB, Addesso V, Schulman L, McGregor C, et al. Bone mass and vitamin D deficiency in adults with advanced cystic fibrosis lung disease. Am J Respir Crit Care Med. 1998;157:1892–9.
29. Sheikh S, Gemma S, Patel A. Factors associated with low bone mineral density in patients with cystic fibrosis. J Bone Miner Metab. 2014;33(2):180–5.
30. Robertson J, Macdonald K. Prevalence of bone loss in a population with cystic fibrosis. Br J Nurs. 2010;19: 636–9.
31. Douros K, Loukou I, Nicolaidou P, Tzonou A, Doudounakis S. Bone mass density and associated factors in cystic fibrosis patients of young age. J Paediatr Child Health. 2008;44:681–5.
32. Grey V, Atkinson S, Drury D, Casey L, Ferland G, Gundberg C, et al. Prevalence of low bone mass and deficiencies of vitamins D and K in pediatric patients with cystic fibrosis from 3 Canadian centers. Pediatrics. 2008;122: 1014–20.
33. Cemlyn-Jones J, Gamboa F, Loureiro M, Fontes BM. Evaluation of bone mineral density in cystic fibrosis patients. Rev Port Pneumol. 2008;14:625–34.
34. Kamen DL, Tangpricha V. Vitamin D and molecular actions on the immune system: modulation of innate and autoimmunity. J Mol Med (Berl). 2010;88:441–50.
35. Adams JS, Rafison B, Witzel S, Reyes RE, Shieh A, Chun R, et al. Regulation of the extrarenal cyp27b1-hydroxylase. J Steroid Biochem Mol Biol. 2014;144, Part A:22–7.
36. Adams JS, Sharma OP, Gacad MA, Singer FR. Metabolism of 25-hydroxyvitamin d3 by cultured pulmonary alveolar macrophages in sarcoidosis. J Clin Invest. 1983;72:1856–60.
37. Liu PT, Stenger S, Li H, Wenzel L, Tan BH, Krutzik SR, et al. Toll-like receptor triggering of a vitamin D-mediated human antimicrobial response. Science. 2006;311:1770–3.
38. Hansdottir S, Monick MM, Hinde SL, Lovan N, Look DC, Hunninghake GW. Respiratory epithelial cells convert inactive vitamin D to its active form: potential effects on host defense. J Immunol. 2008;181:7090–9.
39. Yim S, Dhawan P, Ragunath C, Christakos S, Diamond G. Induction of cathelicidin in normal and cf bronchial epithelial cells by 1,25-dihydroxyvitamin D(3). J Cyst Fibros. 2007;6:403–10.
40. Grossmann RE, Zughaier SM, Liu S, Lyles RH, Tangpricha V. Impact of vitamin D supplementation on markers of inflammation in adults with cystic fibrosis hospitalized for a pulmonary exacerbation. Eur J Clin Nutr. 2012;66:1072–4.
41. Grossmann RE, Zughaier SM, Kumari M, Seydafkan S, Lyles RH, Liu S, et al. Pilot study of vitamin D supplementation in adults with cystic fibrosis pulmonary exacerbation: a randomized, controlled trial. Dermatoendocrinol. 2012;4:191–7.
42. Green D, Carson K, Leonard A, Davis JE, Rosenstein B, Zeitlin P, et al. Current treatment recommendations for correcting vitamin D deficiency in pediatric patients with cystic fibrosis are inadequate. J Pediatr. 2008; 153:554–9.e2.
43. McCauley LA, Thomas W, Laguna TA, Regelmann WE, Moran A, Polgreen LE. Vitamin D deficiency is associated with pulmonary exacerbations in children with cystic fibrosis. Ann Am Thorac Soc. 2013;11:198–204.
44. Pincikova T, Nilsson K, Moen IE, Karpati F, Fluge G, Hollsing A, et al. Inverse relation between vitamin D and serum total immunoglobulin g in the Scandinavian cystic fibrosis nutritional study. Eur J Clin Nutr. 2011;65: 102–9.
45. Marcondes NA, Raimundo FV, Vanacor R, Corte BP, Ascoli AM, de Azambuja AZ, et al. Hypovitaminosis D in patients with cystic fibrosis: a cross-section study in south brazil. Clin Respir J. 2014;8:455–9.
46. Simoneau T, Bazzaz O, Sawicki GS, Gordon C. Vitamin D status in children with cystic fibrosis. Associations with inflammation and bacterial colonization. Ann Am Thorac Soc. 2014;11:205–10.

47. Pincikova T, Nilsson K, Moen IE, Fluge G, Hollsing A, Knudsen PK, et al. Vitamin D deficiency as a risk factor for cystic fibrosis-related diabetes in the Scandinavian cystic fibrosis nutritional study. Diabetologia. 2011;54: 3007–15.

48. Alvarez JA, Ashraf A. Role of vitamin D in insulin secretion and insulin sensitivity for glucose homeostasis. Int J Endocrinol. 2010;2010:351385.

49. Eyles DW, Burne TH, McGrath JJ. Vitamin D, effects on brain development, adult brain function and the links between low levels of vitamin D and neuropsychiatric disease. Front Neuroendocrinol. 2013;34:47–64.

50. Kopp BT, Hayes Jr D, Ratkiewicz M, Baron N, Splaingard M. Light exposure and depression in hospitalized adult patients with cystic fibrosis. J Affect Disord. 2013;150:585–9.

51. Smith BA, Cogswell A, Garcia G. Vitamin D and depressive symptoms in children with cystic fibrosis. Psychosomatics. 2014;55:76–81.

52. Ferguson JH, Chang AB. Vitamin D supplementation for cystic fibrosis. Cochrane Database Syst Rev. 2014;5, CD007298.

53. Sermet-Gaudelus I, Bianchi ML, Garabedian M, Aris RM, Morton A, Hardin DS, et al. European cystic fibrosis bone mineralisation guidelines. J Cyst Fibros. 2011;10 Suppl 2:S16–23.

54. Armas LA, Hollis BW, Heaney RP. Vitamin D2 is much less effective than vitamin D3 in humans. J Clin Endocrinol Metab. 2004;89:5387–91.

55. Khazai NB, Judd SE, Jeng L, Wolfenden LL, Stecenko A, Ziegler TR, et al. Treatment and prevention of vitamin D insufficiency in cystic fibrosis patients: comparative efficacy of ergocalciferol, cholecalciferol, and UV light. J Clin Endocrinol Metab. 2009;94:2037–43.

56. Gronowitz E, Larko O, Gilljam M, Hollsing A, Lindblad A, Mellstrom D, et al. Ultraviolet B radiation improves serum levels of vitamin D in patients with cystic fibrosis. Acta Paediatr. 2005;94:547–52.

57. Vogiatzi MG, Jacobson-Dickman E, DeBoer MD. Vitamin D supplementation and risk of toxicity in pediatrics: a review of current literature. J Clin Endocrinol Metab. 2014;99:1132–41.

58. Cystic fibrosis foundation patient registry 2012 annual data report. Bethesda, MD: Cystic Fibrosis Foundation; 2013.

59. Putman MS, Milliren CE, Derrico N, Uluer A, Sicilian L, Lapey A, et al. Compromised bone microarchitecture and estimated bone strength in young adults with cystic fibrosis. J Clin Endocrinol Metab. 2014;99:3399–407.

60. Aris RM, Renner JB, Winders AD, Buell HE, Riggs DB, Lester GE, et al. Increased rate of fractures and severe Kyphosis: sequelae of living into adulthood with cystic fibrosis. Ann Intern Med. 1998;128:186–93.

61. Rossini M, Del Marco A, Dal Santo F, Gatti D, Braggion C, James G, et al. Prevalence and correlates of vertebral fractures in adults with cystic fibrosis. Bone. 2004;35:771–6.

62. Stalvey MS, Clines GA. Cystic fibrosis-related bone disease: insights into a growing problem. Curr Opin Endocrinol Diabetes Obes. 2013;20:547–52.

63. Latzin P, Griese M, Hermanns V, Kammer B. Sternal fracture with fatal outcome in cystic fibrosis. Thorax. 2005; 60:616.

64. Aris RM, Merkel PA, Bachrach LK, Borowitz DS, Boyle MP, Elkin SL, et al. Guide to bone health and disease in cystic fibrosis. J Clin Endocrinol Metab. 2005;90:1888–96.

65. Saggese G, Baroncelli GI, Bertelloni S. Puberty and bone development. Best Pract Res Clin Endocrinol Metab. 2002;16:53–64.

66. Curran DR, McArdle JR, Talwalkar JS. Diabetes mellitus and bone disease in cystic fibrosis. Semin Respir Crit Care Med. 2009;30:514–30.

67. Rogan MP, Reznikov LR, Pezzulo AA, Gansemer ND, Samuel M, Prather RS, et al. Pigs and humans with cystic fibrosis have reduced insulin-like growth factor 1 (IGF1) levels at birth. Proc Natl Acad Sci U S A. 2010;107: 20571–5.

68. Gordon CM, Binello E, LeBoff MS, Wohl ME, Rosen CJ, Colin AA. Relationship between insulin-like growth factor I, dehydroepiandrosterone sulfate and proresorptive cytokines and bone density in cystic fibrosis. Osteoporos Int. 2006;17:783–90.

69. Hardin DS, Ahn C, Prestidge C, Seilheimer DK, Ellis KJ. Growth hormone improves bone mineral content in children with cystic fibrosis. J Pediatr Endocrinol Metab. 2005;18:589–95.

70. Fulzele K, Clemens TL. Novel functions for insulin in bone. Bone. 2012;50:452–6.

71. Henneicke H, Gasparini SJ, Brennan-Speranza TC, Zhou H, Seibel MJ. Glucocorticoids and bone: local effects and systemic implications. Trends Endocrinol Metab. 2014;25:197–211.

72. Neri AS, Lori I, Festini F, Masi L, Brandi ML, Galici V, et al. Bone mineral density in cystic fibrosis patients under the age of 18 years. Minerva Pediatr. 2008;60:147–54.

73. Weitzmann MN. The role of inflammatory cytokines, the RANKL/OPG axis, and the immunoskeletal interface in physiological bone turnover and osteoporosis. Scientifica (Cairo). 2013;2013:125705.

74. Shead EF, Haworth CS, Condliffe AM, McKeon DJ, Scott MA, Compston JE. Cystic fibrosis transmembrane conductance regulator (cftr) is expressed in human bone. Thorax. 2007;62:650–1.

75. Le Heron L, Guillaume C, Velard F, Braux J, Touqui L, Moriceau S, et al. Cystic fibrosis transmembrane conductance regulator (CFTR) regulates the production of osteoprotegerin (OPG) and prostaglandin (PG) e2 in human bone. J Cyst Fibros. 2010;9:69–72.

76. Ambroszkiewicz J, Sands D, Gajewska J, Chelchowska M, Laskowska-Klita T. Bone turnover markers, osteoprotegerin and rankl cytokines in children with cystic fibrosis. Adv Med Sci. 2013;58:338–43.

77. Stallings VA, Stark LJ, Robinson KA, Feranchak AP, Quinton H. Evidence-based practice recommendations for nutrition-related management of children and adults with cystic fibrosis and pancreatic insufficiency: results of a systematic review. J Am Diet Assoc. 2008;108:832–9.

78. Weaver CM, Heaney RP. Calcium. In: Ross CA, Caballero B, Cousins RJ, Tucker KL, Ziegler TR, editors. Modern nutrition in health and disease. 11th ed. Philadelphia: Lippincott Williams & Wilkins; 2014. p. 133–49.

79. Schulze KJ, O'Brien KO, Germain-Lee EL, Booth SL, Leonard A, Rosenstein BJ. Calcium kinetics are altered in clinically stable girls with cystic fibrosis. J Clin Endocrinol Metab. 2004;89:3385–91.

80. Schulze KJ, O'Brien KO, Germain-Lee EL, Baer DJ, Leonard AL, Rosenstein BJ. Endogenous fecal losses of calcium compromise calcium balance in pancreatic-insufficient girls with cystic fibrosis. J Pediatr. 2003;143:765–71.

81. Schulze KJ, O'Brien KO, Germain-Lee EL, Baer DJ, Leonard A, Rosenstein BJ. Efficiency of calcium absorption is not compromised in clinically stable prepubertal and pubertal girls with cystic fibrosis. Am J Clin Nutr. 2003;78:110–6.

82. Hillman LS, Cassidy JT, Popescu MF, Hewett JE, Kyger J, Robertson JD. Percent true calcium absorption, mineral metabolism, and bone mineralization in children with cystic fibrosis: effect of supplementation with vitamin D and calcium. Pediatr Pulmonol. 2008;43:772–80.

83. Kemi VE, Karkkainen MU, Lamberg-Allardt CJ. High phosphorus intakes acutely and negatively affect ca and bone metabolism in a dose-dependent manner in healthy young females. Br J Nutr. 2006;96:545–52.

84. Kemi VE, Karkkainen MU, Rita HJ, Laaksonen MM, Outila TA, Lamberg-Allardt CJ. Low calcium:phosphorus ratio in habitual diets affects serum parathyroid hormone concentration and calcium metabolism in healthy women with adequate calcium intake. Br J Nutr. 2010;103:561–8.

85. Tucker KL, Rosen CJ. Prevention and management of osteoporosis. In: Ross CA, Caballero B, Cousins RJ, Tucker KL, Ziegler TR, editors. Modern nutrition in health and disease. 11th ed. Philadelphia: Lippincott Williams & Wilkins; 2014. p. 1227–44.

86. Tucker KL, Morita K, Qiao N, Hannan MT, Cupples LA, Kiel DP. Colas, but not other carbonated beverages, are associated with low bone mineral density in older women: the Framingham osteoporosis study. Am J Clin Nutr. 2006;84:936–42.

87. Wyshak G, Frisch RE. Carbonated beverages, dietary calcium, the dietary calcium/phosphorus ratio, and bone fractures in girls and boys. J Adolesc Health. 1994;15:210–5.

88. Kiel DP, Felson DT, Hannan MT, Anderson JJ, Wilson PW. Caffeine and the risk of hip fracture: the Framingham study. Am J Epidemiol. 1990;132:675–84.

89. Hallstrom H, Melhus H, Glynn A, Lind L, Syvanen AC, Michaelsson K. Coffee consumption and cyp1a2 genotype in relation to bone mineral density of the proximal femur in elderly men and women: a cohort study. Nutr Metab. 2010;7:12.

90. Harris SS, Dawson-Hughes B. Caffeine and bone loss in healthy postmenopausal women. Am J Clin Nutr. 1994;60:573–8.

91. Heaney RP. Effects of caffeine on bone and the calcium economy. Food Chem Toxicol. 2002;40:1263–70.

92. Barrett-Connor E, Chang JC, Edelstein SL. Coffee-associated osteoporosis offset by daily milk consumption. The Rancho Bernardo study. JAMA. 1994;271:280–3.

93. Hallstrom H, Wolk A, Glynn A, Michaelsson K. Coffee, tea and caffeine consumption in relation to osteoporotic fracture risk in a cohort of Swedish women. Osteoporos Int. 2006;17:1055–64.

94. Spencer H, Kramer L. Antacid-induced calcium loss. Arch Intern Med. 1983;143:657–9.

95. Spencer H, Kramer L, Norris C, Osis D. Effect of small doses of aluminum-containing antacids on calcium and phosphorus metabolism. Am J Clin Nutr. 1982;36:32–40.

96. Borowitz D, Baker RD, Stallings V. Consensus report on nutrition for pediatric patients with cystic fibrosis. J Pediatr Gastroenterol Nutr. 2002;35:246–59.

97. Devine A, Criddle RA, Dick IM, Kerr DA, Prince RL. A longitudinal study of the effect of sodium and calcium intakes on regional bone density in postmenopausal women. Am J Clin Nutr. 1995;62:740–5.

98. Dougherty KA, Schall JI, Stallings VA. Suboptimal vitamin K status despite supplementation in children and young adults with cystic fibrosis. Am J Clin Nutr. 2010;92:660–7.

99. Conway SP, Wolfe SP, Brownlee KG, White H, Oldroyd B, Truscott JG, et al. Vitamin K status among children with cystic fibrosis and its relationship to bone mineral density and bone turnover. Pediatrics. 2005;115:1325–31.

100. Conway SP. Vitamin K in cystic fibrosis. J R Soc Med. 2004;97 Suppl 44:48–51.

101. Pearson DA. Bone health and osteoporosis: the role of vitamin K and potential antagonism by anticoagulants. Nutr Clin Pract. 2007;22:517–44.

102. Council NR. Dietary reference intakes for vitamin A, vitamin K, arsenic, boron, chromium, copper, iodine, iron, manganese, molybdenum, nickel, silicon, vanadium, and zinc. Washington: The National Academies Press; 2001.

103. Fewtrell MS, Benden C, Williams JE, Chomtho S, Ginty F, Nigdikar SV, et al. Undercarboxylated osteocalcin and bone mass in 8–12 year old children with cystic fibrosis. J Cyst Fibros. 2008;7:307–12.

104. Kratz A, Ferraro M, Sluss PM, Lewandrowski KB. Case records of the Massachusetts general hospital. Weekly clinicopathological exercises. Laboratory reference values. N Engl J Med. 2004;351:1548–63.

105. Jagannath VA, Fedorowicz Z, Thaker V, Chang AB. Vitamin K supplementation for cystic fibrosis. Cochrane Database Syst Rev. 2013;4, CD008482.

106. Nicolaidou P, Stavrinadis I, Loukou I, Papadopoulou A, Georgouli H, Douros K, et al. The effect of vitamin K supplementation on biochemical markers of bone formation in children and adolescents with cystic fibrosis. Eur J Pediatr. 2006;165:540–5.

107. Rizzoli R, Bianchi ML, Garabedian M, McKay HA, Moreno LA. Maximizing bone mineral mass gain during growth for the prevention of fractures in the adolescents and the elderly. Bone. 2010;46:294–305.

108. Castiglioni S, Cazzaniga A, Albisetti W, Maier JA. Magnesium and osteoporosis: current state of knowledge and future research directions. Nutrients. 2013;5:3022–33.

109. Takeda E, Yamamoto H, Yamanaka-Okumura H, Taketani Y. Dietary phosphorus in bone health and quality of life. Nutr Rev. 2012;70:311–21.

110. Sebastian A, Harris ST, Ottaway JH, Todd KM, Morris Jr RC. Improved mineral balance and skeletal metabolism in postmenopausal women treated with potassium bicarbonate. N Engl J Med. 1994;330:1776–81.

111. Guralp O. Effects of vitamin E on bone remodeling in perimenopausal women: mini review. Maturitas. 2014;79:476–80.

112. Chin KY, Ima-Nirwana S. The effects of alpha-tocopherol on bone: a double-edged sword? Nutrients. 2014;6:1424–41.

113. Vacek TP, Kalani A, Voor MJ, Tyagi SC, Tyagi N. The role of homocysteine in bone remodeling. Clin Chem Lab Med. 2013;51:579–90.

114. Herrmann M, Peter Schmidt J, Umanskaya N, Wagner A, Taban-Shomal O, Widmann T, et al. The role of hyperhomocysteinemia as well as folate, vitamin B(6) and B(12) deficiencies in osteoporosis: a systematic review. Clin Chem Lab Med. 2007;45:1621–32.

115. Yamaguchi M. Role of carotenoid beta-cryptoxanthin in bone homeostasis. J Biomed Sci. 2012;19:36.

116. Maurel DB, Boisseau N, Benhamou CL, Jaffre C. Alcohol and bone: review of dose effects and mechanisms. Osteoporos Int. 2012;23:1–16.

117. Melhus H, Michaelsson K, Kindmark A, Bergstrom R, Holmberg L, Mallmin H, et al. Excessive dietary intake of vitamin A is associated with reduced bone mineral density and increased risk for hip fracture. Ann Intern Med. 1998;129:770–8.

118. Michaelsson K, Lithell H, Vessby B, Melhus H. Serum retinol levels and the risk of fracture. N Engl J Med. 2003;348:287–94.

119. Feskanich D, Singh V, Willett WC, Colditz GA. Vitamin A intake and hip fractures among postmenopausal women. JAMA. 2002;287:47–54.

120. Conaway HH, Henning P, Lerner UH. Vitamin A metabolism, action, and role in skeletal homeostasis. Endocr Rev. 2013;34:766–97.

121. Maqbool A, Graham-Maar RC, Schall JI, Zemel BS, Stallings VA. Vitamin A intake and elevated serum retinol levels in children and young adults with cystic fibrosis. J Cyst Fibros. 2008;7:137–41.

122. Gracia-Marco L, Moreno LA, Ortega FB, Leon F, Sioen I, Kafatos A, et al. Levels of physical activity that predict optimal bone mass in adolescents: the Helena study. Am J Prev Med. 2011;40:599–607.

123. Dodd JD, Barry SC, Barry RB, Cawood TJ, McKenna MJ, Gallagher CG. Bone mineral density in cystic fibrosis: benefit of exercise capacity. J Clin Densitom. 2008;11:537–42.

124. Frangolias DD, Pare PD, Kendler DL, Davidson AG, Wong L, Raboud J, et al. Role of exercise and nutrition status on bone mineral density in cystic fibrosis. J Cyst Fibros. 2003;2:163–70.

125. Santos A, Bakker AD, Klein-Nulend J. The role of osteocytes in bone mechanotransduction. Osteoporos Int. 2009;20:1027–31.

126. Bonnet N, Ferrari SL. Exercise and the skeleton: how it works and what it really does. IBMS BoneKEy. 2010;7:235–48.

127. Wardlaw GM. Putting body weight and osteoporosis into perspective. Am J Clin Nutr. 1996;63:433S–6.

128. Shapses SA, Riedt CS. Bone, body weight, and weight reduction: what are the concerns? J Nutr. 2006;136:1453–6.

129. Schoenau E, Neu MC, Manz F. Muscle mass during childhood—relationship to skeletal development. J Musculoskelet Neuronal Interact. 2004;4:105–8.

130. Burr DB. Muscle strength, bone mass, and age-related bone loss. J Bone Miner Res. 1997;12:1547–51.
131. Ionescu AA, Evans WD, Pettit RJ, Nixon LS, Stone MD, Shale DJ. Hidden depletion of fat-free mass and bone mineral density in adults with cystic fibrosis. Chest. 2003;124:2220–8.
132. Bianchi ML, Romano G, Saraifoger S, Costantini D, Limonta C, Colombo C. BMD and body composition in children and young patients affected by cystic fibrosis. J Bone Miner Res. 2006;21:388–96.
133. Conwell LS, Chang AB. Bisphosphonates for osteoporosis in people with cystic fibrosis. Cochrane Database Syst Rev. 2014;3, CD002010.
134. Siwamogsatham O, Stephens K, Tangpricha V. Evaluation of teriparatide for treatment of osteoporosis in four patients with cystic fibrosis: a case series. Case Reports in Endocrinology. 2014;2014:893589.

Chapter 5
Vitamins and Minerals

Suzanne H. Michel and Donna H. Mueller

Key Points
- Persons who have CF are at risk for vitamins and minerals deficiencies.
- Persons who have CF use CF-specific multivitamin supplements with zinc
- CF-specific multivitamin supplements contain higher levels of fat-soluble vitamins when compared to over-the-counter products.
- Published vitamin and mineral screening, annual assessment, and prescription recommendations are available from international CF Foundations and Societies.
- Research and anticipatory guidance for vitamins and minerals are necessary.

Keywords Vitamins • Minerals • Fat-soluble vitamins • Retinol • Alpha-tocopherol • Vitamin K • Water-soluble vitamins • Sodium chloride • Calcium • Iron • Zinc • Magnesium • Copper

Introduction

The importance of vitamin and mineral supplementation for persons who have cystic fibrosis (CF) is well established [1–7]. Prior to the widespread availability of newborn screening, symptoms of overt vitamin or mineral deficiencies often were initial signs indicative of the CF diagnosis [8–11]. Low vitamin serum levels continue to be seen, but signs of overt deficiency are infrequent and descriptions often are published as case reports [1, 12–15]. The introduction of CF-specific multivitamin supplements coupled with improved pancreatic enzyme replacement therapy (PERT) has contributed to the reduction in the incidence and prevalence of deficiencies. Table 5.1 lists the nutrient content of

S.H. Michel, M.P.H., R.D., L.D.N. (✉)
Pulmonary Medicine, Medical University of South Carolina,
PO Box 1674, Folly Beach, SC 29439-1674, USA
e-mail: smichelrd@aol.com

D.H. Mueller, Ph.D., R.D. F.A.D.A., L.D.N., F.C.P.P.
Department of Nutrition Sciences, Drexel University,
2132 Mt. Vernon Street, Philadelphia, Pennsylvania 19130-3134, USA
e-mail: muellerd@drexel.edu

E.H. Yen, A.R. Leonard (eds.), *Nutrition in Cystic Fibrosis: A Guide for Clinicians*, Nutrition and Health, 67
DOI 10.1007/978-3-319-16387-1_5, © Springer International Publishing Switzerland 2015

Table 5.1 Nutrient content of CF-specific multivitamins with zinc and select over-the-counter products

Fat-soluble vitamins[a,b]					
MVW Complete Formulation®, drops, chewables, softgels, D3000 softgels[c]	AQUADEKs®, drops, chewables, softgels	Vitamax®, drops, chewables	ChoiceFul, chewables, softgels, label data	Libertas, ABDEK, drops, chewables, softgels	Poly-Vi-Sol® drops, Centrum®, chewable, tablet
Total vitamin A (IU) (retinol[d] and beta carotene)					
4627/0.5 ml 75% as beta-carotene	5751/1 ml 87% as beta-carotene	3170/1 ml as 100% retinol palmitate	NP	4627/1 ml 100% retinol palmitate	750/ml
9254/1 ml 75% as beta-carotene	11,502/2 ml 87% as beta-carotene	6340/2 ml as 100% retinol palmitate	NP	9254/2 ml 100% retinol palmitate	1500/2 ml
16,000/1 chewable 88% as beta-carotene	18,167/2 chewables 92% as beta-carotene	5000/1 chewable 50% as beta-carotene	13,000/1 chewable 88% as beta-carotene	16,000/1 chewable 100% as beta-carotene	3500/1 chewable 29% as beta-carotene
32,000/2 softgels 88% as beta-carotene	36,334/2 softgels 92% as beta-carotene	NP	28,000/2 softgels 88% as beta-carotene	32,000/2 softgels 88% as beta-carotene	7000/2 tablets 29% as beta-carotene
32,000/2 softgels (D3000) 88% as beta-carotene	NP	NP	NP	NP	NP
Vitamin E (IU)					
50/0.5 ml	50/1 ml[e]	50/1 ml	NP	50/1 ml	5/1 ml
100/1 ml	100/2 ml[e]	100/2 ml	NP	100/2 ml	10/2 ml
200/1 chewable	100/2 chewables[e]	200/1 chewable	180/1 chewable	200/1 chewable	30/1 chewable
400/2 softgels	300/2 softgels[e]	NP	340/2 softgels	400/2 softgels	60/2 tablets
400/2 softgels (D3000)	NP	NP	NP	NP	NP
Vitamin D (IU)					
750/0.5 ml	600/1 ml	400/1 ml	NP	500/1 ml	400/1 ml
1500/1 ml	1200/2 ml	800/2 ml	NP	1000/2 ml	800/2 ml
1500/1 chewable	1200/2 chewables	400/1 chewable	800/1 chewable	1000/1 chewable	400/1 chewable
3000/2 softgels	2400/2 softgels	NP	2000/2 softgels	2000/2 softgels	800/2 tablets
6000/2 softgels (D3000)	NP	NP	NP	NP	NP
Vitamin K (mcg)					
500/0.5 ml	400/1 ml	300/1 ml	NP	400/1 ml	0
1000/1 ml	800/2 ml	600/2 ml	NP	800/2 ml	0
1000/1 chewable	700/2 chewables	200/1 chewable	600/1 chewable	800/1 chewable	10/1 chewable
1600/2 softgels	1400/2 softgels	NP	1400/2 softgels	1600/2 softgels	50/2 tablets
1600/2 softgels (D3000)	NP	NP	NP	NP	NP

(continued)

Table 5.1 (continued)

Water-soluble vitamins & zinc[a,b]					
MVW Complete Formulation™ Drops, Chewables, Softgels, D3000 Softgels	AQUADEKs®, Drops, Softgels	Vitamax® Drops, Chewables	ChoiceFul Chewables, Softgels Label Data	Libertas ABDEK Drops, Chewables, Softgels	Poly-Vi-Sol® Drops Centrum® Chewable, Tablet
Thiamin B1 (mg)					
0.5/0.5 ml	0.6/1 ml	0.5/1 ml	NP	0.5/1 ml	0.5/1 ml
1/1 ml	1.2/2 ml	1/2 ml	NP	1/2 ml	1/2 ml
1.5/1 chewable	1.5/2 chewables	1.5/1 chewable	1.2/1 chewable	1.5/1 chewable	1.5/1 chewable
3/2 softgels or 2 softgels with D3000	3/2 softgels	NP	2/2 softgels	3/2 softgels	3/2 tablets
Riboflavin B2 (mg)					
0.6/0.5 ml	0.6/1 ml	0.6/1 ml	NP	0.6/1 ml	0.6/1 ml
1.2/1 ml	1.2/2 ml	1.2/2 ml	NP	1.2/2 ml	1.2/2 ml
1.7/1 chewable	1.7/2 chewables	1.7/1 chewable	1.4/1 chewable	1.7/1 chewable	1.7/1 chewable
3.4/2 softgels or 2 softgels with D3000	3.4/2 softgels	NP	3/2 softgels	3.4/2 softgels	3.4/2 tablets
Niacin (mg)					
6/0.5 ml	6/1 ml	6/1 ml	NP	6/1 ml	8/1 ml
12/1 ml	12/2 ml	12/2 ml	NP	12/2 ml	16/2 ml
10/1 chewable	10/2 chewables	20/1 chewable	8/1 chewable	10/1 chewable	20/1 chewable
40/2 softgels or 2 softgels with D3000	20/2 softgels	NP	36/2 softgels	40/2 softgels	40/2 tablets
Pyridoxine B6 (mg)					
0.6/0.5 ml	0.6/1 ml	0.6/1 ml	NP	0.6 1 ml	0.4/1 ml
1.2/1 ml	1.2/2 ml	1.2/2 ml	NP	1.2/2 ml	0.8/2 ml
1.9/1 chewable	1.9/2 chewables	2/1 chewable	1.5/1 chewable	1.9/1 chewable	2/1 chewable
3.8/2 softgels or 2 softgels with D3000	3.8/2 softgels	NP	3.8/2 softgels	3.8/2 softgels	4/2 tablets
B12 (mcg)					
4/0.5 ml	0	4/1 ml	NP	4/1 ml	2/1 ml
8/1 ml	0	8/2 ml	NP	8/2 ml	4/2 ml
6/1 chewable	12/2 chewables	6/1 chewable	6/1 chewable	6/1 chewable	6/1 chewable
12/2 softgels or 2 softgels with D3000	24/2 softgels	NP	10/2 softgels	12/2 softgels	12/2 tablets
Biotin (mcg)					
15/0.5 ml	15/1 ml	15/1 ml	NP	15/1 ml	0
30/1 ml	30/2 ml	30/2 ml	NP	30/2 ml	0
100/1 chewable	100/2 chewables	300/1 chewable	80/1 chewable	100/1 chewable	45/1 chewable
200/2 softgels or 2 softgels with D3000	200/2 softgels	NP	160/2 softgels	200/2 softgels	60/2 tablets

(continued)

Table 5.1 (continued)

Water-soluble vitamins & zinc[a,b]					
MVW Complete Formulation™ Drops, Chewables, Softgels, D3000 Softgels	AQUADEKs®, Drops, Softgels	Vitamax® Drops, Chewables	ChoiceFul Chewables, Softgels Label Data	Libertas ABDEK Drops, Chewables, Softgels	Poly-Vi-Sol® Drops Centrum® Chewable, Tablet
Folic acid (mcg)					
0	0	0	NP	0	0
0	0	0	NP	0	0
200/1 chewable	200/2 chewables	200/1 chewable	180/1 chewable	200/1 chewable	400/1 chewable
400/softgels or 2 softgels with D3000	200/2 softgels	NP	360/2 softgels	400/2 softgels	800/2 tablets
Ascorbic acid C (mg)					
45/0.5 ml	45/1 ml	45/1 ml	NP	45/1 ml	35/1 ml
90/1 ml	90/2 ml	90/2 ml	NP	90/2 ml	70/2 ml
100/1 chewable	70/2 chewables	60/1 chewable	60/1 chewable	100/1 chewable	60/1 chewable
200/2 softgels or 2 softgels with D3000	150/2 softgels	NP	60/2 softgels	200/2 softgels	120/2 tablets
Pantothenic acid (mg)					
3/0.5 ml	3/1 ml	3/1 ml	NP	3/1 ml	0
6/1 ml	6/2 ml	6/2 ml	NP	6/2 ml	0
12/1 chewable	12/2 chewables	10/1 chewable	10/1 chewable	12/1 chewable	10/1 chewable
24/2 softgels or 2 softgels with D3000	24/2 softgels	NP	16/2 softgels	24/2 softgels	20/2 tablets
Zinc (mg)					
5/0.5 ml	5/1 ml	7.5/1 ml	NP	5/1 ml	0
10/1 ml	10/2 ml	15/2 ml	NP	10/2 ml	0
15/1 chewable	10/2 chewables	7.5/1 chewable	15/chewable	15/1 chewable	15/1 chewable
20/2 softgels or 2 softgels with D3000	20/2 softgels	NP	30/2 softgels	30/2 softgels	22/2 tablets

[a]The content of this table was confirmed as of October 2014

[b]Created by Suzanne H. Michel, MPH, RD, LDN. Please be aware that companies have copied the look and format of this table. Unless the table has Ms. Michel's name on it, she cannot attest to its accuracy

[c]Tangpricha V, Kelly A, Stephenson A, Maguiness K, Enders J, Robinson KA, Marshall BC, Borowitz D, for the Cystic Fibrosis Foundation Vitamin D Evidence-Based Review Committee. An update on the screening, diagnosis, management, and treatment of vitamin D deficiency in individuals with cystic fibrosis: Evidence-based recommendations from the Cystic Fibrosis Foundation. J Clin Endocrinol Metab. 2012;97(4):1082–93

[d]All products contain retinyl palmitate with the exception of Vitamax Chewable which contains retinol acetate.

[e]Also contains mixed tocopherols

[f]AquADEKs® is a registered trademark of Yasoo Health Inc., Vitamax® is a registered trademark of Shear/Kershman Labs. Inc., Poly-Vi-Sol® is a registered trademark of Mead Johnson and Company, Centrum® is a registered trademark of Wyeth Consumer Care, MVW Complete Formulation is a registered trademark of MVW Nutritionals, LLC

[g]NP no product

currently available CF-specific multivitamins with zinc. The content of CF-specific vitamins has evolved since their introduction over 20 years ago resulting in improvement of targeted micronutrient serum levels [16].

Low serum vitamin and/or mineral levels may reflect maldigestion and malabsorption of CF, inadequate dietary intake, inadequate dosing, inadequate adherence to therapy, incorrect use of supplements and PERT, drug–nutrient interaction, or medical challenges, such as bowel resection or liver disease [17–19]. For optimal absorption fat-soluble vitamins should be taken with a fat-containing food/drink and PERT. Women who have CF, have marginal serum vitamin and mineral levels, and use oral contraceptives may require special attention to optimize micronutrient levels. These women may need additional sources of vitamins B-6, folic acid, riboflavin, ascorbic acid, retinol, and the minerals iron, zinc, and copper [20].

Inadequate serum levels have been reported in pancreatic sufficient patients. Some researchers believe the low levels may reflect challenges at the cellular level, while others postulate that a decline in fat-soluble vitamin serum levels actually may be a sign of developing pancreatic insufficiency [14, 21, 22].

Deficiencies of vitamins A, D, and E and the mineral zinc were identified in infants as young as six weeks of age [23, 24]. Follow-up of the infants up to ten years of age found that despite the use of PERT and vitamin supplementation some children continued to present with low levels of the vitamins, with vitamin E being the most frequent [25]. Treatment with PERT along with zinc containing CF-specific vitamins corrected zinc deficiency in infants [26].

Several of the micronutrients in this chapter are antioxidants, namely beta-carotene, vitamins C and E and the minerals selenium and zinc. The role of antioxidants and CF was reviewed with the conclusion that additional research is necessary prior to recommending supplemental antioxidants beyond what currently is recommended in nutrition consensus reports [27, 28]. Official vitamin recommendations may not reflect currently available evidence. Table 5.2 provides a summary of international CF Foundations' vitamin and mineral recommendations [1–7].

This chapter reviews current knowledge of vitamin and mineral nutrition in CF. Readers are referred to the chapters on pregnancy, lung transplant, and liver disease for vitamin and mineral information specific to those topics. Vitamin D is covered in a separate chapter.

Vitamin A

Vitamin A's role in eye health is well documented but it is also essential for cellular integrity, growth, immune function, and bone and tooth development. Vitamin A deficiency and vitamin A toxicity are of concern in the care of persons who have CF [30]. Serum retinol is homeostatically maintained, while hepatic stores increase indefinitely with increased ingestion [31]. Excessive vitamin A serum level is linked to liver and bone damage [32, 33]. Night blindness has been reported in persons who have CF either prior to or following diagnosis [15, 34, 35]. Vitamin A plays a pivotal role in CF lung health [36, 37]. Rivas-Crespo described better lung function in patients with CF with serum retinol levels up to 110 µg/dL [38]. Although other researchers have noted the relationship of optimal serum vitamin A levels to lung function they have not reported a similar correlation with higher serum levels [39, 40]. Reduced serum retinol levels have been reported in pancreatic sufficient patients [21].

Serum retinol level should be evaluated in the fasting state and is effected by medications, fat malabsorption, liver disease, malnutrition, zinc deficiency, chronic infection, and decreased retinol binding protein [32]. The blood sample should be protected from bright light [41]. Vitamin A status assessed via serum retinol will identify deficiency, while serum retinyl esters as a function of total serum retinol may be more appropriate when concerned about retinol toxicity [30]. Roddy described using molar ratio of retinol to retinol binding protein when providing vitamin A to a deficient patient

Table 5.2 International vitamin and mineral recommendations for CF care[a]

Nutrient	USA-CFF 2002 [2] pediatric	European 2002 [3] All ages	UK CF trust 2002 [7] all ages	USA-CFF 2004 [4] adult	Australasian 2006 [6] all ages	USA CFF newborn 2009 [5] birth to 2 year
	Consensus	Consensus	Evidence and consensus	Consensus	Evidence	Evidence and consensus
Vitamin K mcg/day	300–500	PI and cholestasis 1 mg/day to 10 mg/week	10000	2.5–5 mg/week	0–36 month: 150–500 >4: 300–500	[b]
Vitamin E IU/day	0–12 month: 40–50; 1–3 year: 80–150; 4–8 year: 100–200; >8 year: 200–400	100–400	0–1 year: 10–50 mg; 1–10 years: 50–100 mg; >10 years: 100–200 mg	200–400 IU/day	0–12 month: 40–80; 1–3 year: 50–150; 4–7 year: 150–300; >8 years: 150–500	[b]
Vitamin A IU/day	0–12 month: 1500; 1–3 year: 5000; 4–8 year: 5000–10,000; >8 year: 10,000	PI; 4000–10,000	<1 year: 4000; <1 year: 4000–10,000	10,000	0–12 month: 1500–2000; 1–3 year: 1500–2500; 4-Adult: 2500-5000	[b]
Water Soluble	NI	Supplement if dietary intake is inadequate	NI	NI	Supplement if dietary intake is inadequate or with terminal ileum resection	[b]
Sodium Per day	Infants: 1/8 tsp (12.6 mEq); Others: high salt diet	Infants: PRI: 23–46 mg/kg daily; Breast-fed:supplement with fever or summer mo	Infants: 1–2 mmol/kg/day if urine Na <10; >2 year: additional requirement in warm climates	NI	Infants: 500–1000 mg/day; Children: 4000 mg; >12 year: 6000 mg	0–6 mo: 1/8 tsp/day (12.6 mEq); >6 month: 1/4 t/day (25.2 mEq)
Iron	As indicated	As indicated	NI	As indicated especially women	As indicated	NI
Zinc	Consider for poor growth or refractory vitamin A deficiency. 6 month. zinc trial	Consider with poor growth or severe steatorrhea	NI	If indicated	ND	Consider for inadequate growth despite PERT and sufficient calories. 1 mg/kg/day, 6 month zinc trial.
Calcium	Minimum: 1997 IOM recommendations	Supplement if deficient	NI	NI	Recommended daily intake or 1500 mg/day with low bone density	NI

Abbreviations: *PI* pancreatic insufficient, *PRI* population reference intake, *tsp* teaspoon, *IOM* institute of medicine, *NI* not included in recommendations

[a]Adapted from Table 5.1, reference [31]

[b]Start CF-specific multivitamins shortly after diagnosis

Table 5.3 Retinol activity equivalent (RAE) content of CF-specific vitamins[a]

	MVWComplete formulation µg RAE	AquADEKs µg RAE	Vitamax µg RAE	Choiceful µg RAE	Libertas µg RAE
Liquid	984/0.5 ml	911/1 ml	1744/1 ml	NA	2545/1 ml
Chewable	2464/1	2470/2	1100/1[b]	2002/1	1600/1
Softgels	4928/2	4940/2	NA	4312/2	4928/2

See Table 5.1 for retinol and beta-carotene content of each product
• Beta-carotene IU×0.10
• Retinyl palmitate IU×0.55
• Retinol acetate IU×0.34
[a]Conversion factors from reference [43]
[b]Retinol acetate all others retinyl palmitate

[15]. In a patient with liver disease better serum retinol level was achieved in response to a higher retinol product [15]. Patients refractory to vitamin A supplementation may require zinc supplements [32]. Vitamin A is an acute phase reactant, therefore serum levels should not be checked during a pulmonary exacerbation. CRP and IgG are used to identify inflammation [42]. Providing vitamin A supplementation based on individualized needs, which reflect evaluation of serum levels, is integral to avoid deficiency and toxicity [42].

Development of CF-specific multivitamins has aided in the reduction of vitamin A deficiency. Vitamin A content of the early products was predominantly retinol, while later products contain a combination of retinol and beta-carotene [16]. Table 5.3 provides the retinol activity equivalents (RAE) of currently available CF-specific multivitamins using conversion factors found in reference 43. In a series of studies on similar CF patients and using similar methods, changes in vitamin A intake from food and supplements and serum retinol levels were noted [16, 43, 44]. When compared to the DRI and NHANES, retinol intake and serum levels were found to be greater than recommended, yet lower than suggested by Rivas-Crespo [16, 38, 43, 44]. Serum retinol was lower, and the increase in the number of subjects with low serum levels in the Bertolas study may reflect the increase in beta-carotene content of CF-specific vitamins [16].

Vitamin A deficiency or excess are teratogenic and associated with adverse reproductive outcomes [45]. Increased serum retinol levels have been reported in patients, CF and non-CF, post-lung transplant [46]. The reader is referred to the chapters on pregnancy and on transplant for greater detail.

Vitamin E

Vitamin E is essential for normal development, cell membrane stability, and prevention of hemolysis. It is an antioxidant. Overt symptoms of vitamin E deficiency presenting as peripheral neuropathy or cerebellar ataxia were seen prior to the use of enteric-coated enzymes and routine vitamin supplementation [8, 47–49]. Neurological symptoms of vitamin E deficiency are seen less frequently today but case reports can still be found [50, 51]. Low plasma vitamin E levels were reported in patients taking multivitamins not formulated for person who have CF [52, 53]. In a study of 69 children who had CF, Huang found that following current standards of care resulted in normal to high levels of vitamin E [54]. Little evidence is available describing the impact of polyunsaturated fatty acids on serum tocopherol levels of persons who have CF [55–57]. Liver disease, short bowel syndrome, failure to thrive, and bacterial overgrowth may result in vitamin E deficiency.

Evaluation of serum vitamin E in infants diagnosed through newborn screening revealed vitamin E deficiency that was corrected in the majority of infants with use of CF-specific multivitamins containing vitamin E along with the use of PERT [39, 49]. During a ten-year follow-up in one study 11.8% of the subjects were found to be deficient in vitamin E while in another study vitamin E deficiency was corrected in all infants [25, 39]. Correcting vitamin E deficiency early in infancy is critical to prevent detrimental effect of prolonged deficiency on cognitive function [58].

Varying results have been reported describing the impact of vitamin E on lung function [22, 39, 59]. Limited reports describe hemorrhagic effects of excessive vitamin E (1000 IU or more daily) supplementation on PIVKA [60]. Individuals deficient in vitamin K may be at increased risk of coagulation defects with excessive supplementation with vitamin E [61]. Vitamin E may demonstrate a dual role in relationship to bone health, that is at appropriate doses beneficial but at excessive doses may be harmful [62].

Increased serum vitamin E levels have been reported in patients, CF and non-CF, post-lung transplant [46]. Please see the transplant chapter for additional information. Vitamin E deficiency has been found in pancreatic sufficient persons who have CF [21].

The efficacy of various forms of vitamin E has been evaluated [63–67]. One study described vitamin E absorption with the use of d-alpha-tocopherol polyethylene glycol 1000 succinate (TPGS) [67]. When taken with PERT, the fat-soluble form of vitamin E is equally well absorbed as the water-soluble form [63, 65]. In a series of studies with the same subjects, using similar methods little change was seen in vitamin E status, with 13% of the subjects deficient [16].

Since vitamin E is transported throughout the body with serum lipids, serum vitamin E levels are dependent on serum lipid levels. Clinically, vitamin E serum levels may be assessed using either of the two calculations based on serum levels: serum/plasma concentration as a ratio to total cholesterol or as a ratio to total lipids (cholesterol, triglycerides, and phospholipids combined) [54, 68]. Although total lipids commonly are not available, some researchers prefer to use it to assess vitamin E (α-tocopherol) status in patients who have CF, others believe that the vitamin E:cholesterol is appropriate [54, 69]. A patient is considered vitamin E deficient when: vitamin E:total lipids is less than 0.8 mg/dL or vitamin E:cholesterol is less than 2.47 mg/g [54]. James suggested a vitamin E:cholesterol ratio of less than 5.4 mg/g is deficient in those who have CF [70]. Vitamin E evaluation is performed fasting and the tube of blood should be protected from light [41].

Vitamin K

Vitamin K was first identified in 1929 and its role in coagulation was quickly defined [71]. It wasn't until the late seventies that the relationship of vitamin K to bone health was reported [72]. Individuals who have CF are at risk for vitamin K deficiency due to maldigestion and resultant malabsorption, bile salt deficiency, liver disease, bowel resection, bacterial overgrowth, chronic antibiotic use, diet low in vitamin K, insufficient PERT, and/or lack of suitable vitamin K supplementation [73]. Excessive vitamins A and E may antagonize vitamin K absorption or function [60, 74].

Vitamin K refers to similar fat-soluble compounds, with different chemical structures, sources, and biologic actions including blood clotting and bone metabolism. Phytonadione (Vitamin K_1) commonly is found in plants, especially dark green leafy vegetables and is commercially manufactured for supplemental use. The menaquinones (vitamin K_2) are synthesized by obligate anaerobic bacteria in the ileum and colon.

In the 1960s Shwachman and Di Sant'Agnese reported vitamin K deficiency and resultant bleeding was so frequently seen in CF that it could be an early sign of CF [75, 76]. Reports of severe life-threatening bleeding were frequently reported in the literature [77, 78]. Case reports of diagnosis based on severe bleeding or cerebral hemorrhage continue to be found in the literature [79–81]. Sokal did not find increased PIVKA in infants identified through newborn screening, perhaps reflecting prophylactic vitamin K provided by injection versus oral dose [23, 80]. Lack of normalization of vitamin K by oral doses may reflect malabsorption of the vitamin prior to diagnosis of CF [80].

Although overt symptoms of vitamin K deficiency may no longer be seen following diagnosis, using more sensitive markers of vitamin K nutrition, reports of deficiency continue to be published [82]. Elevated PIVKA and suboptimal bone health related to vitamin K deficiency has been reported in persons who have CF [83–86]. Liver disease and frequent or chronic antibiotic use will influence vitamin K status [41].

Vitamin K nutritional status is difficult to determine clinically since there is no single index or biomarker indicative of adequacy versus deficiency [87]. Plasma concentrations of phylloquinone reflect intake during the previous 24 h. Customary laboratory tests such as for prothrombin/international normalized ratio (PT/INR) reflect blood clotting times, rather than actual vitamin K status and is insensitive to mild deficiency. Only 50% of the normal prothrombin concentration is necessary for normal test results [84]. PIVKA or DCP (protein induced in vitamin K absence or des-gamma-carboxy prothrombin) and undercarboxylated OC (osteocalcin) are more specific and sensitive markers of vitamin K deficiency when compared to prothrombin concentration [87]. PIVKA and gamma-carboxy prothrombin are more widely available than they were some years ago.

Little evidence is available to guide vitamin K treatment in CF [83, 88–92]. Recommended doses of vitamin K from international CF societies range from 0.5 mg daily to 10 mg weekly, including one recommendation of 10 mg daily, see Table 5.2 [2–4, 6, 7]. At one point the need for supplemental vitamin K in healthy persons with CF was questioned [93]. Daily versus weekly supplementation may be more effective [88, 94]. There are no reports of toxicity from intakes of excessive amounts of vitamin K1 or K2 [95]. Based on currently available evidence vitamin K supplementation is necessary for all persons who have CF.

Water-Soluble Vitamins

There are no specific intake recommendations for water-soluble vitamins in CF. This may reflect the assumption that persons who have CF and consume a balanced diet do not develop overt symptoms of deficiencies [11, 96]. Deficiencies may be related to inappropriate diet, acute illness, liver or renal disease, or medications. McCabe reported riboflavin deficiency in three patients who presented with angular stomatitis. All of the children were ill and required supplementation [97]. Deficiencies of vitamin B_{12} and folic acid were reported in persons who have CF presenting with peripheral neuropathy [51]. Preliminary work with CF patients receiving 5-methyltetrahydrofolate (the active form of folic acid) and vitamin B_{12} demonstrated improved inflammatory response [98]. Plasma ascorbic acid decreases with age, the explanation for this is unclear [99]. CF-specific vitamins contain a full complement of the water-soluble vitamins. Thus, in general, overt symptoms of deficiencies are prevented. However, research describing the more subtle role of the water-soluble vitamins and CF is needed.

Minerals: Sodium Chloride, Calcium, and Magnesium

Sodium Chloride

Sodium chloride is central to both the diagnosis and to the care of persons who have CF. Genotype may influence sodium chloride losses through the skin, although at this time there are no recommendations to adjust dietary salt intake based on sweat test results [100–102]. There are many reports of hypoelectrolytemia in infants and older patients who are not supplemented with salt or insufficient salt

[101–105]. Infants who have CF need supplemental salt as human milk and infant formulas do not contain sufficient sodium chloride to meet needs. When salt was removed from commercially available infant foods some infants with CF experienced electrolyte depletion [103]. Without added dietary salt, persons who have CF are at risk of electrolyte abnormalities and compromised growth [106, 107]. Patients who, in addition to CF, have an ileostomy require additional salt [107].

Assessing sodium status is challenging and a patient may develop symptoms of sodium chloride depletion (decreased appetite, nausea, vomiting, muscle cramps, fatigue, poor concentration, headaches, poor growth) prior to the development of decreased plasma or urine sodium levels [105, 108]. Urine sodium to creatinine may be a more informative measure of sodium nutrition for infants [108].

Persons who have CF may be at risk for electrolyte abnormalities during excessive sweating, which may blunt the trigger to drink and cause "voluntary dehydration" [104, 106]. Extra care is needed to consume optimal sodium chloride when exercising [104]. United States' CFF salt recommendations for infants are: 1/8 teaspoon of table salt for the stable, growing infant from birth to 6 months of age, increased to 1/4 teaspoon at 6 months of age [5]. To avoid complications of over or under dosing, parents need to demonstrate that they understand the recommendations. Older patients are encouraged to eat a high salt diet while those active in warm environments should add 0.125 (1/8) teaspoon of salt to every 12 oz of sports drink to avoid voluntary dehydration [109]. International sodium recommendations for children, adolescents, and adults who have CF range from 1000 to 6000 mg daily and reflect usual versus extreme conditions. Extreme conditions include very high ambient temperature, excessive exercise, or illness with fever, vomiting, and/or diarrhea [6, 7].

Calcium

Although there are numerous papers describing bone health in persons who have CF, limited studies are available that specifically assess calcium needs. Calcium nutrition in CF is compromised by endogenous fecal and urinary losses; the specific mechanism is not clear and may be more complex than saponification with intestinal fat [110, 111]. Persons with CF using high doses of supplemental pancreatic enzymes are small for age, young, and use gastric acid inhibitors may have limited calcium availability for bone mineralization [112].

Optimizing calcium intake at times of greatest bone calcium deposition is paramount [111, 113–115]. Both US and European CFF recommend a minimum calcium intake as described by the Food and Nutrition Board [115, 116]. Optimal calcium intake may play a role in preventing kidney stones [117]. If a review of the usual diet reveals inadequate intake, calcium supplementation may be necessary. Calcium carbonate is best absorbed when taken with food. Calcium citrate and calcium maleate do not require food for optimal absorption.

Magnesium

Magnesium plays an important role in bone health and cardiorespiratory function. Persons who have CF may be at risk for magnesium deficiency due to inadequate intake, malabsorption, and drug/nutrient interaction [118]. Medications such as aminoglycosides and immunosuppressants used with transplant patients may interfere with magnesium nutrition [73]. Monitoring serum levels is difficult since only 1 % of the body's magnesium is found in the blood, yet necessary for patients on specific medications, or who have renal insufficiency, low bone mineral density, or CF-related diabetes [74, 119]. Magnesium supplementation has been shown to improve respiratory muscle strength in children and adolescents and to play an important role in the effectiveness of rhDNase therapy [120, 121].

Trace Minerals: Zinc, Iron, Selenium, Copper, Fluoride

Zinc

Zinc is involved in over 300 body functions including many related to pulmonary health, immunity, and growth [123]. Its role in health for the person who has cystic fibrosis is critical, especially for the lungs and pancreas [124]. Zinc absorption is influenced by the zinc content of the diet and fat malabsorption, thereby making persons who have CF at risk for zinc deficiency [26, 125]. Prior to initiation of PERT, infants who have CF are at risk for zinc deficiency due to malabsorption and endogenous losses [24, 126]. Case reports of acrodermatitis enteropathica-like rash due to zinc deficiency prior to diagnosis are described in the literature [127, 128]. In trials of zinc supplementation, subjects deficient in zinc demonstrated improved outcomes as seen by improved appetite, weight, and lung function [124, 129–132]. Plasma and serum zinc laboratory measures are not informative for marginal zinc levels. Results are influenced by inflammation, food intake, and time of day that the study sample is obtained [133]. Contamination from the skin at the time of phlebotomy or zinc in collection materials may result in an inaccurate result [133]. Careful evaluation of dietary zinc intake in addition to clinical assessment is important in making the diagnosis of zinc deficiency. Empiric zinc supplementation for 6 months is recommended for those with CF exhibiting growth failure, vitamin A deficiency, or night blindness refractory to vitamin A supplementation [2, 29]. Dose is based on the elemental content of the zinc compound. The various elemental zinc compounds of supplements and their elemental zinc content are: zinc sulfate 23%, zinc gluconate 14%, zinc acetate 30%, zinc oxide 80%.

Iron

Iron nutrition involves a complex system including: dietary intake, absorption, transport, storage, and excretion. In CF, iron status also may be impacted by increased losses in sputum and the GI tract, and the severity of suppurative lung disease [134, 135]. Iron may facilitate *pseudomonas aeruginosa* growth and iron loss through the airway may contribute to iron deficiency [134, 136]. The incidence of iron deficiency anemia ranges from 33% in children to 74% in adults who have CF and is associated with poorer lung function and vitamin deficiency [13, 137–139]. The progression of iron status from normal, through iron deficiency, to iron deficiency anemia usually is gradual and subtle. Assessing iron status and treating iron deficiency in persons who have CF is challenging [140–142]. Interpreting the laboratory results of each change can be formidable [138]. There are numerous laboratory methods to identify anemia. The tests usually obtained for annual assessment (hemoglobin, mean corpuscular volume, and hematocrit) can identify late stages of anemia. Ferritin, which can identify early and diminished iron stores, is an acute phase reactant and is not informative during periods of inflammation [138]. Soluble transferrin receptor levels has been recommended in addition to iron, transferrin, and ferritin levels, although in work by Uijterschout, hepcidin was more useful in identifying early deficient iron stores [74, 143]. Skikne has suggested the calculation of soluble transferrin receptor to log ferritin ratio as an accurate method of identifying true iron deficiency in CF [144].

Concern about iron supplementation and increased lung disease in persons who have CF has made treatment decisions challenging. Finding the optimal treatment route of delivery has yet to be identified [145]. Treating a group of CF patients identified with iron deficiency with low dose oral iron supplementation for six weeks did not change markers of iron deficiency, but did not cause worsening of lung disease [141]. Intravenous iron supplementation is another possible route for treating iron deficiency but may result in complications including allergic phenomenon [142, 145].

As noted by Hoo et al. there may be a risk of respiratory deterioration if oral iron supplementation is continued after the patient has become iron replete. Therefore careful identification of the truly iron deficient patient is necessary as is optimal repletion [140]. Preventing iron deficiency through optimal dietary intake may be the best option.

Selenium

Selenium is an antioxidant and vital for the proper functioning of the immune system and is a catalyst for the production of active thyroid hormone. It is required for sperm motility in males and may reduce the risk for miscarriage in females [147]. In CF there was a great deal of interest in selenium in the 1970s reflecting a veterinary pathologist's claim that selenium supplementation could cure CF. No evidence was found that confirmed his assertion [148]. One death was reported in a child with CF who was given selenium supplements [149]. Mislabeling and manufacturing of selenium and of vitamin supplements resulted in reports of selenium poisoning in the non-CF population [150]. Some research specific to selenium's role in CF was published in the 1980s–1990s. Those studies identified low serum levels in persons who have CF [27, 151, 152]. Supplementation with PERT resulted in increased plasma serum selenium and glutathione peroxidase activity [151]. The enzymes in PERT are obtained from animal pancreas and reflect selenium content of the animal's diet. In studies to improve antioxidant levels in persons who have CF, selenium supplementation alone was not effective [153]. However, when combined with other antioxidants improved serum selenium levels and improved $FEV_1\%$ were noted [154]. Reviews of the role of antioxidants, including selenium, concluded that selenium supplementation was not recommended [27, 28].

Copper

Copper plays a role in iron metabolism and antioxidant activity, yet little is known about copper metabolism in persons who have CF. Assessing copper status in humans is challenging since physiological stress raises serum copper laboratory values [155]. Few studies are available describing copper nutrition and CF. Percival found altered copper status in children and adult males who have CF and noted the results may reflect poor copper absorption, inadequate dietary intake, chronic inflammation, or defect in ion transport [156, 157]. Copper combined with or without zinc supplementation did not change serum copper levels suggesting moderate copper deficiency in CF may reflect abnormal copper metabolism [155]. Reduced copper enzyme activity was noted in patients who have CF, suggesting a functional deficiency not easily corrected by increased copper intake [155, 157].

Fluoride

Fluoride is critical for preventing dental caries. Vitamin supplements designed for persons who have CF do not contain fluoride. Due to the wide variation in the fluoride content of community drinking water infants, toddlers, and children who have CF are best referred to their primary care provider for individualized fluoride supplementation recommendation [5, 158].

Conclusion

Optimal vitamin and mineral nutrition is essential for overall health of persons who have CF. A diet varied in food intake contributes to overall nutrient intake. The use of vitamin and mineral supplements reflective of need identified through laboratory assessment avoids deficiencies or toxicities. Assessment of vitamin and mineral supplementation adherence along with PERT is crucial to care. Healthcare providers are encouraged to use available resources to educate families and persons who have CF about the importance of vitamin and mineral nutrition. Future research is necessary to inform healthcare providers regarding optimal form and dose of vitamins and minerals in CF.

References

1. Ramsey BW, Farrell PM, Pencharz P, The Consensus Committee. Nutritional assessment and management in cystic fibrosis: a consensus report. Am J Clin Nutr. 1992;55:108–16.
2. Borowitz D, Baker RD, Stallings V. Consensus report on nutrition for pediatric patients with cystic fibrosis. J Pediatr Gastroenterol Nutr. 2002;35:246–59.
3. Sinaasappel M, Stern M, Littlewood J, Wolfe S, Steinkamp G, Harry GM, Heijerman HGM, Robberecht E, Döring G. Nutrition in patients with cystic fibrosis: a European consensus. J Cyst Fibros. 2002;1:51–75.
4. Yankaskas JR, Marshall BC, Sufian B, Simon RH, Rodman D. Cystic fibrosis adult care: consensus conference report. Chest. 2004;125:1S–39.
5. Borowitz D, Robinson KA, Rosenfeld M, Davis SD, Sabadosa KA, Spear SL, Michel SH, Parad RB, White TB, Farrell PM, Marshall BC, Accurso FJ. Cystic fibrosis foundation evidence-based guidelines for management of infants with cystic fibrosis. J Pediatr. 2009;155:S73–93.
6. Australasian clinical practice guidelines for nutrition in cystic fibrosis. daa.asn.au/wp-content/uploads/2012/09/Guidelines_CF-Final.pdf. Accessed July 2014.
7. Nutritional management of cystic fibrosis. www.cysticfibrosis.org.uk/media/82052/nutritional-management-of-cystic-fibrosis-apr02.pdf. Accessed July 2014.
8. Farrell PM, Bieri JG, Fratononi JF, Wood RE, di Sant'Agnese PA. The occurrence and effects of human vitamin E deficiency-a study in patients with cystic fibrosis. J Clin Invest. 1977;60:233–41.
9. Palin D, Underwood BA, Denning CF. The effect of oral zinc supplementation on plasma levels of vitamin A and retinol-binding protein in cystic fibrosis. Am J Clin Nutr. 1979;32:1253–9.
10. Hubbard VS, Farrell PM, di Sant'Agnese PA. 25-Hydroxy cholecalciferol levels in patients with cystic fibrosis. J Pediatr. 1979;94:84–6.
11. Solomons NW, Wagonfield JB, Rieger C, Jacob RA, Bolt M, Horst JV, Rothberg R, Sandstead H. Some biochemical indices of nutrition in treated cystic fibrosis patients. Am J Clin Nutr. 1981;34:462–74.
12. Leung M, Bayliff CD, Patersn NA, Leggatt P. Night blindness secondary to vitamin A deficiency in a patient with cystic fibrosis and short gut syndrome. Can J Hosp Pharm. 2006;59(2):74–5.
13. Obeid M, Price J, Sun L, Scantlebury MH, Overby P, Sidhu R, et al. Facial palsy and idiopathic intracranial hypertension in twins with cystic fibrosis and hypovitaminosis A. Pediatr Neurol. 2011;44:150–2.
14. Rana M, Wong-See D, Katz T, Gaskin K, Whitehead B, Jaffe A, Coakley J, Lochhead A. Fat-soluble vitamin deficiency in children and adolescents with cystic fibrosis. J Clin Pathol. 2014;14(7):1–4. doi:10.1136/jclinpath-2013-201787.
15. Roddy MF, Greally P, Clancy G, Leen G, Feehan S, Elnazir B. Night blindness in a teenager with cystic fibrosis. Nutr Clin Pract. 2011;26:718–21.
16. Bertolaso C, Groleau V, Schall JI, Maqbool A, Mascarenhas M, Latham NE, Dougherty KA, Stallings VA. Fat-soluble vitamins in cystic fibrosis and pancreatic insufficiency: efficacy of a nutrition intervention. J Pediatr Gastroenterol Nutr. 2014;58(4):443–8.
17. Hollander FM, de Roos NM, Dopheide J, Hoekstra T, van Berkhout FT. Self-reported use of vitamins and other nutritional supplements in adult patients with cystic fibrosis. Is daily practice in concordance with recommendations? Int J Vitam Nutr Res. 2010;80(6):408–15.
18. Palmery M, Saraceno A, Vaiarelli A, Carlomagno G. Oral contraceptives and changes in nutritional requirements. Eur Rev Med Pharmacol Sci. 2013;17:1804–13.
19. Siwamogsatham O, Dong W, Binongo JN, Chowdhury R, Alvarez JA, Feinman SJ, Enders J, Tangpricha V. Relationship between fat-soluble vitamin supplementation and blood concentrations in adolescent and adult patients with cystic fibrosis. Nutr Clin Pract. 2014;29:491–7.

20. Wilson SMC, Bivins BN, Russell KA, Bailey LB. Oral contraceptive use: impact on folate, vitamin B6 and vitamin B12 status. Nutr Rev. 2011;69:572–83.
21. Lancellotti L, D'Orazio C, Mastella G, Mazzi G, Lippi U. Deficiency of vitamins E and A in cystic fibrosis is independent of pancreatic function and current enzyme and vitamin supplementation. Eur J Pediatr. 1996;155:281–5.
22. Hakim F, Kerem E, Rivlin J, Bentur L, Stankiewicz H, Bdolach-Abram T, Wilschanski M. Vitamins A and E and pulmonary exacerbations in patients with cystic fibrosis. J Pediatr Gastroenterol Nutr. 2007;45:347–53.
23. Sokol RJ, Reardon MC, Accurso FJ, Stall C, Narkewicz M, Abman SH, Hammond KB. Fat-soluble-vitamin status during the first year of life in infants with cystic fibrosis identified by screening of newborns. Am J Clin Nutr. 1989;50:1064–71.
24. Krebs NF, Sontag M, Accurso FJ, Hambidge KM. Low plasma zinc concentrations in young infants with cystic fibrosis. J Pediatr. 1998;133:761–4.
25. Feranchak AP, Sontag MK, Wagerer JS, Hammond KB, Accurso FJ, Sokol RJ. Prospective, long-term study of fat-soluble vitamin status in children with cystic fibrosis identified by newborn screen. J Pediatr. 1999;135:601–10.
26. Easley D, Krebs N, Jefferson M, Miller L, Erskine J, Accurso F, Hambidge KM. Effect of pancreatic enzymes on zinc absorption in cystic fibrosis. J Pediatr Gastroenterol Nutr. 1998;26:136–9.
27. Cantin AM, White TB, Cross CE, Forman HJ, Sokol RJ. Borowitz. Antioxidants in cystic fibrosis: conclusions from the CF antioxidant workshop, Bethesda, Maryland, November 11–12, 2003. Free Radic Biol Med. 2007;42:15–31.
28. Shamseer L, Adams D, Brown N, Johnson JA, Vohra S. Antioxidant micronutrients for lung disease in cystic fibrosis. Cochrane Database Syst Rev. 2010;12, CD007020.
29. Tinley CG, Withers NJ, Sheldon CD, Quinn AG, Jackson AA. Zinc therapy for night blindness in cystic fibrosis. J Cyst Fibros. 2008;7:333–335.

Vitamin A

30. James DR, Owen G, Campbell IA, Goodchild MC. Vitamin A absorption in cystic fibrosis: risk of hypervitaminosis A. Gut. 1992;33:707–10.
31. Maqbool A, Dougherty K, Rovner AJ, Michel S, Stallings VA. Nutrition. In: Allen JL, Panitch HB, Rubenstein RC, editors. Nutrition. New York: Informa healthcare; 2010. p. 308–27.
32. Institute of Medicine. Dietary reference intakes for vitamin A, vitamin K, arsenic, boron, chromium, copper, iodine, iron, manganese, molybdenum, nickel, silicon, vanadium and zinc. Washington: National Academy Press, 2001. p 82–161.
33. Michaëlsson K, Lithell H, Vessby B, Melhus H. Serum retinol levels and the risk of fracture. N Engl J Med. 2003;348:287–94.
34. Huet F, Semama DM, Maingueneau C, Charavel A, Nivelon JL. Vitamin A deficiency and nocturnal vision in teenagers with cystic fibrosis. Eur J Pediatr. 1997;156:949–51.
35. Schupp C, Olano-Martin E, Gerth C, Morrissey BM, Cross CE, Werner JS. Lutein, zeazanthin, macular pigment, and visual function in adult cystic fibrosis patients. Am J Clin Nutr. 2004;79:1045–52.
36. Greer RM, Buntain HM, Lewindon PJ, Wainwright CE, Potter JM, Wong JC, Francis PW, Batch JA, Bell SC. Vitamin A levels in patients with CF are influenced by the inflammatory response. J Cyst Fibros. 2004;3:143–9.
37. Aird FK, Greene SA, Ogston SA, Macdonald TM, Mukhopadhyay S. Vitamin A and lung function in CF. J Cyst Fibros. 2006;5:129–31.
38. Rivas-Crespo MR, Jiménez DG, Acuña Quirós MD, Aguirre AS, González SH, Martin JJD, Otero JMG, Almarza AL, Bousoño-Garcia C. High serum retinol and lung function in young patient with cystic fibrosis. J Pediatr Gastroenterol Nutr. 2013;56(6):657–62.
39. Bines JE, Truby HD, Armstrong DS, Carzino R, Grimwood K. Vitamin A and E deficiency and lung disease in infants with cystic fibrosis. J Paediatr Child Health. 2005;41:663–8.
40. Bonifant CM, Shevill E, Chang AB. Vitamin A supplementation for cystic fibrosis. Cochrane Database Syst Rev. 2014;(5): CD006751.
41. Krause's food & the nutrition care process. 13th ed. In: Mahan LK, Escott-Stump S, Raymond JL, editors. Elsevier Saunders, St Louis, Missouri, 2012. p 1089–94.
42. Brei C, Simon A, Krawinkel MB, Naehrlich L. Individualized vitamin A supplementation for patients with cystic fibrosis. Clin Nutr. 2013;32:805–10.
43. Graham-Maar RC, Schall JI, Stettler N, Zemel BS, Stallings VA. Elevated vitamin A intake and serum retinol in preadolescent children with cystic fibrosis. Am J Clin Nutr. 2006;84:174–82.
44. Maqbool A, Graham-Maar RC, Schall JI, Zemel BS, Stallings VA. Vitamin A intake and elevated serum retinol levels in children and young adults with cystic fibrosis. J Cyst Fibros. 2008;7:137–41.

45. World Health Organization. Vitamin A dosage during pregnancy and lactation: recommendations and report of a consultation. 1998. Document NUT/98.4.
46. Ho T, Gupta S, Brotherwood M, Robert R, Cortes D, Verjee Z, Tullis E, Keshavjee S, Chaparro C, Stephenson A. Increased vitamin A and E levels after lung transplant. Transplantation. 2011;92:601–6.

Vitamin E

47. Farrell PM, Mischler EH, Gutcher G. Evaluation of vitamin E deficiency in children with lung disease. Ann N Y Acad Sci. 1982;393:96–106.
48. Cynamon HA, Milov DE, Valenstein E, Wagner M. Effect of vitamin E deficiency on neurologic function in patients with cystic fibrosis. J Pediatr. 1988;113:637–40.
49. Sokol RJ, Butler-Simon N, Heubi JE, Iannaccone ST, McClung HJ, Accurso F, Hammond K, Heyman M, Sinatra F, Riely C, Perrault J, Levy J, Siverman A. Vitamin E deficiency neuropathy in children with fat malabsorption. Studies in cystic fibrosis and chronic cholestasis. Ann N Y Acad Sci. 1989;570:156–69.
50. Sitrin MD, Lieberman F, Jensen WE, Noronha A, Milburn C, Addington W. Vitamin E deficiency and neurologic disease in adults with cystic fibrosis. Ann Intern Med. 1987;107:51–4.
51. Chakrabarty B, Kabra SK, Gulati S, Toteja GS, Lodha R, Kabra M, Pandey RM, Srivastava A. Peripheral neuropathy in cystic fibrosis: a prevalence study. J Cyst Fibros. 2013;12:754–60.
52. Kelleher J, Miller MG, Littlewood JM, McDonald AM, Losowsky MS. The clinical effect of correction of vitamin E depletion in cystic fibrosis. Int J Vitam Nutr Res. 1987;57:253–9.
53. Leonard DH, Roos-Wilson C, Smyth AR, Polnay J, Range SP, Knowx AJ. A study of a single high potency multivitamin preparation in the management of cystic fibrosis. J Hum Nutr Diet. 1998;11:490–500.
54. Huang SH, Schall JI, Zemel BS, Stallings VA. Vitamin E status in children with cystic fibrosis and pancreatic insufficiency. J Pediatr. 2006;148:556–9.
55. Van Biervliet S, Vanbillemont G, Van Biervliet JP, Declercq D, Robberecht E, Christophe A. Relation between fatty acid composition and clinical status or genotype in cystic fibrosis patients. Ann Nutr Metab. 2007;51:541–9.
56. Van Biervliet BS, Devos M, Delhaye T, Van Biervliet JP, Robberecht E, Christophe A. Oral DHA supplementation in delta F508 homozygous cystic fibrosis patients. Prostaglandins Leukot Essent Fatty Acids. 2008;78:109–15.
57. Wood LG, Gitzgerald DA, Garg ML. Hypothesis: vitamin E complements polyunsaturated fatty acids in essential fatty acid deficiency in cystic fibrosis. J Am Coll Nutr. 2003;22:253–7.
58. Kosick RL, Lai HC, Laxova A, Zaremba KM, Losorok MR, Douglas JA, Rock MJ, Splaingard ML, Farrell PM. Preventing early, prolonged vitamin E deficiency: an opportunity for better cognitive outcomes via early diagnosis through neonatal screening. J Pediatr. 2005;147:S51–6.
59. Oudshoorn JH, Klijn PH, Hofman Z, Voorbji HA, van der Ent CK, Berger R, Houwen RH. Dietary supplementation with multiple micronutrients: no beneficial effects in pediatric cystic fibrosis patients. J Cyst Fibros. 2007;6:35–40.
60. Booth SL, Golly I, Sacheck JM, Roubenoff R, Dallal GE, Hamada K, Blumberg JB. Effect of vitamin E supplementation on vitamin K status in adults with normal coagulation status. Am J Clin Nutr. 2004;80(1):143–8.
61. Institute of Medicine. Dietary reference intakes for vitamin C, vitamin E, selenium, and carotenoids. Washington: National Academy Press; 2000.
62. Chin KY, Ima-Nirwana S. The effects of alpha-tocopherol on bone: a double-edged sword? Nutrients. 2014;6: 1424–41.
63. Nasir SZ, O'Leary H, Hillermeier C. Correction of vitamin E deficiency with fat-soluble versus water-miscible preparations of vitamin E in patients with cystic fibrosis. J Pediatr. 1993;122:810–2.
64. Winklhofer-Roob BM, van't Hof MA, Shmerling DH. Long-term oral vitamin E supplementation in cystic fibrosis patients: RRR-alpha-tocopherol compared with all-rac-alpha-tocopheryl acetate preparations. Am J Clin Nutr. 1996;63(5):722–8.
65. Soltani-Frisk S, Gronowitz E, Andersson H, Strandvik B. Water-miscible tocopherol is not superior to fat-soluble preparation for vitamin E absorption in cystic fibrosis. Acta Paediatr. 2001;90(10):1112–5.
66. Back EI, Frindt C, Ocenaskova E, Nohr D, Stern M, Biesalski HK. Can changes in hydrophobicity increase the bioavailability of alpha-tocopherol? Eur J Nutr. 2006;45:1–6.
67. Papas K, Kalbfleisch J, Mohon R. Bioavailability of a novel, water-soluble vitamin E formulation in malabsorbing patients. Dig Dis Sci. 2007;52:347–52.
68. Sokol RJ, Heubi JE, Iannaccone ST, Bove KE, Balistreri WF. Vitamin E deficiency with normal serum vitamin E concentrations in children with chronic cholestasis. N Engl J Med. 1984;310:1209–12.
69. Sokol R. Selection bias and vitamin E status in cystic fibrosis. J Pediatr. 2007;150(5):e85–6.
70. James DR, Alfaham M, Goodchild MC. Increased susceptibility to peroxide-induced haemolysis with normal vitamin E concentrations in cystic fibrosis. Clin Chim Acta. 1991;204:279–90.

Vitamin K

71. Dam H. The antihaemorrhagic vitamin of the chick. Biochemistry. 1935;29:1273–85.
72. Nelsestuen GL, Zytkovica TH, Howard JB. The mode of action of vitamin K. Identification of gamma-carboxyglutamic acid as a component of protrombin. J Biol Chem. 1974;249:6347–50.
73. Michel SH, Maqbool A, Hanna MD, Mascarenhas M. Nutrition management of pediatric patients who have cystic fibrosis. Pediatr Clin N Am. 2009;56:1123–41.
74. Alexander G, Suttie J. The effects of vitamin E on vitamin K activity. FASEB J. 1999;13:A535.
75. Shwachman H. Therapy of cystic fibrosis of the pancreas. Pediatrics. 1960;25:155–63.
76. Di Sant'Agnese P, Vidaurreta A. Cystic fibrosis of the pancreas. J Am Med Assoc. 1960;172:2065–72.
77. Torstenson OL, Humphrey GB, Edson JR, Warwick WJ. Cystic fibrosis presenting with severe hemorrhage due to vitamin K malabsorption: a report of 3 cases. Pediatrics. 1970;45:857–61.
78. Walters TR, Koch HF. Haemorrhagic diathesis and cystic fibrosis in infancy. Am J Dis Child. 1972;124:641–2.
79. Hamid B, Khan A. Cerebral hemorrhage as the initial manifestation of cystic fibrosis. J Child Neurol. 2007;22:114–5.
80. Verghese T, Beverley D. Vitamin K deficient bleeding in cystic fibrosis. Arch Dis Child. 2003;88:553–5.
81. Ngo B, Van Pelt K, Labarque V, Van De Casseye W, Penders J. Late vitamin K deficiency bleeding leading to a diagnosis of cystic fibrosis: a case report. Acta Clin Belg. 2011;66(2):142–3.
82. Rashid M, Durie P, Andrew M, Kalnins D, Shin J, Corey M, Tullis E, Pencharz PB. Prevalence of vitamin K deficiency in cystic fibrosis. Am J Clin Nutr. 1999;70:378–82.
83. Beker LT, Ahrens RA, Fink RJ, O'Brien ME, Davidson KW, Sokoll LJ, Sadowski JA. Effect of vitamin K1 supplementation on vitamin K status in cystic fibrosis patients. J Pediatr Gastroenterol Nutr. 1997;24:512–7.
84. Conway SP, Wolfe SP, Brownlee KG, White H, Oldroyd B, Truscott JG, Harvey JM, Shearer MJ. Vitamin K status among children with cystic fibrosis and its relationship to bone mineral density and bone turnover. Pediatrics. 2005;115:1325–31.
85. Nicolaidou P, Stavrinadis I, Loukou I, Papadopoulou A, Georgouli H, Douros K, Priftis KN, Gourgiotis D, Matsinos YG, Doudounakis S. The effect of vitamin K supplementation on biochemical markers of bone formation in children and adolescents with cystic fibrosis. Eur J Pediatr. 2006;165:540–5.
86. Fewtrell MS, Benden C, Williams JE, Chomtho S, Ginty F, Nigdikar SV, Jaffe A. Undercarboxylated osteocalcin and bone mass in 8–12 year old children with cystic fibrosis. J Cyst Fibros. 2008;7:307–12.
87. Mosler K, von Kries R, Vermeer C, Saupe J, Schmitz T, Schoster A. Assessment of vitamin K deficiency in CF-how much sophistication is useful? J Cyst Fibros. 2003;2:91–6.
88. Wilson DC, Rashid M, Durie PR, Tsang A, Kalnins D, Andrew M, Corey M, Shin J, Tullis E, Pencharz PB. Treatment of vitamin K deficiency in cystic fibrosis: effectiveness of a daily fat-soluble vitamin combination. J Pediatr. 2001;138:851–5.
89. van Hoorn JH, Hendriks JJ, Vermeer C, Forgot PP. Vitamin K supplementation in cystic fibrosis. Arch Dis Child. 2003;88:974–5.
90. Drury D, Grey VL, Ferland G, Gunberg C, Lands LC. Efficacy of high dose phylloquinone in correcting vitamin K deficiency in cystic fibrosis. J Cyst Fibros. 2008;7:457–9.
91. Dougherty KA, Schall JI, Stallings VA. Suboptimal vitamin K status despite supplementation in children and young adults with cystic fibrosis. Am J Clin Nutr. 2010;92:660–7.
92. Jagannath VA, Fedorowicz Z, Thaker V, Chang AB. Vitamin K supplementation for cystic fibrosis (Review). Cochrane Database Syst Rev. 2013;(4). CD008482.
93. Durie PR. Vitamin K, and the management of patients with cystic fibrosis. Can Med Assoc J. 1994;151:933–6.
94. Olsen RE. Vitamin K. In: Shils ME, Olson JA, Shike M, editors. Modern nutrition in health and disease. 8th ed. Baltimore: Williams and Wilkins; 1994. p. 343–58.
95. Food and Nutrition Board, Institute of Medicine. Dietary reference intakes for vitamin A, vitamin K, arsenic, boron, chromium, copper, iodine, iron, manganese, molybdenum, nickel, silicon, vanadium and zinc. Washington: National Academy Press, 2001. p. 162–96.

Water-Soluble Vitamins

96. Carr SB, McBratney J. The role of vitamins in cystic fibrosis. J R Soc Med. 2000;93 Suppl 38:14–9.
97. McCabe H. Riboflavin deficiency in cystic fibrosis: three case reports. J Hum Nutr Diet. 2001;14:365–70.

98. Scambi C, DeFranceschi L, Gurini P, Poli F, Siciliano A, Pattini P, et al. Preliminary evidence for cell membrane amelioration in children with cystic fibrosis by 5-MTHF and vitamin B12 supplementation: a single arm trial. PLoS One. 2009;4, e4782.
99. Back EL, Frindt C, Nohr D, Frank J, Ziebach R, Stern M, Ranke M, Biesalski HK. Antioxidant deficiency in cystic fibrosis: when is the right time to take action. Am J Clin Nutr. 2004;80:374–84.

Sodium chloride

100. Leoni GB. A specific cystic fibrosis mutation (T3381) associated with phenotype of isolated hypotonic dehydration. J Pediatr. 1995;127:281–3.
101. Fustik S, Pop-Jordanova N, Slaveska N, Koceva S, Efremov G. Metabolic alkalosis with hypoelectrolytemia in infants with cystic fibrosis. Pediatr Int. 2002;44:289–92.
102. Yalcin E. Clinical features and treatment approaches in cystic fibrosis with pseudo-Bartter syndrome. Ann Trop Paediatr. 2005;25:119–24.
103. Laughlin JJ, Brady MS, Eigen H. Changing feeding trends as a cause of electrolyte depletion in infants with cystic fibrosis. Pediatrics. 1981;68:203–7.
104. Bar-Or O, Blimkie CJR. Voluntary dehydration and heat intolerance in cystic fibrosis. Lancet. 1992;339:696–9.
105. Scurati-Manzoni E, Fossali EF, Agostoni C, Riva E, Simonetti GD, Zanolari-Calderari M, Bianchetti MG, Lava SA. Electrolyte abnormalities in cystic fibrosis: systematic review of the literature. Pediatr Nephrol. 2014;29:1015–23.
106. Orenstein DM, Henke KG, Costill DL, Doershuk CF, Lemon PJ, Stern RC. Exercise and heat stress in cystic fibrosis patients. Pediatr Res. 1983;17:267–9.
107. Bower TR, Pringle KC, Soper RT. Sodium deficit causing decreased weight gain and metabolic acidosis in infants with ileostomy. J Pediatr Surg. 1988;23:567–72.
108. Coates AJ, Crofton PM, Marshall T. Evaluation of salt supplementation in CF infants. J Cyst Fibros. 2009;8:382–5.
109. Kriemler S, Wilk B, Schurer W, Wilson WM, Bar-Or O. Preventing voluntary dehydration in children with cystic fibrosis who exercise in the heat. Med Sci Sports Exerc. 1999;31:774–9.

Calcium

110. Schulze KJ, O'Brien KO, Germain-Lee EL, Baer DJ, Leonard AL, Rosenstein BJ. Efficiency of calcium absorption is not compromised in clinically stable prepubertal and pubertal girls with cystic fibrosis. Am J Clin Nutr. 2003;78:110–6.
111. Schulze KJ, O'Brien KO, Germain-Lee EL, Booth SL, Leonard AL, Rosenstein BJ. Calcium kinetics are altered in clinically stable girls with cystic fibrosis. J Clin Endocrinol Metab. 2004;89:3385–91.
112. Schulze KJ, O'Brien KO, Germain-Lee EL, Baer DJ, Leonard AL, Rosenstein BJ. Endogenous fecal losses of calcium compromise calcium balance in pancreatic-insufficient girls with cystic fibrosis. J Pediatr. 2003;143:765–71.
113. Schulze KJ, Cutchins C, Rosenstein BJ, Germain-Lee EL, Obrien KO. Calcium acquisition rates do not support age-appropriate gains I total body bone mineral content in prepuberty and late puberty in girls with cystic fibrosis. Osteoporos Int. 2006;17:731–40.
114. Hillman LS, Cassidy JT, Popescu MF, Hewett JE, Kyger J, Robertson JD. Percent true calcium absorption, mineral metabolism, and bone mineralization in children with cystic fibrosis: effect of supplementation with vitamin D and calcium. Pediatr Pulmonol. 2008;43:772–80.
115. Sermet-Gaudelus I, Bianchi ML, Garabédian M, Aris RM, Morton A, Hardin DS, Elkin SL, Compston JE, Conway SP, Castanet M, Wolfe S, Saworth CS. European cystic fibrosis bone mineralization guidelines. J Cyst Fibros. 2011;10 Suppl 10:16–23.
116. Aris RM, Merkel PA, Bachrach LK, Borowitz DS, Boyle MP, Elkin SL, Guise TA, Hardin DS, Haworth CS, Holick MF, Joseph PM, O'Biren K, Tullis E, Watts NB, White TB. Consensus statement: guide to bone health and disease in cystic fibrosis. J Clin Endocrinol Metab. 2005;90:1888–96.
117. Sorensen MD, Kahn AJ, Reiner AP, Tseng TY, Shikany JM, Wallace RB, Chi T, Wactawski-Wend J, Jackson RD, O'Sullivan MJ, Sadetshy N, Stoller ML, WHI Working Group. Impact of nutritional factors on incident kidney stone formation: a report from the WHI OS. J Urol. 2012;187:1645–49.

Magnesium

118. Hersh T, Siddiqui DA. Magnesium and the pancreas. Am J Clin Nutr. 1973;26:362–6.
119. Saris NEL, Mervaala E, Karppanen H, Khawaja JÁ, Lewenstam A. Magnesium: an update on physiological, clinical and analytical aspects. Clin Chim Acta. 2000;294:1–26.
120. Sanders NN, Franckx H, DeBoeck K, Haustraete J, DeSmedt SC, Demeester J. Role of magnesium in the failure of rhDNase therapy in patients with cystic fibrosis. Thorax. 2006;61:962–8.
121. Gontijo-Amaral C, Guimarães EV, Camargos P. Oral magnesium supplementation in children with cystic fibrosis improves clinical and functional variables: a double-blind, randomized, placebo-controlled crossover trial. Am J Clin Nutr. 2012;96:50–6.
122. Atsmon J, Dolev E. Drug-induced hypomagnesaemia: scope and management. Drug Saf. 2005;28:763–88.

Zinc

123. Prasad AS. Zinc deficiency in women, infants, and children. J Am Coll Nutr. 1996;15:113–20.
124. Damphousse V, Mailhot M, Berthiaume Y, Rabasa-Lhoret R, Mailhot G. Plasma zinc in adults with cystic fibrosis: correlations with clinical outcomes. J Trace Elem Med Biol. 2014;28:60–4.
125. Krebs NF. Overview of zinc absorption and excretion in the human gastrointestinal tract. J Nutr. 2000;130 Suppl 5:1374–7.
126. Krebs NF, Westcott JE, Arnold TD, Kluger BM, Accurso FJ, Miller LV, Hambidge KM. Abnormalities in zinc homeostasis in young infants with cystic fibrosis. Pediatr Res. 2000;48:256–61.
127. Crone J, Huber WD, Eichler I, Granditsch G. Acrodermatitis enteropathica-like eruption as the presenting sign of cystic fibrosis and review of the literature. Eur J Pediatr. 2002;161:475–8.
128. Bernstein ML, McCusker MM, Grant-Kels JM. Cutaneous manifestations of cystic fibrosis. Pediatr Dermatol. 2008;25:150–7.
129. Abdulhamid I, Beck FW, Millard S, Chen X, Prasad A. Effect of zinc supplementation on respiratory tract infections in children with cystic fibrosis. Pediatr Pulmonol. 2008;43:281–7.
130. Van Biervliet S, Van Biervliet JP, Robberecht E. Serum zinc in patients with cystic fibrosis at diagnosis and after one year of therapy. Biol Trace Elem Res. 2006;112:205–11.
131. Van Biervliet S, VandeVelde S, Van Biervliet JP, Robberecht E. The effect of zinc supplements in cystic fibrosis patients. Ann Nutr Metab. 2008;52:152–6.
132. Ataee P, Najafi M, Gharagozlou M, Aflatounian M, Khodadad A, Farahmand F, Motamed F, Fallahi GH, Kalantari N, Soheili H, Modarresi V, Sabbaghian M, Rezaei N. Effect of supplementary zinc on body mass index, pulmonary function and hospitalization in children with cystic fibrosis. Turk J Pediatr. 2014;56:127–32.
133. Krebs NF. Update on zinc deficiency and excess in clinical pediatric practice. Ann Nutr Metab. 2013;62 Suppl 1:19–29.

Iron

134. Reid DW, Withers NJ, Francis L, Wilson JW, Kotsimbos TC. Iron deficiency in CF: relationship to lung disease severity and chronic pseudomonas aeruginosa infection. Chest. 2002;121:48–54.
135. Reid DW, Lam QT, Schneider H, Walter EH. Airway iron and iron-regulatory cytokines in CF. Eur Respir J. 2004;24:286–91.
136. Uljterschout L, Nuijsink M, Hendriks D, Rimke V, Brus F. Iron deficiency occurs frequently in children with cystic fibrosis. Pediatr Pulmonol. 2013;136:458–462.
137. Von Drygalski A, Biller J. Anemia in CF: incidence, mechanisms, and association with pulmonary function and vitamin deficiency. Nutr Clin Pract. 2008;23:557–63.
138. Keevil B, Rowlands D, Burton I, Webb AK. Assessment of iron status in cystic fibrosis patients. Ann Clin Biochem. 2000;37(Pt 5):662–5.
139. Fischer R, Simmerlein R, Huber RM, Schiffl H, Lang SM. Lung disease severity, chronic inflammation, iron deficiency and erythropoietin response in adults with CF. Pediatr Pulmonol. 2007;42:1193–7.
140. Hoo ZH, Wildman MJ. Regarding the article entitled "Iron supplementation does not worsen respiratory health or alter the sputum microbiome in cystic fibrosis." J Cyst Fibros. 2014. doi:10.1016/j.jcf2014.06.002.

141. Gifford AH, Alexandru DM, Zhigang L, Dorman DB, Moulton LA, Price KE, Hampton TH, Sogin ML, Zuckerman JB, Parker HW, Stanton BA, O'Toole GA. Iron supplementation does not worsen respiratory health or alter the sputum microbiome in cystic fibrosis. J Cyst Fibros. 2014;13(30):311–8.
142. Hoo ZH, Wildman MJ. Intravenous iron among cystic fibrosis patients. J Cyst Fibros. 2012;11:560–2.
143. Uijterschout L, Swinkels DW, Akkermans MD, Zandstra T, Nuijsink M, Hendriks D, Hudig C, Tjalsma H, Vos R, van Goudoever JB, Brus F. The value of soluble transferrin receptor and hepcidin in the assessment of iron status in children with cystic fibrosis. J Cyst Fibros. 2014. doi:10.1016/j.jcf.2014.03.007.
144. Skikne BS, Punnonen K, Caldron PH, Bennett MT, Rehu M, Gasior GH, et al. Improved differential diagnosis of anemia of chronic disease and iron deficiency anemia: a prospective multicenter evaluation of soluble transferrin receptor and the sTfR/log ferritin index. Am J Hematol. 2011;86(11):923–7.
145. Smith DJ, Anderson GJ, Lamont IL, Mael P, Bell SC, Reid DW. Accurate assessment of systemic iron status in cystic fibrosis will avoid the hazards of inappropriate iron supplementation. J Cyst Fibros. 2013;12:303–4.
146. Khalid S, McGrowder D, Kemp M, Johnson P. The use of soluble transferrin receptor to assess iron deficiency in adults with cystic fibrosis. Clin Chim Acta. 2007;378:194–200.

Selenium

147. Rayman MP. The importance of selenium to human health. Lancet. 2000;356:233–41.
148. Hubbard VS, Barbero G, Chase HP. Selenium and cystic fibrosis. J Pediatr. 1980;96:421–2.
149. Snodgrass W, Rumack BH, Sullivan Jr JB, Peterson RG, Chase HP, Cotton EK, Sokol R. Selenium: childhood poisoning and cystic fibrosis. Clin Toxicol. 1981;18:211–20.
150. MacFarquhar JK, Broussard DL, Melstrom P, Hutchinson R, Wolkin A, Martin C, Burk RF, Dunn JR, Green AL, Hammond R, Schaffner W, Jones TF. Acute selenium toxicity associate a dietary supplement. Arch Intern Med. 2010;170:256–61.
151. Winklhofer-Roob BM, Tiran B, Tuchschmid PE, van't Hof MA, Shmerling DH. Effects of pancreatic enzyme preparations on erythrocyte glutathione peroxidase activities and plasma selenium concentrations in CF. Free Radical Biol Med. 1998;25:242–9.
152. Michalke B. Selenium speciation in human serum of cystic fibrosis patients compared to serum from healthy persons. J Chromatogr A. 2004;1058:203–8.
153. Portal B, Richard MJ, Coudray C, Arnaud J, Favier A. Effect of double-blind cross-over selenium supplementation on lipid peroxidation markers in cystic fibrosis patients. Clin Chim Acta. 1995;234:137–46.
154. Wood LG, Fitzgerald DA, Lee AK, Garg ML. Improved antioxidant and fatty acid status of patients with cystic fibrosis after antioxidant supplementation is linked to improved lung function. Am J Clin Nutr. 2003;77:150–9.

Copper

155. Best K, McCoy K, Gemma S, DiSilvestro RA. Copper enzyme activities in cystic fibrosis before and after copper supplementation plus or minus zinc. Metabolism. 2004;53:37–41.
156. Percival SS, Bowser E, Wagner M. Reduced copper enzyme activities in blood cells of children with cystic fibrosis. Am J Clin Nutr. 1995;62:633–8.
157. Percival SS, Kauwell GPA, Bower E, Wagner M. Altered copper status in adult men with cystic fibrosis. J Am Coll Nutr. 1999;18:614–9.

Fluoride

158. Clark MB, Slayton RL, Section on Oral Health. Fluoride use in caries prevention in the primary care setting. Pediatrics. 2014;134:626–33.

Chapter 6
Nutrition in Infancy

Evans Machogu and Tami Miller

Key Points

- Nutritional deficiencies are usually the earliest manifestations in the infant with cystic fibrosis with over 85% of infants being pancreatic insufficient.
- Left untreated or undertreated pancreatic insufficiency will lead to chronic malnutrition.
- A comprehensive, yet individualized nutrition plan for the infant newly diagnosed with CF requires a team approach and includes initiation of pancreatic enzymes (PERT), fat-soluble vitamins, salt supplementation as well as breast milk and/or infant formula and complementary foods
- Most pancreatic insufficient infants require up to 150% of the dietary reference values for age to maintain appropriate growth
- Gastrostomy tube placement should be considered early for children not gaining adequate weight in spite of adequate or suboptimal intake due to a suppressed appetite.
- The goals of management are to attain and maintain normal growth and development comparable to healthy infants and frequent assessments through the first 2 years of life are required to assure optimal growth.
- Nutritional status in cystic fibrosis has been associated with progression of pulmonary disease as well as survival.

Keywords Cystic fibrosis • Nutrition • Malnutrition • Failure to thrive • Pancreatic enzyme replacement therapy

E. Machogu, M.B.Ch.B., M.S.
Section of Pediatric Pulmonology, Allergy, and Sleep Medicine, Indiana University Health,
705 Riley Hospital Drive/ROC 4270, Indianapolis, IN 46202, USA
e-mail: emachogu@iupui.edu

T. Miller, R.D., C.S.P., C.D. (✉)
Cystic Fibrosis Program, Children's Hospital of Wisconsin, 9000 W. Wisconsin Ave.,
Milwaukee, WI 53201, USA
e-mail: tmiller@chw.org

E.H. Yen, A.R. Leonard (eds.), *Nutrition in Cystic Fibrosis: A Guide for Clinicians*, Nutrition and Health,
DOI 10.1007/978-3-319-16387-1_6, © Springer International Publishing Switzerland 2015

Abbreviations

BMI   Body mass index
CDC   Center for Disease Control and Prevention
CF   Cystic fibrosis
CFA   Coefficient of fat absorption
CFF   Cystic fibrosis foundation
CFTR   Cystic fibrosis transmembrane regulator
FEV_1 Forced expiratory volume in 1 second
g   Gram
kcal   Kilocalorie
kg   Kilogram
MI   Meconium ileus
mmol   Millimoles
PERT   Pancreatic enzyme replacement therapy
PI   Pancreatic insufficiency
PS   Pancreatic sufficient
WFA   Weight for age
WFL   Weight for length

Introduction

Nourishing the infant with cystic fibrosis (CF) through the first years of life is of utmost importance and requires a team approach to optimize the growth and overall health of the infant. A comprehensive, yet individualized nutrition plan for the infant newly diagnosed with CF often includes initiation of pancreatic enzymes (PERT), fat-soluble vitamins, salt supplementation as well as breast milk, infant formula, and complementary foods. The Cystic Fibrosis Foundation (CFF) evidenced-based guidelines for management of infants with CF provide a framework of recommendations to address the nutritional challenges in the early years of life. In addition to the medical and nutritional therapies, an understanding of the correlation of early nutritional status and long-term CF outcomes is essential for caregivers of the infant. This chapter will review many of these recommendations and expound on some practical strategies to enhance the nutritional care of the infant with CF.

Choice of Feeding Method

The CF Foundation recommends that human milk be used as the initial type of feeding for infants with CF. If infants are fed formula, standard infant formulas (as opposed to hydrolyzed protein formulas) should be used and calorie-dense feedings should be used if weight loss or inadequate weight gain is identified [1].

The benefits of human milk feeding for healthy infants are well recognized. Reduction in respiratory and diarrheal infections [2, 3], reduction in risk for sudden infant death syndrome [4], better neurodevelopment, prevention or delay of the occurrence of atopic dermatitis, cow milk allergy, and wheezing in early childhood [5, 6], enhanced maternal infant bonding, among others are well documented.

Despite the known benefits of breastfeeding, infants with CF are more likely to receive formula compared to breast milk [7, 8]. A 2004 survey of US accredited CF centers showed that, among respondents, only 49% ever received breast milk [9]. In a cohort of infants born and diagnosed through newborn screening in Wisconsin between 1994 and 2006, only 51% of them ever received breast milk [10], while the most recent study of infants in five US CF Centers reveals 72% received breast milk at birth; however, breast milk intake was reduced to 25% by 2 months of age and 13% by 5 months of age [11]. In comparison of infants born in the USA in 2011, 49% were breastfeeding at 6 months and 27% at 12 months [12].

Although breastfeeding should be encouraged for all infants with CF, parental choice should be considered, and all mothers should be supported in their decision to breastfeed or not. The diagnosis of CF often occurs during the first couple of weeks of life when breast feeding is becoming established. The stress of diagnosis and additional infant care requirements could contribute to a rapid decline in breast feeding in the infant with CF. Strategies to promote breast feeding include lactation support services, emotional support during the time of diagnosis, and encouragement to seek help for the caregivers of newly diagnosed infants with CF from extended family and friends.

Clinicians may be concerned with meeting the energy requirements of infants with CF who breastfeed. Few studies have compared growth between breast-fed and formula-fed infants. In the Wisconsin retrospective study, exclusive breastfeeding for <2 months did not compromise growth and was associated with fewer infections with Pseudomonas aeruginosa [10]. In another single-center study patients with a history of prolonged breastfeeding showed higher values of Forced Expiratory Volume in 1 second (FEV_1) and fewer infections in the first 3 years of life [7].

When formula feeding is used for infants with CF, cow milk-based formulas are recommended. In one study, with enzyme replacement in pancreatic insufficient patients, fat absorption was equivalent for both semi-elemental and non-elemental formulas [13]. In another prospective randomized study, growth velocity was similar in infants fed either a hydrolysate formula or a standard cow milk-based formula [14].

The use of fortified breast milk and high-calorie infant formulas is indicated when growth rates are not optimal. Fortified breast milk and formulas ranging from 22 to 30 cal/oz (73–100 cal/100 mL) can be used to promote catch-up weight gain, meet increased energy expenditure related to illness, and provide concentrated calories if the infant is only able to consume a limited volume of breast milk or formula. Calorie concentration can be achieved with the addition of powdered infant formula to standard formula or breast milk. Occasionally, modular products (Microlipid®, medium chain triglyceride oil) can be used to increase the calorie content of infant formula or breast milk, but the cost of these products and the lack of additional nutrients besides fat and calories usually limit their use.

Beginning at about 6 months, complementary foods should be introduced to the infant with CF. Higher calorie food choices should be emphasized particularly for infants with poor weight gain. Mixing infant cereal with breast milk or formula, the addition of fat to infant foods, and selecting food sources that contain higher amounts of calories are all strategies to maximize the calorie intake of solid foods and promote normal growth rates in the infant with CF. Dietitians can counsel caregivers on strategies to advance the texture and nutrient content of complementary foods as the infant progresses to table foods later in the first year of life (Table 6.1).

Assessment of Pancreatic Status and Initiation of PERT

As soon as a diagnosis of CF is suspected or proven, the need for supplemental pancreatic enzymes should also be determined. This is covered in Chapter 7 in more detail. Pancreatic insufficiency (PI) is diagnosed in up to 60% of infants with CF diagnosed through newborn screening

Table 6.1 Feeding guide for the infant/toddler with CF. Feeding guide for the infant/toddler with CF

Age of baby	Foods to offer	Special instructions
Birth to 6 months	• Breast milk or iron-fortified formula • 1/8 teaspoon salt per day	• Provide lactation support to optimize the success of breast feeding (as indicated) • Fortified breast milk and/or calorie-dense formula to maximize growth rates (as indicated) • Cow milk-based formula is recommended for infants with CF. Modify type of formula to meet individual needs of the infant • The American Academy of Pediatrics recommends delaying solid foods until 6 months of age
6–8 months	• Breast milk or iron-fortified formula • Single-grain infant cereal • High-calorie strained fruits and vegetables • Strained meats • ¼ teaspoon salt per day	• Spoon feed cereal mixed with breast milk or formula • Strained foods can be given in any order • Select foods with the most calories (sweet potatoes and bananas) most often • Add ½ teaspoon melted butter, margarine, or oil to 2 oz. (60 gm) strained foods when extra calories are needed • Offer foods 1–3 times a day; increase as the baby gets older • Feed the baby in an infant seat or high chair

8–10 months	• Breast milk or iron-fortified formula
	• Multigrain infant cereals
	• Mashed avocado
	• Combination foods
	• Whole milk yogurt, vanilla pudding, and ice cream
	• Mashed table foods
	• Hummus
	• Finger foods
	  – Dry cereal soaked in milk or formula
	  – Buttered toast bites
	  – Buttery snack crackers
	  – Muffin bites
	  – Soft fruits or vegetables
	  – Cheese
	  – Pancakes or waffles with butter and syrup
	• ¼ teaspoon salt per day
		• Offer a variety of food 3 times a day; gradually add new foods and increase the amount and texture of the food
		• Add extra strained meat to combination foods or baby food "dinners"
		• Continue to add extra fats to food to increase calories; add 2–3 teaspoons whipping cream to yogurt or pudding
		• "Puffs" are very low in calories and nutrients and should be given infrequently
		• Feed the baby in a high chair
		• Start to offer breast milk or formula in a cup
		• Avoid juice or sweetened drinks

[15]. However, even in children with mutations associated with pancreatic insufficiency, PI may not be present at the time of diagnosis [16, 17] but gradually develops in infancy with over 90% of children diagnosed within the first year.

The CF Foundation recommends that pancreatic enzyme replacement should be initiated in all infants with two CFTR mutations associated with PI and in infants with objective evidence of PI including a low fecal elastase <200 µg/g or Coefficient of Fat Absorption (CFA) <85% and in infants with unequivocal signs or symptoms of malabsorption, while awaiting confirmatory test results [1]. Furthermore, PERT should be started in patients with PI even in absence of signs and symptoms of fat malabsorption. Pancreatic enzymes should not be started in infants with one or two CFTR mutations associated with pancreatic sufficiency unless there are unequivocal signs or symptoms of malabsorption while awaiting confirmatory results unless there is an objective test of pancreatic function indicating fat malabsorption [1].

Enzyme Administration and Dosing

Current consensus guidelines recommend that PERT should be initiated at a dose of 2000–5000 lipase units at each feeding, adjusted up to a dose of no greater than 2500 lipase units per kg per feeding with a maximum daily dose of 10,000 lipase units per kg per day due to the risk of fibrosing colonopathy [18–20]. In 2013, Borowitz et al. reported that the upper limit of enzyme dosing for infants with CF is not evidence based, but rather extrapolated from an older child or adult's usual intake of 3 meals and 1–2 snacks. Infants, particularly neonates, may eat as frequently as every 2–3 h and may easily exceed the previously recommended daily dose of PERT. Young infants have not shown evidence of fibrosing colonopathy; therefore, exceeding the upper limit of PERT to greater than 10,000 units lipase/kg per day may be tolerated during early infancy [21].

Recent analysis of CF Registry data reveals a strong association of improved growth rates when infants with CF received initial PERT doses of 1750–2000 lipase units/kg per largest meal. A statistically significant linear relationship between PERT dose and weight-for-length percentile occurred for doses 0–2000 units lipase/kg per largest meal, but did not continue for doses beyond that [22].

Enzyme capsules should be opened and the contents mixed with small amounts of applesauce and administered orally at the beginning of the feeding. Once administered, pancreatic enzymes are effective for about 45 minutes and should be repeated when the next feeding falls after this time frame. Parents should watch for stray enzyme microspheres in the infant's mouth and/or on mother's breast, as irritation could occur. With the initiation of PERT, parents should be advised to protect the perianal skin from potential irritation from frequent stooling as active enzymes may be contained in the stool.

As the infant with CF begins to eat complementary foods with moderate amounts of fat and protein, PERT will be necessary to aid in the absorption of these nutrients. Initially, the infant's diet is limited to single-grain cereals, fruits, and vegetables all of which are low in fat and protein. However, when the cereal is mixed with breast milk or formula, as well as the addition of fat in the form of oil or butter to enhance the calorie content of these foods, then PERT should be administered. When these foods and breast milk or formula are given within the 45-minute window of PERT dosing, additional enzymes may not be necessary. However, if offered separately from breast or bottle feedings, small amounts of PERT may be needed when fortified foods are given. As the infant grows and his/her diet expands to include more food sources that contain fats and proteins, additional PERT is often required to digest these nutrients. Clinicians may need to specify PERT doses for breast/bottle feedings alone versus feedings which combine breast milk/formula as well as fat and protein containing foods. As the infant grows and the volume of intake increases, PERT dose should be adjusted.

Rapid Growth Change

Infants with CF should experience rapid growth when they are able to consume sufficient calories and do not have significant malabsorption. However, this is also a period of high metabolic demand, and regular assessments are required to ensure adequate growth is occurring [1]. To closely assess growth and the health of the newly diagnosed infant with CF, the CFF recommends monthly follow-up in an accredited CF center until the age of 6 months and every 2 months from 6 months until the first birthday. Thereafter, patients should be seen every 2–3 months for routine care and more frequently if warranted due to ongoing or acute issues.

The CF Registered Dietitian should conduct a thorough nutrition assessment and provide anticipatory guidance to the infant and caregivers. An evaluation should include calculation of intake, calorie needs, average daily weight gain, PERT dose, and vitamin and mineral supplementation. The CFF consensus report provides guidelines for expected daily weight gain, calorie requirements, and an algorithm to address suboptimal growth and intake. Of utmost importance is close follow-up to

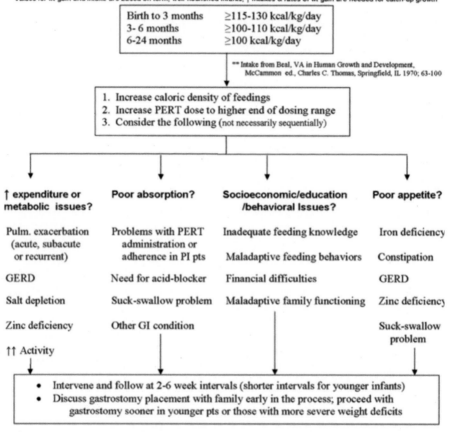

Calculate average daily weight gain since last visit and compare to expected *

Age range	Males (gm/day)	Females (gm/day)	Age range	Males (gm/day)	Females (gm/day)
Birth–1 month	30	26	4 - 5 months	17	16
1 - 2 months	35	29	5 - 6 months	15	14
2 - 3 months	26	23	6 - 9 months	10-13	10
3 - 4 months	20	19	9-24 months	7-10	7-10

* Based on expected rate of wt gain at the 50th %ile
  for age   (Guo et al. J Pediatr 1991;119:355-362)

Expected wt gain not achieved: refer for dietitian evaluation and assess intake **
Values for wt gain and intake are based on term, well-nourished infants; ↑ intakes & rates of wt gain are needed for catch-up growth

Birth to 3 months	≥115-130 kcal/kg/day
3- 6 months	≥100-110 kcal/kg/day
6-24 months	≥100 kcal/kg/day

** Intake from Beal, VA in Human Growth and Development,
   McCammon ed., Charles C. Thomas, Springfield, IL 1970; 63-100

1. Increase caloric density of feedings
2. Increase PERT dose to higher end of dosing range
3. Consider the following (not necessarily sequentially)

↑ expenditure or metabolic issues?	Poor absorption?	Socioeconomic/education /behavioral Issues?	Poor appetite?
Pulm. exacerbation (acute, subacute or recurrent)	Problems with PERT administration or adherence in PI pts	Inadequate feeding knowledge	Iron deficiency
GERD	Need for acid-blocker	Maladaptive feeding behaviors	Constipation
Salt depletion	Suck-swallow problem	Financial difficulties	GERD
Zinc deficiency	Other GI condition	Maladaptive family functioning	Zinc deficiency
↑↑ Activity			Suck-swallow problem

- Intervene and follow at 2-6 week intervals (shorter intervals for younger infants)
- Discuss gastrostomy placement with family early in the process; proceed with gastrostomy sooner in younger pts or those with more severe weight deficits

Fig. 6.1 Evaluation of infants with weight loss or inadequate weight gain (based on consensus opinion)

monitor the impact of the interventions made and to make early interventions to maximize the growth and nutritional status of the infant with CF. A guide for anticipated rates of growth and calorie needs is presented in Fig. 6.1.

Micronutrient Needs

Infants with CF are at risk for deficiency of fat-soluble vitamins including vitamins A, D, E, and K [23–27]. Despite widespread newborn screening, at diagnosis, many infants with CF show deficiency in one or more fat-soluble vitamins [23, 28] with development of symptoms reported in some children

Table 6.2 Tips for CF vitamin administration

Tips for CF vitamin administration
• Divide the vitamin dose into two-half volumes to help the newborn tolerate the CF vitamin if emesis occurs. Transition to one-full dose as tolerated.
• Mix the CF vitamin into 1 ounce of breast milk or formula in a bottle and feed as the first part of the feeding. Complete the feeding with additional breast milk or formula.
• CF vitamins are known to stain clothing. Let parents know that this can happen. Castile soap can be helpful in removing stains. Do not use water. Pour the soap directly on the stain and scrub. When the stain is faded, the item can be washed.

[29, 30]. Therefore, supplementation of CF-specific vitamin drops should be started in pancreatic insufficient infants at the time of diagnosis (see Table 6.2).

The CFF recommends measurement of vitamin levels A, D, and E within the first 2-3 months of diagnosis and thereafter yearly [1]. Supplemental vitamins should be adjusted to achieve optimum levels and further testing for vitamin levels should be performed sooner if levels are found to be low. Most often, additional vitamin D supplementation may be required to achieve normal levels.

At the age of one year, guidelines for vitamin supplementation often imply that the dose should be doubled; however, when vitamin levels are normal or slightly elevated, the additional supplementation may not be necessary. Doses of fat soluble vitamins, like many CF therapies, should be tailored to the individual needs of the patient.

For infants who consume breast milk, iron supplementation is recommended beginning at 4 months of age. Multiple studies have shown the association of iron deficiency anemia and later cognitive deficits [31, 32]. The American Academy of Pediatrics (AAP) recommends that exclusively breast-fed term infants receive an iron supplementation of 1 mg/kg/day starting at 4 months of age which should be continued until appropriate iron-containing complementary foods have been introduced [33].

The CFF Consensus Report on Nutrition for Pediatric Patients recommends that zinc levels not be measured. Empiric zinc supplementation as a treatment trial for a period of 6 months can be considered for CF patients who are failing to thrive or have short stature despite adequate calorie intake and PERT [34]. Fluoride is both safe and effective in preventing and controlling dental caries. Patients aged 6 months to 2 years whose community water supply contains less than 0.3 parts per million of fluoride should be supplemented with 0.25 mg/day regardless of mode of feeding. A comprehensive review of micronutrient requirements in CF is covered in Chapter 4 and this chapter.

Salt Supplementation

CF is characterized by increased electrolyte loss in sweat and other epithelial surfaces, especially in infants who have a larger relative body surface area compared to adults. Furthermore, infants with CF have much higher rates of unstimulated sweating than normal infants and are at risk of losing substantial amounts of sodium and chloride even in the absence of extraneous high temperatures [35]. Up to 80 mEq of sodium and chloride may be lost per day with profuse sweating [36]. Risk factors for the development of metabolic acidosis and hypoelectrolytemia include early infant age, breast feeding, delayed CF diagnosis, heat exhaustion, and more severe CFTR mutations. Evidence of salt loss in extreme weather is limited to case reports and case series and metabolic alkalosis can be the initial presentation in newly diagnosed children [37–40]. Acute salt depletion, especially in high ambient temperature, may often lead to lethargy, irritation, vomiting, loss of appetite, and dehydration, while infants with chronic salt depletion may exhibit anorexia and failure to thrive (FTT) [39].

The total daily sodium requirements in normal healthy infants are 5 and 16 mEq for 0–6 and 7–12 month olds, respectively [41]. Due to the relatively low salt content of human breast milk and infant formula, and no added salt in commercial baby foods, infants with CF are at risk of receiving inadequate amounts of salt through their diet [42]. Current CF Consensus guidelines recommend that infants with CF should be supplemented with 1/8 teaspoon of table salt daily (equivalent to about 12.5 mEq sodium) until 6 months of age and increased to ¼ teaspoon daily until one year of age but not exceeding 4 mEq/kg/day [34, 43]. Additional amounts should be considered in children living in hot climates, during periods of illness and high environmental temperatures. This is especially important prior to introduction of complementary feeds. Measuring spoons should be used to dispense accurate amounts. Sodium chloride solution preparations are available from pharmacies and provide more accurate measurements.

The salt should be distributed in feeds in small amounts throughout the day to avoid aversion due to taste. For bottle-fed infants, small amounts of salt should be added to 3–4 bottles per day until the total daily amount is distributed. Options to provide the salt to a breast-fed infant include adding it to the fruit puree used for pancreatic enzyme dosing or adding it to expressed breast milk which is fed in a bottle. The increased dosing at age 6 months usually corresponds to the initiation of solid food which is a good vehicle for the additional salt supplementation. Measured salt supplementation can be discontinued at the end of the first year of life and when the child is consuming mostly table foods. At that time, caregivers should be instructed to sprinkle salt on foods several times each day; they should also be educated on the need for additional salt supplementation during extreme conditions likely to produce perspiration such as during warm weather conditions, illness, or exercise.

Laboratory Assessment of Micronutrients

Vitamin levels including vitamin A, D, and E should be assessed approximately 2-3 months after starting vitamin supplementation. Repeat testing is then done yearly and more frequently if adequate vitamin levels are not achieved with the standard recommended doses. Alongside vitamin levels, a complete blood count, serum electrolytes, BUN and creatinine, liver enzymes, GGT and albumin, bilirubin as well as alkaline phosphatase are measured at the initial visit and yearly. More frequent monitoring is dictated by vitamin levels, the patient's clinical status, nutritional status, and assessment of risk for deficiencies [43].

Early Intervention and Long-Term Pulmonary Outcomes

Malnutrition is usually the earliest manifestation in infants with CF [44]. However, widespread newborn screening for CF has reduced the time until both the diagnosis and nutritional therapies are implemented. As a result, improvements in nutritional status have been demonstrated over the past decade. Early treatment with pancreatic enzyme replacement therapy (PERT), fat-soluble vitamin supplementation, as well as medical nutrition therapy frequently results in improved growth rates in infants with CF.

Several studies have demonstrated the correlation between improved nutritional status and pulmonary function as measured by FEV_1, progression of lung disease, and survival in CF [44–47]. For infants diagnosed early, recovery of birth weight z-score within 2 years of diagnosis of CF [48] and a higher weight for length (WFL) have been shown to be positively associated with better lung function status at 6 years [46, 49–51]. After the age of 2 years, a higher baseline body mass index (BMI), weight for age (WFA) maintenance above the 10th percentile and/or a slower rate of decline in BMI are associated with a slower rate of decline in lung function [50, 52]. Konstan et al. demonstrated in a cohort of 931 patients that nutritional status at 3 years correlated with pulmonary outcomes at 5.5–7.5 years [50]. A recent study also demonstrated that patients who achieved a WFA percentile >50% at age 4 years attained a much higher height-for-age (HFA) percentile early in life which was also associated with fewer pulmonary exacerbations and higher FEV$_1$ [53]. Thus, lung functions at later ages are variably dependent on nutritional status and growth beyond two years [52, 54, 55].

In 2008, the CFF issued a clinical practice guideline recommending early detection and aggressive treatment of under-nutrition [56]. The Foundation currently recommends monitoring growth in children with CF using the WFL measurements on the traditional 2000 Centers for Disease Control and Prevention (CDC) growth charts for children under the age of two, and thereafter using BMI percentile for age. The AAP recommends the use of World Health Organization (WHO) growth charts for measuring infant growth until the age of 24 months. Most electronic medical record (EMR) systems utilize the WHO growth charts making the use of CDC charts outdated. The 2013 CFF Center Specific Registry Reports first used WHO data to report infant outcomes as an initial step towards a transition away from CDC growth charts.

Based on registry data, better FEV$_1$ status at about 80% predicted or above was associated with BMI percentiles at the 50th percentile and higher. For children diagnosed before age 2 years, the Foundation recommends that children reach a weight-for-length status of ≥50th percentile by age 2 years [57]. For children and adolescents aged 2–20 years, the CF Foundation recommends that weight-for-stature assessment use the BMI percentile method, and that children and adolescents maintain a BMI at or above the 50th percentile.

A recent analysis of the CF Registry data demonstrates that WFL at 55–70 percentile on the WHO charts at 2 years resulted in slightly higher FEV$_1$ measurements age 6 than when WFL was less than the 50th percentile on the WHO growth chart. Infants with WFL below the 50th percentile on the CDC chart but greater than 50th percentile on the WHO chart had lower FEV$_1$ compared to those measuring above the 50th percentile on both charts [58]. Regardless of growth chart used, the goal for infant growth rates is to maximize the WFL ratio to optimize lung function later in life. Nutritional interventions made earlier in life can result in overall higher growth rates and improved lung function.

Special Considerations

Meconium Ileus

Approximately 10–20% of infants with CF present with simple or complex meconium ileus at birth. These infants require a variety of invasive and noninvasive strategies to decompress the bowel and relieve the obstruction [59–62]. Some infants with simple meconium ileus will respond to hyperosmolar enemas; however, a recent review suggests decreased effectiveness of the use of contrast enemas resulting in more surgical interventions [6]. Strategies reported to improve success of non-surgical interventions include repeated attempts with enemas, radiologist experience, and use of Gastrografin as the contrast agent. Infants with complex meconium ileus or those who fail to respond to contrast enemas require a laparotomy with resection and primary anastomosis, enterotomy, and/or stoma formation [61, 63].

While the operative management for meconium ileus is beyond the scope of this chapter, nutritional management of newborns with meconium ileus is relevant to all providers. Infants with both simple and complex meconium ileus may require parenteral nutrition from the time of admission to the Neonatal Intensive Care Unit until full volume enteral feeds have been reached, bowel function has normalized, and the infant demonstrates appropriate weight gain.

Once the patient shows readiness for enteral feedings, trophic feedings of expressed breast milk or infant formula can gradually be transitioned to bolus feedings, while monitoring for signs of abdominal distention, emesis, and/or constipation which may signal intolerance. While no specific guidelines are available, common practice is to initiate PERT when feeding volumes reach 30 mL per bolus feeding. Doses of 1500–3000 units of lipase per feeding are typically used and are increased as enteral feedings reach the volumes necessary to promote age-appropriate weight gain. Enzymes are usually administered orally with small amounts of applesauce at the beginning of the feeding. CF-specific vitamin drops and salt supplementation should be introduced at the time parenteral nutrition is discontinued.

For infants requiring ostomies, the aim is for closure as soon as possible. Closure times are variable and range from 3 to 6 weeks with variable times to full enteral nutrition [61, 63].

In spite of the early complications of meconium ileus including the need for surgery, frequent hospitalizations and earlier acquisition of Pseudomonas aeruginosa infection, long-term outcomes of lung function have been reported to be similar to infants without meconium ileus [59, 62].

Long-term (10–17 years) case-controlled follow-up revealed similar nutritional and pulmonary outcomes of CF patients presenting with meconium ileus with early-diagnosed symptomatic CF without meconium ileus [7]. A comparison of infants diagnosed through newborn screening in 2000, however, showed children born with meconium ileus and who required surgical intervention were more likely to be shorter and thinner than those who did not require surgery. Abnormal fatty acid profiles were also more prevalent in infants with meconium ileus before the age of 3 years. Daily intake of calories was generally higher in infants with meconium ileus than babies with CF but without meconium ileus [8].

Nutritional Requirements and Failure to Thrive

Nutritional and growth monitoring are vital in CF and are part of each clinic visit assessment. Although most infants with CF have a normal birth weight, it is usually significantly lower compared to healthy infants at the initial evaluation [64]. As previously mentioned, the goal of treatment is to achieve normal growth comparable to healthy infants. For children diagnosed before age 2 years, the CF Foundation recommends that infants reach a weight-for-length status of 50th percentile by age 2 years. Figure 6.1 shows the expected weight gain and growth velocity for infants of different age groups based on expected rate of weight gain at the 50th percentile for age [65]. Chapters 2 and 8 discuss in detail nutritional requirements as well as interventions for different age groups.

In certain circumstances, infants may fail to achieve adequate growth and would, therefore, be deemed to have FTT. Several factors may individually or collectively contribute to impaired nutritional status including pancreatic insufficiency with inadequate PERT, chronic malabsorption, recurrent sinopulmonary infections, chronic inflammation, increased metabolic needs, and energy expenditure as well as suboptimal intake. Poor appetite from chronic or recurrent infections may suppress adequate intake and contribute to malnutrition. Nutritional assessment should be performed at diagnosis and at each clinic visit and growth carefully monitored with early aggressive intervention. Infants not meeting the expected growth should be evaluated for causes for poor weight gain as documented in the algorithm in Table 6.1 in no particular order. Energy needs should be tailored to individual patient needs with most pancreatic insufficient infants requiring up to 150% of the dietary reference values for age [66]. Estimating energy needs based on ideal WFL rather than actual weight will establish energy goals to result in catch-up weight gain. For children unable to increase their calorie intake through volume, increased caloric density up to 30 cal/oz (100 cal/100 mL) should be considered. Infant formulas can be fortified to increase the caloric density by revising the ratio of formula and water and/or the addition of glucose polymers and/or medium chain triglyceride oil. Multiple studies have demonstrated that higher energy intake resulted in improved weight gain. Many infants demonstrate catch-up growth with initiation of appropriate nutritional intervention [67].

Additional considerations to address FTT in infancy include introducing the concept of enteral tube feelings as a component of CF care. Gastrostomy tube placement should be considered early for children not gaining adequate weight in spite of adequate or suboptimal intake due to a suppressed appetite. Gastrostomy tube feeding will provide extra calories to compensate for the high energy expenditure [68]. It has been established that supplemental gastrostomy tube feedings result in improvement in nutritional status and stabilization of the pulmonary function [69–71]. Despite the nutritional advantages, parents are often reluctant and fearful about feeding tube placement. Thorough education, emotional support, and involvement of sub-specialists such as pediatric gastroenterologists may help parents cope with these difficult decisions.

For families unable to provide adequate nutrition due to financial constraints, referral to community-based programs such as Supplemental Nutrition Assistance Program (SNAP) and Women, Infants and Children (WIC) should be made early. The CF team social worker can be a valuable resource for families dealing with an infant with FTT and should be involved with the family early. Collaborative follow-up care with the pediatrician, public health nurse, or home health care nurse can also allow the CF team to closely monitor the infant when travel to the CF center is cost or time prohibited for frequent weight checks and assessments that are necessary for an infant with FTT. Children with poor weight gain and FTT should be seen in follow-up at 2–6 week intervals and often shorter intervals for younger infants.

Appetite supplements are not usually prescribed for infants, but older toddlers and preschoolers with a suppressed intake may benefit from appetite supplements. Some appetite stimulants have been used and shown to be effective in children and adults in improving enteral intake and ultimately weight gain [72–74].

Several nutrition strategies can be put into place to maximize the calorie content of foods and liquids consumed in the first 2 years of life. First and foremost, parents should be taught early on that their child's need for high calorie diets begins in infancy and will likely continue throughout his/her lifetime. Education regarding label reading, consistent practices of adding fats to foods, and high calorie beverages will allow the family to maximize the caloric intake of the infant's diet and maximize weight gain.

Due to the simple nature of complementary foods in the infant's early diet, the addition of vegetable oils or softened butter or margarine is common practice to optimize calories in these foods. As the child's diet progresses to more finger foods and a wider variety of foods, including more calorie-dense foods becomes easier to incorporate, but still requires intent on the part of the parents to include them in the child's diet. As the child weans from breast milk or formula around the first birthday, whole milk, whole milk with added whipping cream, or commercially available pediatric nutrition beverages can continue provide a high energy source from beverages to the toddler with CF. Table 6.1 offers suggestions and strategies for increasing the calorie content of the diet in the first 2 years of life.

Conclusion

Nourishing the infant newly diagnosed with CF through the first 2 years of life requires a team approach with frequent assessments to assure optimal growth and provision of medical nutrition therapy, PERT, vitamin, and mineral supplementation. The CF Foundation Consensus Guidelines provide recommendations to enhance the care of these high-risk infants. Care teams should carefully implement these guidelines while at the same time provide support and education to the caregivers. Newborn screening for CF allows care teams to provide early and aggressive nutrition support to the infant which is essential to the long-term health of the individual with CF.

References

1. Cystic Fibrosis F, Borowitz D, Robinson KA, Rosenfeld M, Davis SD, Sabadosa KA, et al. Cystic Fibrosis Foundation evidence-based guidelines for management of infants with cystic fibrosis. J Pediatr. 2009;155(6 Suppl): S73–93.
2. Duijts L, Jaddoe VW, Hofman A, Moll HA. Prolonged and exclusive breastfeeding reduces the risk of infectious diseases in infancy. Pediatrics. 2010;126(1):e18–25. Epub 2010/06/23.
3. Quigley MA, Kelly YJ, Sacker A. Breastfeeding and hospitalization for diarrheal and respiratory infection in the United Kingdom Millennium Cohort Study. Pediatrics. 2007;119(4):e837–42. Epub 2007/04/04.
4. Hauck FR, Thompson JM, Tanabe KO, Moon RY, Vennemann MM. Breastfeeding and reduced risk of sudden infant death syndrome: a meta-analysis. Pediatrics. 2011;128(1):103–10. Epub 2011/06/15.
5. Greer FR, Sicherer SH, Burks AW. Effects of early nutritional interventions on the development of atopic disease in infants and children: the role of maternal dietary restriction, breastfeeding, timing of introduction of complementary foods, and hydrolyzed formulas. Pediatrics. 2008;121(1):183–91. Epub 2008/01/02.
6. Thygarajan A, Burks AW. American Academy of Pediatrics recommendations on the effects of early nutritional interventions on the development of atopic disease. Curr Opin Pediatr. 2008;20(6):698–702. Epub 2008/11/14.
7. Colombo C, Costantini D, Zazzeron L, Faelli N, Russo MC, Ghisleni D, et al. Benefits of breastfeeding in cystic fibrosis: a single-centre follow-up survey. Acta Paediatr. 2007;96(8):1228–32. Epub 2007/06/26.
8. Tluczek A, Clark R, McKechnie AC, Orland KM, Brown RL. Task-oriented and bottle feeding adversely affect the quality of mother-infant interactions after abnormal newborn screens. J Dev Behav Pediatr. 2010;31(5):414–26. Epub 2010/05/25.
9. Parker EM, O'Sullivan BP, Shea JC, Regan MM, Freedman SD. Survey of breast-feeding practices and outcomes in the cystic fibrosis population. Pediatr Pulmonol. 2004;37(4):362–7. Epub 2004/03/17.
10. Jadin SA, Wu GS, Zhang Z, Shoff SM, Tippets BM, Farrell PM, et al. Growth and pulmonary outcomes during the first 2 y of life of breastfed and formula-fed infants diagnosed with cystic fibrosis through the Wisconsin Routine Newborn Screening Program. Am J Clin Nutr. 2011;93(5):1038–47. Epub 2011/03/25.
11. Huebner J, Oldroyd HBL, Andrade O, Horn B, Laxova A, Greer F, Lai HJ. Breastfeeding characteristics during the first six months of life in infants with CF diagnosed through newborn Screening in 2012–13. Pediatr Pulmonol. 2014;49(Supp 38):406.
12. Prevention CfDCa. Breastfeeding Report Card 2014. 2014.
13. Erskine JM, Lingard CD, Sontag MK, Accurso FJ. Enteral nutrition for patients with cystic fibrosis: comparison of a semi-elemental and nonelemental formula. J Pediatr. 1998;132(2):265–9. Epub 1998/03/20.
14. Ellis L, Kalnins D, Corey M, Brennan J, Pencharz P, Durie P. Do infants with cystic fibrosis need a protein hydrolysate formula? A prospective, randomized, comparative study. J Pediatr. 1998;132(2):270–6. Epub 1998/03/20.
15. Borowitz D. Update on the evaluation of pancreatic exocrine status in cystic fibrosis. Curr Opin Pulm Med. 2005;11(6):524–7. Epub 2005/10/12.
16. Bronstein MN, Sokol RJ, Abman SH, Chatfield BA, Hammond KB, Hambidge KM, et al. Pancreatic insufficiency, growth, and nutrition in infants identified by newborn screening as having cystic fibrosis. J Pediatr. 1992;120(4 Pt 1):533–40. Epub 1992/04/01.
17. Walkowiak J, Sands D, Nowakowska A, Piotrowski R, Zybert K, Herzig KH, et al. Early decline of pancreatic function in cystic fibrosis patients with class 1 or 2 CFTR mutations. J Pediatr Gastroenterol Nutr. 2005;40(2):199–201. Epub 2005/02/09.
18. Borowitz DS, Grand RJ, Durie PR. Use of pancreatic enzyme supplements for patients with cystic fibrosis in the context of fibrosing colonopathy. Consensus Committee. J Pediatr. 1995;127(5):681–4. Epub 1995/11/01.
19. Schwarzenberg SJ, Wielinski CL, Shamieh I, Carpenter BL, Jessurun J, Weisdorf SA, et al. Cystic fibrosis-associated colitis and fibrosing colonopathy. J Pediatr. 1995;127(4):565–70. Epub 1995/10/01.
20. FitzSimmons SC, Burkhart GA, Borowitz D, Grand RJ, Hammerstrom T, Durie PR, et al. High-dose pancreatic-enzyme supplements and fibrosing colonopathy in children with cystic fibrosis. N Engl J Med. 1997;336(18):1283–9. Epub 1997/05/01.
21. Borowitz D, Gelfond D, Maguiness K, Heubi JE, Ramsey B. Maximal daily dose of pancreatic enzyme replacement therapy in infants with cystic fibrosis: a reconsideration. J Cyst Fibros. 2013;12(6):784–5. Epub 2013/07/03.
22. Schechter M, Michel SH, Haupt M, Seo B, Khurmi R, Liu S, Kapoor M. Relationship of initial pancreatic enzyme replacement therapy dose and growth in young children with cystic fibrosis. Pediatr Pulmonol. 2014;49(Supp 38):420.
23. Feranchak AP, Sontag MK, Wagener JS, Hammond KB, Accurso FJ, Sokol RJ. Prospective, long-term study of fat-soluble vitamin status in children with cystic fibrosis identified by newborn screen. J Pediatr. 1999;135(5):601–10. Epub 1999/11/05.
24. Rovner AJ, Stallings VA, Schall JI, Leonard MB, Zemel BS. Vitamin D insufficiency in children, adolescents, and young adults with cystic fibrosis despite routine oral supplementation. Am J Clin Nutr. 2007;86(6):1694–9.

25. Drury D, Grey VL, Ferland G, Gundberg C, Lands LC. Efficacy of high dose phylloquinone in correcting vitamin K deficiency in cystic fibrosis. J Cyst Fibros. 2008;7(5):457–9.
26. Neville LA, Ranganathan SC. Vitamin D in infants with cystic fibrosis diagnosed by newborn screening. J Paediatr Child Health. 2009;45(1–2):36–41.
27. Bines JE, Truby HD, Armstrong DS, Carzino R, Grimwood K. Vitamin A and E deficiency and lung disease in infants with cystic fibrosis. J Paediatr Child Health. 2005;41(12):663–8.
28. Marcus MS, Sondel SA, Farrell PM, Laxova A, Carey PM, Langhough R, et al. Nutritional status of infants with cystic fibrosis associated with early diagnosis and intervention. Am J Clin Nutr. 1991;54(3):578–85. Epub 1991/09/01.
29. Rayner RJ, Tyrrell JC, Hiller EJ, Marenah C, Neugebauer MA, Vernon SA, et al. Night blindness and conjunctival xerosis caused by vitamin A deficiency in patients with cystic fibrosis. Arch Dis Child. 1989;64(8):1151–6.
30. Sitrin MD, Lieberman F, Jensen WE, Noronha A, Milburn C, Addington W. Vitamin E deficiency and neurologic disease in adults with cystic fibrosis. Ann Intern Med. 1987;107(1):51–4.
31. Lozoff B, De Andraca I, Castillo M, Smith JB, Walter T, Pino P. Behavioral and developmental effects of preventing iron-deficiency anemia in healthy full-term infants. Pediatrics. 2003;112(4):846–54.
32. Logan S, Martins S, Gilbert R. Iron therapy for improving psychomotor development and cognitive function in children under the age of three with iron deficiency anaemia. Cochrane Database Syst Rev. 2001;2, CD001444.
33. Baker RD, Greer FR. Committee on Nutrition American Academy of P. Diagnosis and prevention of iron deficiency and iron-deficiency anemia in infants and young children (0–3 years of age). Pediatrics. 2010;126(5):1040–50.
34. Borowitz D, Baker RD, Stallings V. Consensus report on nutrition for pediatric patients with cystic fibrosis. J Pediatr Gastroenterol Nutr. 2002;35(3):246–59.
35. Sibinga MS, Barbero GJ. Studies in the physiology of sweating in cystic fibrosis. II. Elevated night sweating rates. Arch Dis Child. 1961;36:537–9. Epub 1961/10/01.
36. Gottlieb RP. Metabolic alkalosis in cystic fibrosis. J Pediatr. 1971;79(6):930–6. Epub 1971/12/01.
37. Ballestero Y, Hernandez MI, Rojo P, Manzanares J, Nebreda V, Carbajosa H, et al. Hyponatremic dehydration as a presentation of cystic fibrosis. Pediatr Emerg Care. 2006;22(11):725–7. Epub 2006/11/18.
38. Laughlin JJ, Brady MS, Eigen H. Changing feeding trends as a cause of electrolyte depletion in infants with cystic fibrosis. Pediatrics. 1981;68(2):203–7. Epub 1981/08/01.
39. Fustik S, Pop-Jordanova N, Slaveska N, Koceva S, Efremov G. Metabolic alkalosis with hypoelectrolytemia in infants with cystic fibrosis. Pediatr Int. 2002;44(3):289–92. Epub 2002/05/02.
40. Beckerman RC, Taussig LM. Hypoelectrolytemia and metabolic alkalosis in infants with cystic fibrosis. Pediatrics. 1979;63(4):580–3. Epub 1979/04/01.
41. National Research Council. Dietary Reference Intakes for Water, Potassium, Sodium, Chloride, and Sulfate. Washington, DC: The National Academies Press, 2005.
42. Coates AJ, Crofton PM, Marshall T. Evaluation of salt supplementation in CF infants. J Cyst Fibros. 2009;8(6):382–5. Epub 2009/10/06.
43. Cystic Fibrosis F, Borowitz D, Parad RB, Sharp JK, Sabadosa KA, Robinson KA, et al. Cystic Fibrosis Foundation practice guidelines for the management of infants with cystic fibrosis transmembrane conductance regulator-related metabolic syndrome during the first two years of life and beyond. J Pediatr. 2009;155(6 Suppl):S106–16.
44. Matel JL, Milla CE. Nutrition in cystic fibrosis. Semin Respir Crit Care Med. 2009;30(5):579–86.
45. Kraemer R, Rudeberg A, Hadorn B, Rossi E. Relative underweight in cystic fibrosis and its prognostic value. Acta Paediatr Scand. 1978;67(1):33–7.
46. Hankard R, Munck A, Navarro J. Nutrition and growth in cystic fibrosis. Horm Res. 2002;58 Suppl 1:16–20.
47. Rosenfeld M, Davis R, FitzSimmons S, Pepe M, Ramsey B. Gender gap in cystic fibrosis mortality. Am J Epidemiol. 1997;145(9):794–803.
48. Lai HJ, Shoff SM, Farrell PM. Recovery of birth weight z score within 2 years of diagnosis is positively associated with pulmonary status at 6 years of age in children with cystic fibrosis. Pediatrics. 2009;123(2):714–22.
49. Rosenfeld M, Casey S, Pepe M, Ramsey BW. Nutritional effects of long-term gastrostomy feedings in children with cystic fibrosis. J Am Diet Assoc. 1999;99(2):191–4.
50. Konstan MW, Butler SM, Wohl ME, Stoddard M, Matousek R, Wagener JS, et al. Growth and nutritional indexes in early life predict pulmonary function in cystic fibrosis. J Pediatr. 2003;142(6):624–30.
51. Steinkamp G, Wiedemann B. Relationship between nutritional status and lung function in cystic fibrosis: cross sectional and longitudinal analyses from the German CF quality assurance (CFQA) project. Thorax. 2002;57(7):596–601.
52. McPhail GL, Acton JD, Fenchel MC, Amin RS, Seid M. Improvements in lung function outcomes in children with cystic fibrosis are associated with better nutrition, fewer chronic pseudomonas aeruginosa infections, and dornase alfa use. J Pediatr. 2008;153(6):752–7.
53. Yen EH, Quinton H, Borowitz D. Better nutritional status in early childhood is associated with improved clinical outcomes and survival in patients with cystic fibrosis. J Pediatr. 2013;162(3):530–5.

54. Peterson ML, Jacobs Jr DR, Milla CE. Longitudinal changes in growth parameters are correlated with changes in pulmonary function in children with cystic fibrosis. Pediatrics. 2003;112(3 Pt 1):588–92.
55. Walkowiak J, Przyslawski J. Five-year prospective analysis of dietary intake and clinical status in malnourished cystic fibrosis patients. J Hum Nutr Diet. 2003;16(4):225–31.
56. Ramsey BW, Farrell PM, Pencharz P. Nutritional assessment and management in cystic fibrosis: a consensus report. The Consensus Committee. Am J Clin Nutr. 1992;55(1):108–16.
57. Stallings VA, Stark LJ, Robinson KA, Feranchak AP, Quinton H. Evidence-based practice recommendations for nutrition-related management of children and adults with cystic fibrosis and pancreatic insufficiency: results of a systematic review. J Am Diet Assoc. 2008;108(5):832–9.
58. Machogu E, Cao Y, Miller T, Simpson P, Levy H, Quintero D, Goday PS. Comparison of the WHO and CDC growth charts in predicting pulmonary outcomes in cystic fibrosis. JPGN. doi:10.1097/MPG.0000000000000610.
59. Kappler M, Feilcke M, Schroter C, Kraxner A, Griese M. Long-term pulmonary outcome after meconium ileus in cystic fibrosis. Pediatr Pulmonol. 2009;44(12):1201–6. Epub 2009/11/17.
60. Gorter RR, Karimi A, Sleeboom C, Kneepkens CM, Heij HA. Clinical and genetic characteristics of meconium ileus in newborns with and without cystic fibrosis. J Pediatr Gastroenterol Nutr. 2010;50(5):569–72. Epub 2010/04/14.
61. Farrelly PJ, Charlesworth C, Lee S, Southern KW, Baillie CT. Gastrointestinal surgery in cystic fibrosis: a 20-year review. J Pediatr Surg. 2014;49(2):280–3. Epub 2014/02/18.
62. Carlyle BE, Borowitz DS, Glick PL. A review of pathophysiology and management of fetuses and neonates with meconium ileus for the pediatric surgeon. J Pediatr Surg. 2012;47(4):772–81. Epub 2012/04/14.
63. Escobar MA, Grosfeld JL, Burdick JJ, Powell RL, Jay CL, Wait AD, et al. Surgical considerations in cystic fibrosis: a 32-year evaluation of outcomes. Surgery. 2005;138(4):560–71. discussion 71–2. Epub 2005/11/05.
64. Farrell PM, Kosorok MR, Laxova A, Shen G, Koscik RE, Bruns WT, et al. Nutritional benefits of neonatal screening for cystic fibrosis. Wisconsin Cystic Fibrosis Neonatal Screening Study Group. N Engl J Med. 1997;337(14):963–9.
65. Guo SM, Roche AF, Fomon SJ, Nelson SE, Chumlea WC, Rogers RR, et al. Reference data on gains in weight and length during the first two years of life. J Pediatr. 1991;119(3):355–62. Epub 1991/09/01.
66. Davies PS. Energy requirements for growth and development in infancy. Am J Clin Nutr. 1998;68(4):939S–43. Epub 1998/10/15.
67. Pederzini F, D'Orazio C, Tamiazzo G, Faraguna D, Giglio L, Mastella G. Growth evaluation at one year of life in infants with cystic fibrosis diagnosed by neonatal screening. Pediatr Pulmonol Suppl. 1991;7:64–8.
68. Marin VB, Velandia S, Hunter B, Gattas V, Fielbaum O, Herrera O, et al. Energy expenditure, nutrition status, and body composition in children with cystic fibrosis. Nutrition. 2004;20(2):181–6.
69. Williams SG, Ashworth F, McAlweenie A, Poole S, Hodson ME, Westaby D. Percutaneous endoscopic gastrostomy feeding in patients with cystic fibrosis. Gut. 1999;44(1):87–90.
70. Bradley GM, Carson KA, Leonard AR, Mogayzel Jr PJ, Oliva-Hemker M. Nutritional outcomes following gastrostomy in children with cystic fibrosis. Pediatr Pulmonol. 2012;47(8):743–8.
71. Best C, Brearley A, Gaillard P, Regelmann W, Billings J, Dunitz J, et al. A pre-post retrospective study of patients with cystic fibrosis and gastrostomy tubes. J Pediatr Gastroenterol Nutr. 2011;53(4):453–8.
72. Homnick DN, Marks JH, Hare KL, Bonnema SK. Long-term trial of cyproheptadine as an appetite stimulant in cystic fibrosis. Pediatr Pulmonol. 2005;40(3):251–6.
73. Homnick DN, Homnick BD, Reeves AJ, Marks JH, Pimentel RS, Bonnema SK. Cyproheptadine is an effective appetite stimulant in cystic fibrosis. Pediatr Pulmonol. 2004;38(2):129–34.
74. Epifanio M, Marostica PC, Mattiello R, Feix L, Nejedlo R, Fischer GB, et al. A randomized, double-blind, placebo-controlled trial of cyproheptadine for appetite stimulation in cystic fibrosis. J Pediatr (Rio J). 2012;88(2):155–60.

Chapter 7
Nutritional Assessment: Age 2–20 Years

Karen Maguiness and Molly Bozic

Key Points

- An accurate nutritional assessment for the 2 to 20-year-old child with cystic fibrosis is essential.
- Anthropometric measures, biochemical data, clinical evaluation, and diet history comprise the nutritional assessment for the 2- to 20-year-old child with cystic fibrosis.
- Related diseases (such as CF liver disease, CF-related diabetes), stool and gastrointestinal history, vitamin/mineral history, and pancreatic enzyme replacement history should also be obtained in the nutritional assessment of the 2- to 20-year-old child with cystic fibrosis.
- Short- and long-term weight goals should be established for the 2- to 20-year-old child with cystic fibrosis. Standard yearly labs should be obtained for the 2- to 20-year-old child with cystic fibrosis with additional labs obtained as indicated by the patient's individual medical condition.

Keywords Nutritional assessment • Anthropometric data • Biochemical • Clinical assessment • Diet history • Vitamin history • Stool history

Introduction

A thorough and comprehensive nutritional assessment performed by the combined efforts of a dietitian and physician is essential for the management of the child with cystic fibrosis (CF). The primary purpose of a nutritional assessment in CF is to evaluate diet, clinical status, growth velocity, and body measurements while concomitantly monitoring the additional therapy required as a result of having CF (e.g. pancreatic enzyme replacement and fat-soluble vitamin therapy). Based on these evaluations,

K. Maguiness, M.S., R.D., C.S.P.
Pediatric Pulmonology, Riley Hospital for Children,
ROC Room 4270, 705 Riley Hospital Drive, Indianapolis, IN 46202, USA
e-mail: kmaguine@iu.edu

M. Bozic, M.D. (✉)
Pediatric Gastroenterology, Riley Hospital for Children,
ROC Room 4210, 705 Riley Hospital Drive, Indianapolis, IN 46202, USA
e-mail: mbozic@iu.edu

E.H. Yen, A.R. Leonard (eds.), *Nutrition in Cystic Fibrosis: A Guide for Clinicians*, Nutrition and Health, DOI 10.1007/978-3-319-16387-1_7, © Springer International Publishing Switzerland 2015

one can assess if the current nutrition regimen is adequate, or if intervention or modification is required. Properly assessing and interpreting the nutritional status of patients with CF requires skill, experience, and knowledge of the latest standards of care, clinical guidelines, and evidence-based research. This chapter will detail what should be performed as part of a clinic nutrition evaluation for individuals with CF who are 2–20 years of age.

The primary nutritional goal for a child with cystic fibrosis is the same as a child who does not have CF; to be well-nourished! Without a doubt, children with CF present distinct challenges regarding attaining and maintaining optimal nutrition. Food jags, maldigestion with resultant malabsorption secondary to pancreatic insufficiency; intestinal resection due to meconium ileus, poorly controlled CF-related diabetes, and impaired bile flow in cases of severe CF-related liver disease all present potential unique nutritional challenges [1]. Recurrent pulmonary infections and increased oxidative stress, fevers, and increased metabolic rates also further complicate nutritional optimization [2].

Setting accurate and attainable nutritional goals is important in cystic fibrosis. The Cystic Fibrosis Foundation (CFF) recommends a BMI of ≥50th percentile for 2- to 20-year-olds [3], as this is associated with better pulmonary status as measured by FEV_1. Additionally, a weight for age of >10th percentile by age 4 years is associated with improved short- and long-term pulmonary outcomes [4]. Families and patients with CF typically want to know "where they are" and "where they should be at" in terms of their nutritional status. Nutrition goals may be short term and simple: such as daily calorie goals or monthly weight gain goals, or long term: such as an eventual weight goal based on either a previous weight for age percentile or on a weight that corresponds with a BMI of ≥50th percentile.

Once nutrition goals are established, frequent and routine monitoring are necessary. The most effective way to use growth charts diagnostically is through serial measurements [2]. The CFF mandates that patients be seen in clinic every 3 months [1]; more often if indicated. The availability of these frequent body measurements provides a certain luxury for dietitians and physicians; it allows for close monitoring of nutritional status in a timely manner and permits early detection and intervention when decline in nutritional status is noted. When performing a thorough and comprehensive nutritional assessment in a child with CF, the following sentence with abbreviations may be of help: "Remember **ABC&D and don't forget to RSVP**" (Tables 7.1 and 7.2).

Anthropometric Data

A reliable nutritional assessment requires that the health professionals who obtain the body measurements have been properly trained and that the measuring equipment being used is appropriate and correctly calibrated [2]. A clinic serving those with CF can have the latest, state-of-the-art devices to measure weights and heights; however, if the individual obtaining these measures does so incorrectly (for example, does not ask patients to take off their shoes, or carelessly obtains these measures), not only will the weight and height measurements be incorrect, but there will also be a ripple effect leading to incorrect body mass index (BMI) calculation as well as incorrect estimation of rates of growth between clinic visits. In addition to relying on accurate measurements, members of the CF team who evaluate the weights and heights need to use the appropriate resources and possess the skill set to accurately interpret the data to make recommendations in the context of CF. If any of these components are lacking, the quality of the nutritional assessment is diminished. Comparison of an individual to an established norm provides the basis for objective recommendations and evaluation of nutritional care [5].

Table 7.1 Nutritional assessment of the patient with CF A, B, C, D Nutrition Evaluation

ABC&D evaluation	
A—Anthropometric	Weight (kg and NCHS percentile)
	Height (cm and NCHS percentile)
	Body mass index (percentile and kg/m^2)
	Goal weight (kg) Goal Weight (weight at which BMI would be equivalent to the 50th %tile)
	Previous weight (kg)
	Rate of weight gain in grams/day (or % weight loss)
	Mid-arm circumference, skinfold measurements
B—Biochemical	Fat-soluble vitamin levels:
	A—serum plasma retinol
	D—25-OH vitamin D
	E—alpha tocopherol
	K—PIVKA-II (preferred) or PT/INR
	Other—see biochemical section
C—Clinical evaluation	Evaluation of clinical status: skin, nails, face, neck, mouth, tongue, eyes, hair, teeth, and abdomen
D—Diet history	Diet recall, food records, food frequency
	Specific interventions to increase calories
	Oral nutrition supplement history
	Enteral feeding history
	Any nutritional issues such as skipping meals, slow eating, food refusal, texture aversion, binge eating, "fad" diets

A Anthropometric Data
B Biochemical Data
C Clinical Assessment
D Diet History

Weight, Height, and Body Mass Index

Gathering anthropometric data including weight, height, and BMI and plotting each on appropriate growth curves should be performed at every clinic visit. The American Academy of Pediatrics (AAP) [6] and the CFF [1] both recommend use of the Center for Disease Control (CDC) 2000 National Center for Health Statistics growth charts for plotting weight, height, and BMI of the 2 to 20-year-old. These may be found online at http://www.cdc.gov/growthcharts/.

Accurate Measurement of Weight

Scales should be regularly calibrated and checked for accuracy. The clinic scale(s) should be kept in an area that is protected, thus, decreasing the potential for it to be treated in a rough manner which could lead to poor calibration and thus inaccurate weights. Children should be weighed in light clothing or an exam gown, with shoes removed [2]. For toddlers or preschoolers not yet potty trained, a clean and dry diaper may be worn. The best weight and height measurements are done when a child is calm and willing to cooperate. The scale should be zeroed prior to the child standing on it. Once zeroed, the patient should be instructed to stand in the middle of the scale platform until an accurate reading has been obtained. Weight measurements should be made to the nearest 0.1 kg [7]. Prior to obtaining a patient's weight, it is helpful to review previous measurements to ensure that the new weight aligns with previous weights.

Table 7.2 Nutritional assessment of the patient with CF (RSVP)

"RSVP" Nutrition evaluation	
R—Related Disease/Illness/Genetics/Previous Medical history	Possible impact on nutrition from: CF related diabetes CF liver disease Degree of pulmonary involvement Presence of infection Genetic mutations Intestinal resection Other
S—Stool/GI history	Number of stools/day Color of stools Consistency of stools Caliber of stools Visible oil or mucous in stools Significant foul (ripe) smell to stools Floating stools Gassiness Stomach pain Stomach distention Constipation Use of H_2 blocker or PPI Use of polyethylene glycol/fiber/stool softener
V—Vitamin history	Name/form/dose of multivitamin(s) (liquid/gummy/chewable/gel cap) Name/form/dose fat-soluble vitamins(A, D, E, K) Use of non-prescribed vitamins or supplements Any financial difficulties affording vitamin(s)? Frequency of administration
P—Pancreatic enzymes	Name and strength of enzyme Number of enzymes/meal and snack Number of enzymes with glass of milk or supplement Number of enzymes with before/after tube feedings Total number or enzymes taken in 24 Hours Lipase units/kg/meal and Lipase units/kg/day "Any nutrition issues" with eating or taking enzymes at school, daycare, and so forth.

Related illnesses history
Stool history
Vitamin and mineral history
Pancreatic enzyme replacement history

Accurate Measurement of Height

The words "height" or "stature" imply a linear measurement obtained when a child is standing, as opposed to "length," which indicates a measurement when a child is in a recumbent or lying down. All children 2 years and older should be measured in a standing position [2].

The use of the "sliding" measuring devices commonly attached to standing scales is not recommended for measurement of height as they do not consistently yield an accurate measurement. A wall mounted stadiometer is the most precise instrument to measure height. A stadiometer has a moveable headboard positioned at a 90° angle to a wall mounted fixed incremental linear measurement readout [7]. The child should be in bare feet or thin socks and with removal of any hair adornment that would affect height. The best height measurements are done when the child is calm and willing to cooperate. The patient should be instructed to stand with his or her back, bottom, and shoulders against the wall, hands at their side, feet flat on the floor with heels close together, head and chin level and with eyes looking forward, and standing as tall as possible (with heels still flat on the ground) [2]. Asking the patient to take a deep breath and hold it prior to the measurement assists them in "standing tall." The sliding headboard is then gently positioned atop of the child's head, with the height measurement made to the nearest 0.1 cm [7]. It is good practice to review previous height measurements prior to obtaining a new one to ensure that the updated measurement corresponds with previous measurements.

Weight for Age and Height for Age Percentiles

Weight and height for age percentiles may be plotted by hand on a growth chart, or by using a reliable computerized program or smart device app. If plotting by hand, it is essential that the patient's age be accurately calculated (in years, months, and days) such that both the weight and the height percentiles may be precisely plotted. If plotting by hand, the use of a page-size clear sturdy plastic template, with perfectly centered edge-to-edge horizontal and vertical lines, and a small hole at their intersection in the center can be a useful tool for accurate plotting.

Growth charts provide a useful visual depiction of weights and heights over time and allow one to easily monitor trends. It may be beneficial for the clinician to place noteworthy "landmarks" on growth charts, for example, when a gastrostomy tube was placed or removed. Where "one is" versus where "one should be" on a growth chart requires discernment for the patient with CF. Of primary importance is that children attain and maintain their highest potential for weight and height for age and that any downward trending to a lower percentile be identified in a timely manner with appropriate intervention.

A weight for age of >10th percentile by 4 years of age is associated with improved short- and long-term pulmonary outcomes in CF [4]; thus, it should be of paramount importance to strive for this in the preschool years. Consideration of mid-parental height may be used when evaluating the height percentile of the child [1] and [8]. Mid-parental height may be calculated using the following equation [9]:

$$\text{Boys}: \left[\text{Parental height} + \left(\text{maternal height} + 5 \text{ in. or } 13 \text{ cm} \right) \right] / 2$$

$$\text{Girls}: \left[\text{Maternal height} + \left(\text{paternal height} + 5 \text{ in. or } 13 \text{ cm} \right) \right] / 2$$

When calculating mid-parental height, an actual measurement of each parent, using a stadiometer, will yield much more reliable results than a verbal report or estimate of the parent's height.

"Weight age equivalent" is a term that can also provide descriptive information for patients who are underweight. This may be defined as the age at which the patient's present weight plots at the 50th percentile on a growth chart. For example, if an 18-year-old male weighs just 43 kg, he is the "weight age equivalent" of a 12.5-year-old male. A "height age equivalent" may be similarly calculated.

Calculation of BMI

Calculating BMI is straightforward; the *accuracy of the BMI* depends upon the precision of the weight and height measurements inputted into the BMI equation. BMI may be reported as kg/m^2 as well as in percentiles for those aged 2-20 years, and should be plotted on the 2000 CDC BMI growth charts (Table 7.3) [7].

Table 7.3 Calculating BMI (kg/m^2)

	OR	
$\dfrac{\text{Weight}(\text{kg})}{\left[\text{Height}(\text{m})\right]^2}$ (Centimeters divided by 100 = meters)		$\dfrac{\left[\text{Weight}(\text{pounds})\right]}{\left[\text{Height}(\text{in})\right]^2} \times 703$

An inaccurate height measurement is more likely to occur than an inaccurate weight measurement due to the nature of how these two measurements are obtained. An accurate weight essentially requires only a properly calibrated scale and the patient standing still on the scale platform. A precise height, however, necessitates a cooperative patient who is properly positioned and aligned (feet, legs, back, shoulders, and head), as well as the health care professional who is obtaining this measure to carefully position the headboard and to view the measurement readout at eye level. Because weight goals, nutritional classification, and registry data are often based on BMI percentiles, accurate heights are especially important in CF. If in doubt, re-measure the patient's height.

Calculating Short- and Long-Term Goal Weights

For patients who are underweight, it is often helpful to mutually establish feasible, and achievable, weight goals so that interim progress may be acknowledged and celebrated. For patients in need of a substantial amount of "catch-up" weight gain, it may be useful to set "in between" or incremental weight goals equivalent to a BMI at, for example, the 10th and 25th percentiles. Setting an immediate weight goal for a BMI at the 50th percentile that is too discrepant from the present weight can seem unattainable and be disheartening to the patient and their family.

Calculating Percent of Goal Weight

Percent of goal weight may simply be calculated by dividing actual weight by goal weight and multiplying by 100.

Calculating Rate of Weight Gain or Growth Velocity

Rate of weight gain may be easily calculated by dividing the number of grams of weight the patient gained by the number of days between visits (Tables 7.4 and 7.5).

Mid-Upper Arm Circumference

Mid-upper arm circumference is another measure that may be used to evaluate nutritional status by measuring soft tissue. Using a marker and a non-stretchable tape measurer (metallic tape or insert tape), the midpoint on the right upper arm is marked half way between the acromion process (bony protrusion on the upper shoulder) and the olecranon process (tip of the elbow) [7]. The *marking* of the arm should occur with the elbow bent at a 90° angle. The *measurement* of the mid-arm circumference

Table 7.4 Example of calculating rate of weight gain between visits

Age: 11 years 6 months

Sex: Male

Today's date: July 13th

Today's weight: 38.2 kg

Date of last clinic visit: April 20th

Weight on April 20th: 37.0 kg

Number of days between April 20th and July 13th:

10 days (remaining in April)+**31** days (May)+**30** days (June)+**13** days (July 13)=**84** days

Amount of weight gain:

38.2−37.0 kg=1.2 kg×1000 g/kg=**1200 g in 84 days**

Divide 1200 g by 84 days=**13.7 g/day**

Table 7.5 Expected rate of rate gain (g/day) for Age (50th to 97th percentile rate of gain)

Age range (years)	Male	Female
2–3	4.7–6.7	5.2–8.2
3–4	5.2–8.1	5.3–9.0
4–5	5.9–9.5	5.9–10.0
5–6	6.3–10.4	6.3–10.9
6–7	6.5–11.7	6.9–12.2
7–8	7.1–13.4	7.9–14.2
8–9	8.0–15.5	9.4–16.6
9–10	9.3–17.4	10.7–18.8
10–11	10.9–18.8	11.9–20.0
11–12	12.6–19.3	12.2–19.7
12–13	14.1–19.1	11.4–17.7
13–14	14.8–18.3	9.5–14.6
14–15	14.4–17.2	7.2–10.8
15–16	12.6–15.7	5.0–7.4
16–17	9.9–13.2	3.4–4.9
17–18	7.1–9.5	2.9–3.5
18–19	5.2–5.3	2.7–3.1
19–20	3.8–4.4	1.7–2.4

Reference: Please note that higher rates of weight gain than those listed in this reference chart may be indicated for those children requiring "catch up" weight gain. NCHS 2000 growth charts

should be done with the arm hanging relaxed at the side with fingertips facing the ground. The tape measure should be snug, but not so tight as to compress the skin around the arm to the extent that an indentation is made. Standards for values based on age are well documented [7].

Skinfold Measurements

Tricep and subscapular skinfold measurements may also be used to evaluate nutritional status in cystic fibrosis. To be done accurately, proper equipment and training is required (e.g. correct measuring tape and "accurate calipers). Specific knowledge of appropriate body landmarks, precise application of calipers, and knowledge of normative values is essential [7]. Serial measures of skinfold measurements are needed to document depletion or repletion of fat stores.

Biochemical Data

Anthropometric data is only one aspect of the nutritional evaluation. Laboratory data is an essential aspect of determining nutritional status in the cystic fibrosis patient. The following provides guidelines for measurement of laboratory data.

Standard Yearly Labs

Standard yearly labs are recommended in all patients with cystic fibrosis (see Table 7.6). Current guidelines recommend yearly evaluation of fat-soluble vitamins including Vitamin D (25-OH Vitamin D), Vitamin A (retinol), Vitamin E (alpha-tocopherol), and Vitamin K (prothrombin time (PT)/ International Normalized Ratio (INR) [3]. For those patients with severe CF-related liver disease, PIVKA-II (protein induced by vitamin K absence-II) may be helpful to determine Vitamin K stores. It is not uncommon for patients with cystic fibrosis, and especially those with CF-related liver disease, to require large amounts of fat-soluble vitamin supplementation [10]. Yearly measurements of complete blood counts (CBC) allow for monitoring of anemia which may be secondary to iron deficiency, low hemoglobin, low hematocrit, low MCV (mean corpuscular volume) or overt blood loss; e.g. from bleeding esophageal/rectal varices in the cirrhotic CF patient or mucosal blood loss, e.g., in the CF patient with Crohn's disease. High MCV in the context of anemia may be indicative of a Vitamin B_{12} deficiency. Yearly comprehensive metabolic profiles allow for evaluation of protein stores (albumin) and screening for potential CF-related liver disease (abnormal alanine aminotransferase test (ALT), aspartate aminotransferase test (AST), and bilirubin), which may place them at further risk for nutritional deficiencies.

There are unique circumstances for some patients with cystic fibrosis which require additional laboratory evaluation.

Table 7.6 Standard *Yearly* lab evaluation recommended in all patients with cystic fibrosis

Measurement	What to order	If abnormal
Comprehensive metabolic profile	CMP	• Elevated AST, ALT, bilirubin may indicate CF liver disease (though poor predictor). Consider GI referral • Low albumin may be secondary to impaired liver synthetic function (consider GI referral) or may indicate poor nutritional status. • Elevated fasting glucose may be concerning for CF related diabetes. (Consider HgbA1c and/or glucose tolerance test) • Low bicarbonate (in context of failure to thrive—consider renal tubular acidosis)
Complete blood count with differential	CBC with differential	• Microcytic anemia—consider checking iron studies for iron deficiency; obtain Hemoccult to evaluate for possible GI sources of blood loss.
Gamma glutamyl transferase	GGT	• Elevation may be indicative of CF related liver disease (though poor predictor). Consider GI referral.
Vitamin A	Retinol	• Deficiency—monitor for vision problems (e.g. night blindness)
Vitamin D	25 (OH) Vitamin D	• Severe deficiency consider evaluation for osteoporosis/ osteopenia
Vitamin E	Alpha tocopherol	• Deficiency—monitor for peripheral neuropathy
Vitamin K	PT/INR	• Elevation may be secondary to nutritional deficiency or impaired liver synthetic function

Stool Labs

In addition to serum laboratory evaluation, stool evaluation can also assess a patient's nutritional status. All patients diagnosed with cystic fibrosis should have a fecal elastase performed to assess pancreatic sufficiency/insufficiency. A spot fecal elastase is an easy, quick, and reliable assessment of pancreatic sufficiency. Formed stool may be placed in a specimen cup and frozen until taken to the labs. Stool should be placed on ice and brought to the lab within 24 h of collection.

The 72 h fecal fat study is another method, albeit quite burdensome to do accurately, to diagnose steatorrhea. A coefficient of fat absorption study may be done using stool markers taken 72 h apart. The diet history should start and finish at the same time the stool markers are ingested (72 h timeframe). The stools should be collected from the initial stool marker stain through the second stool marker stain. The stool collection may take longer than 72 h due to variability in intestinal transit time. The result is calculated by using the following equation:

$$\frac{\left[\text{Grams fat consumed} - \text{Grams fat excreted}\right]}{\left[\text{Grams fat consumed}\right]}$$

This result should then be multiplied by 100 to obtain percent fat absorption during the 72 h time frame.

The validity of the results of 72 h fecal fat collection rests upon meticulous measurement of food intake, exact knowledge of fat content of foods and beverages consumed, and precise collection of stool output for the entire duration of the study.

While a 72 h fecal fat test can evaluate for fat malabsorption, a fecal hydrolysis stool study can evaluate for carbohydrate malabsorption by evaluating the stool for reducing substances. This test is ordered when there is a suspicion that a disaccharidase deficiency may be the cause of diarrhea. This stool usually should be water to loose and placed in a specimen cup. A fresh specimen may be submitted to the lab but needs to be submitted within 2 h of collection. Fecal hydrolysis stool specimen may also be a frozen specimen that is submitted to the lab within 24 h of collection.

If there is a concern for possible protein malabsorption, a fecal alpha-1 antitrypsin stool study can be useful in diagnosing protein-losing enteropathies especially when used in conjunction with serum alpha-1-antitrypsin (A1A) levels as part of A1A clearance studies. This stool specimen should also be a frozen specimen which is submitted within 24 h of collection.

Persistent Failure to Thrive Despite Optimal Caloric Intake/Other Gastrointestinal Disorders Which May Contribute to Poor Nutrition

For those patients with cystic fibrosis that have persistent failure to thrive despite adequate caloric intake, attention should be made to other conditions outside of cystic fibrosis that could contribute to persistent failure to thrive. Good clinical exam skills and history taking can provide clues to other reasons for poor growth. For instance, in a child with poor linear growth, providers may consider obtaining a free thyroxine (T4) and thyroid-stimulating hormone (TSH) to evaluate for possible thyroid disease. In the child with poor growth, abdominal pain, persistent loose stools with blood, inflammatory bowel disease should be considered; sending an erythrocyte sedimentation rate (ESR), C-reactive protein (CRP) albumin, CBC, and a stool calprotectin may be appropriate. The patient with persistent failure to thrive, abdominal distension and bloating, loose stools and abdominal pain should be evaluated for possible celiac disease with a Tissue Transglutaminase Immunoglobulin A (TTg IgA) and Total serum immunoglobulin A (total IgA). Table 7.7 provides a summary of potential gastrointestinal diseases that may be considered in the patient with cystic fibrosis and persistent malnutrition/failure to thrive.

Table 7.7 Other conditions that may result in malnutrition/failure to thrive

Condition	Clinical symptoms	Laboratory evaluation	Signs of disease
Inflammatory bowel disease	Abdominal pain, diarrhea, blood in stool, nocturnal stooling, perianal disease	CBC with d/p, CMP, ESR, CRP, Iron Studies, Fecal calprotectin	• Anemia, low albumin, elevated inflammatory makers, marked elevation of calprotectin, consider IBD
Celiac disease	Abdominal pain, abdominal bloating/distension, diarrhea, rash	TTg IgA, Total IgA, Celiac Genetic Screen	• Elevated TTg with normal levels of total IgA—consider celiac disease
Thyroid disease	Poor linear growth, temperature intolerance, rapid heart rate, sweating	T3, T4, TSH	• Low T3/T4 with elevated TSH consider hypothyroidism
Liver disease	Jaundice, hepatosplenomegaly, ascites, hematemesis, hematochezia	AST, ALT, GGT, albumin, PT/INR, CBC with d/p	• Thrombocytopenia, leukopenia may indicate portal hypertension. Low albumin or elevated INR may indicate impaired liver synthetic function
Renal tubular acidosis	Failure to thrive with persistent acidosis	Serum, bicarbonate, urine pH, urine electrolytes,	• Unexplained normal anion gap metabolic acidosis may be suggestive of RTA
Disaccharidase deficiency	Failure to thrive with chronic diarrhea	Fecal hydrolysis or disaccharidase analysis at endoscopy	• Elevated post fecal hydrolysis possible disaccharidase deficiency
Protein losing enteropathy	Failure to thrive, diarrhea, marked hypoalbuminemia	Fecal alpha-1-antitrypsin level	• High fecal alpha-1 antitrypsin may be suggestive of protein losing enteropathy.
Cardiac disease	Failure to thrive, hypoxia, heart murmur	Cardiac ECHO	• Consider cardiology referral for congenital heart disease
Metabolic disease	Failure to thrive, HSM, acidosis, developmental delay, abnormal muscle tone	Lactate, pyruvate, carnitine/acylcarnitine profile, serum amino acids, urine genetic screen	• High lactate/pyruvate ratio, abnormal carnitine/acylcarnitine, UGS may suggest mitochondrial/metabolic disorder.

Clinical Assessment

The clinical exam can provide many clues to the nutritional status and evidence of nutritional deficiencies. A complete and thorough physical exam is essential at each clinical visit. Attention should be made not only to the pulmonary and gastrointestinal exam but to a full physical exam to monitor for specific nutritional deficiencies. Table 7.8 provides a comprehensive overview of physical exam findings and potential nutritional deficiencies.

Diet History

To assess eating patterns as well as nutrient and caloric intake, a thorough diet history is required. The type of diet history and the amount of desired detail can vary from for each patient. For example, for a well-nourished individual who is gaining weight appropriately and who enjoys most foods, obtaining a "usual" daily intake or a "24-hour recall" may be sufficient. In the case of patients who struggle to gain weight despite their best efforts, a comprehensive review of intake using a food record is warranted to more accurately capture an understanding of feeding patterns and nutritional intake [2].

Table 7.8 Physical exam findings suggestive of possible nutritional deficiency[a]

	Finding	Suggestive nutritional deficiency
Skin	Pallor	Iron deficiency
	Dermatitis	Zinc deficiency
Neck	Enlarged thyroid	Iodine deficiency
Mouth	Dry, cracked, red lips	Riboflavin, niacin, or vitamin B6 deficiency
	Bleeding gums	Vitamin C deficiency
	Poor taste	Zinc deficiency
Eyes	Night blindness	Vitamin A deficiency
Hair	Thin or sparse hair	Zinc deficiency
Teeth	Excessive dental carries	Excessive simple carbohydrate intake
	Enamel hypoplasia	May be suggestive of celiac disease

[a]This table adapted from ASPEN Pediatric Nutrition Support Core Curriculum. 6th edition—editor in chief Mark Corkins, MD, CNSP, SPR, FAAP. ASPEN 8630 Fenton Street, Suite 412, Silver Spring, MD 20910-3805 [2]

This should include type and measured amounts of food eaten and beverages consumed; location, time, and duration of meal or snack; brand name or label of the food if available; preparation methods; amount served and amount actually eaten; and the number of enzymes taken at each time. Supplements and tube feedings should also be included in this history. The duration of the food record should be for at least 3 consecutive days, with one of those days being a weekend for an accurate reflection of average intake. There are also apps for smart phones which can assist patient's and their famililes in recording food intake food intake, or patients may record intake using computer programs. Food records submitted electronically increase the potential for "real-time" communication between the patient and the dietitian.

Asking patients and families about any adverse eating behaviors such as pain or difficulty swallowing, coughing, or choking with eating, abdominal pain or vomiting after eating, early satiety, and constipation may provide additional insight of factors that may contribute to poor caloric intake.

Related Diseases

A thorough medical history and knowledge of past medical history is important as related diseases can have a large impact on a child's nutritional status. For instance, surgical resection from meconium ileus in infancy can have a marked impact on nutritional status throughout a child's lifetime. A child with poorly controlled diabetes will have additional challenges in establishing good weight gain.

CF-Related Liver Disease

The vast majority of patients with cystic fibrosis will have elevation of transaminases at some point in their lifetime. Only a small percentage, 5–10% of patients with CF, will develop severe CF-related liver disease characterized by cirrhosis, portal hypertension, and decreased liver synthetic function [11]. The patient with severe CF-related liver disease is at increased risk for malnutrition given impaired bile flow. Fat-soluble vitamin levels should be monitored at least yearly in all patients with CF liver disease [10, 12]. If a patient requires additional vitamin supplementation, monitoring levels 1–2 months after starting supplementation ensures adequate levels have been obtained. Patients should have CBC with differential and platelets. Thrombocytopenia and leukopenia may be an indication of hypersplenism and/or portal hypertension. Iron deficiency anemia may be a result of

Table 7.9 Laboratory evaluation in the patient with severe CF related liver disease

Evaluation	Comment	Further work up/evaluation
CBC with differential and platelets (d/p)	• Anemia—consider blood loss from bleeding esophageal, gastric, rectal varices. • Thrombocytopenia—may be sign of portal hypertension/splenic sequestration • Leukopenia—may be sign of portal hypertension/splenic sequestration	• Hemoccult stool • Obtain iron studies • Consider endoscopy • Evaluate liver/spleen size on physical exam • Consider abdominal ultrasound with Dopplers • GI referral
CMP	• Hypoalbuminemia—may be sign of malnutrition and/or impaired synthetic function • Elevated AST, ALT, bilirubin—may be sign of worsening liver disease (although poor predictor)	• GI referral • Routine laboratory evaluation every 4–12 months
PT/INR	• Elevation indicative of impaired liver synthetic function or vitamin K deficiency	• Replacement with Vitamin K 1 mg/kg/year of age to max of 10 mg p.o. once daily.
GGT	• Elevation may be sign of obstructive liver disease (although poor predictor in CF)	• GI referral • Routine laboratory evaluation every 4–12 months
Fat-soluble vitamins	• Often low and require higher doses of supplementation compared to the CF patient without liver disease	• Supplement as necessary with follow up evaluation to ensure normal/improving levels.
Zinc	• Often low in liver disease	• Supplement as necessary with follow up evaluation to ensure normal/improving levels.

bleeding esophageal/rectal varices or bleeding portal hypertensive gastropathy. GGT is often elevated in the patient with CF and may be an indication of further impaired bile flow. Albumin and PT/INR evaluation allows for monitoring of impaired liver synthetic function which often does not occur until late in the disease process (Table 7.9).

CF-Related Diabetes

Cystic fibrosis-related diabetes is a common comorbidity in patients with cystic fibrosis affecting almost 20% of adolescent children [13]. Poorly controlled CF-related diabetes can further impact the nutritional status of the patient with cystic fibrosis. The CFF and American Diabetes Association have published clinical care guidelines for cystic fibrosis-related diabetes [14]. Screening for CF-related diabetes should begin at 10 years of age in all patients who do not have CF-related diabetes already diagnosed. HgbA$_1$c is not considered sufficiently sensitive and should not be used as a screening modality for CF related diabetes. Screening for CFRD should be performed using a 2 hour, 75 g oral glucose tolerance test [14]. Refer to Chapter 10 for more detailed information on CF-related diabetes.

Bone Disease

Clinical evaluation of bone health and monitoring for evidence of bone disease is important in the patient with cystic fibrosis. Pancreatic insufficient patients with CF are at further risk for poor bone health secondary to malabsorption of fat-soluble vitamins. Risk factors for poor bone health include

Table 7.10   Risk factors for poor bone health

Risk factors for poor bone health
Patients with CF who are candidates for organ transplantation
Post organ transplantation
End-stage lung disease
End-stage liver disease
Bone fracture secondary to low-impact activity
Chronic use of corticosteroids
Delayed pubertal development
Nutritional failure

patients that are candidates for organ transplantation, post-organ transplantation, end-stage lung disease, bone fracture with a low-impact activity, chronic corticosteroid use, delayed pubertal development, and nutritional failure (Table 7.10) [15]. Children 8 years and older who are at risk for poor bone health should have an assessment of bone mass by lumbar spine DEXA. In addition to the DEXA, children at risk for poor bone health should have annual serum calcium, phosphorous, intact parathyroid hormone, and 25-hydroxy vitamin D measured [15]. Dietary intake of calcium and vitamin D should be determined by dietary history at clinic visits [15]. See Chapter 4 for more detailed information on CF and Bone Health.

Stool History

A thorough stool history is as important as a good diet history (see Table 7.11). Providers should inquire as to how many stools a patient has in 24 hours. Consistency and caliber the stool should be ascertained (e.g. hard, soft, loose, watery, mushy, wide, difficult to pass). Presence of grease, oil, or mucous may represent suboptimal pancreatic enzyme replacement. Stooling patterns such as nocturnal stooling may be a clue to an underlying gastrointestinal disorder such as inflammatory bowel disease. Presence of blood in stool may also be indicative of an inflammatory process or could indicate presence of bleeding esophageal or rectal varices. It is important, especially in the pediatric population, to inquire about dietary history when taking a stool history. For instance, a child consuming 40 ounces of fruit juice a day could clearly lead to problems with diarrhea.

Vitamin and Mineral History

Since the first CF specific vitamin was introduced in 1991, there has been continued development of new vitamin products and periodic reformulation of existing ones. Creation and modification of CF specific vitamins reflects current research and knowledge of the specialized nutritional needs of individuals with CF. Vitamins specific for CF not only undergo periodic modification in their actual vitamin amounts, but also in the form in which specific vitamins are delivered. For example, vitamin A is provided in several of the products as a combination of beta-carotene and retinol, whereas earlier formulations and some of the current formulations are entirely from retinol (as a result, retinol activity equivalents may be a more prudent way to compare vitamin A content between products). Because CF specific vitamin products frequently change, specific product names and content have been purposely omitted from this section.

Table 7.11 Stool history and associated conditions with suggestive interventions

Stool quality	Potential condition	Suggestive intervention
Grease/oil in stool	• Pancreatic Insufficiency	• Review pancreatic enzyme supplementation and adherence • Obtain repeat fecal elastase if pancreatic sufficient patient with CF
Blood in stool	• Rectal Prolapse • Perianal fissure from constipation • Inflammatory bowel disease • Hemorrhoids	• Review pancreatic enzyme dosing • Soften stools with stool softener if hard stools/straining with toileting • Obtain laboratory evaluation (CBC with d/p, CMP, ESR, CRP) if concern for IBD • Soften stools if external hemorrhoids seen on exam
Acholic stools	• Biliary obstruction, liver disease	• Obtain AST, ALT, bilirubin, GGT, PT/INR • Consider abdominal ultrasound with Dopplers
Loose stools	• Pancreatic Insufficiency • Infectious • Malabsorption e.g. celiac) • Inflammatory (e.g. IBD)	• If acute and associated with prodromal symptoms consider infectious stool workup • If chronic and failure to thrive, consider evaluation for celiac, IBD, disaccharidase deficiency, adherence with pancreatic enzyme supplementation
Infrequent stools	• Constipation • DIOS	• Consider TTg IgA, IgA if associated failure to thrive. • Consider T4/TSH if poor linear growth • Consider stool softener and/or colonic motility agent
Hard stools	• Constipation • DIOS	• Consider stool softener and/or colonic motility agent

To obtain a reliable vitamin history, it is often useful to encourage patients to photograph the vitamin products they take (including all label information) or to ask them to bring their vitamin bottles with them to their clinic appointments. This helps eliminate the "guesswork" as many vitamin products have similar names which patients (as well as providers) can understandably have difficulty recalling the *exact* name or formulation of the product.

Adherence with vitamins in CF has been demonstrated to be variable [16]. It is helpful to ask open-ended questions such as, "How many times a week do your take your vitamin?" rather than "Do you take your vitamin every day?" It is important to know specifically what products your patient takes, as well as the dose and degree of frequency, in order to provide appropriate recommendations when updated serum lab values are known.

Pancreatic Enzyme Replacement Therapy History

A good pancreatic enzyme replacement history involves thorough knowledge of all enzyme products currently available on the market. The brand, strength, and dose of pancreatic enzyme replacement the patient is taking with all meals, snacks, and with supplements or tube feedings should be recorded at each clinic appointment. There should also be discussion regarding any difficulty taking or "remembering" enzymes. The time spent obtaining this history not only provides useful information to the clinician, but also affords the opportunity to assess patient knowledge and provide a refresher on the rationale and function of pancreatic enzyme replacement therapy. Inquiring about specific practices such as how many or even if enzymes are taken with a glass of milk, when and how enzymes are given with tube feedings, and the number of total enzymes taken in a day provides valuable information in assessing the adequacy of the present enzyme dosing regimen. Total comprehension of individual enzyme practice is essential in the context of weight, BMI, calorie, and stool/GI history.

For some families, showing the different enzyme products available by using a laminated picture or a pill case that contains all of the different pancreatic enzyme replacement capsules helps confirm the product being taken as well as provide visual depiction of capsule size. Calculation of dosing enzymes may be found in the chapter on pancreatic enzymes, but typically is estimated by lipase units/kg/meal; lipase units/kg/day; or lipase units/gram of fat.

Conclusion

There are multiple considerations in executing a thorough nutritional assessment for the patient with cystic fibrosis in the 2 to 20-year-old age group. Weight, height, and BMI are certainly key factors, but only when taken into consideration along with biochemical and clinical data; diet and gastrointestinal history; pancreatic enzyme replacement and vitamin supplementation practices; in addition to consideration of past and present medical conditions. As we continue to learn more about the association between nutrition and health outcomes, it is prudent to attain and maximize nutritional status early in childhood and maintain through adulthood.

References

1. Borowitz D, Baker RD, Stallings V. Consensus report on nutrition for pediatric patients with cystic fibrosis. J Pediatr Gastroenterol Nutr. 2002;35(3):246–59.
2. Corkins MR, Balint J. American Society for P, Enteral N. A.S.P.E.N. pediatric nutrition support core curriculum. Silver Spring: American Society for Parenteral and Enteral Nutrition; 2010.
3. Stallings VA, Stark LJ, Robinson KA, Feranchak AP, Quinton H. Evidence-based practice recommendations for nutrition-related management of children and adults with cystic fibrosis and pancreatic insufficiency: results of a systematic review. J Am Diet Assoc. 2008;108(5):832–9.
4. Yen EH, Quinton H, Borowitz D. Better nutritional status in early childhood is associated with improved clinical outcomes and survival in patients with cystic fibrosis. J Pediatr. 2013;162(3):530–5.e1.
5. Hendricks KM. Manual of pediatric nutrition. In: Walker WA, editor. 2nd ed. Ontario: B.C. Decker; 1990.
6. Pediatric nutrition: policy of the American Academy of Pediatrics. In: Kleinman RE, Greer FR, editors. 7th ed.
7. Frisancho AR. Anthropometric standards for the assessment of growth and nutritional status. Ann Arbor: University of Michigan Press; 1990.
8. Zhang Z, Shoff SM, Lai HJ. Incorporating genetic potential when evaluating stature in children with cystic fibrosis. J Cyst Fibros. 2010;9(2):135–42.
9. Himes JH, Roche AF, Thissen D, Moore WM. Parent-specific adjustments for evaluation of recumbent length and stature of children. Pediatrics. 1985;75(2):304–13.
10. Debray D, Kelly D, Houwen R, Strandvik B, Colombo C. Best practice guidance for the diagnosis and management of cystic fibrosis-associated liver disease. J Cyst Fibros. 2011;10 Suppl 2:S29–36.
11. Colombo C. Liver disease in cystic fibrosis. Curr Opin Pulm Med. 2007;13(6):529–36.
12. Sokol RJ, Durie PR. Recommendations for management of liver and biliary tract disease in cystic fibrosis. Cystic Fibrosis Foundation Hepatobiliary Disease Consensus Group. J Pediatr Gastroenterol Nutr. 1999;28 Suppl 1:S1–13.
13. Moran A, Dunitz J, Nathan B, Saeed A, Holme B, Thomas W. Cystic fibrosis-related diabetes: current trends in prevalence, incidence, and mortality. Diabetes Care. 2009;32(9):1626–31.
14. Moran A, Brunzell C, Cohen RC, Katz M, Marshall BC, Onady G, et al. Clinical care guidelines for cystic fibrosis-related diabetes: a position statement of the American Diabetes Association and a clinical practice guideline of the Cystic Fibrosis Foundation, endorsed by the Pediatric Endocrine Society. Diabetes Care. 2010;33(12):2697–708.
15. Aris RM, Merkel PA, Bachrach LK, Borowitz DS, Boyle MP, Elkin SL, et al. Guide to bone health and disease in cystic fibrosis. J Clin Endocrinol Metab. 2005;90(3):1888–96.
16. Modi AC, Lim CS, Yu N, Geller D, Wagner MH, Quittner AL. A multi-method assessment of treatment adherence for children with cystic fibrosis. J Cyst Fibros. 2006;5(3):177–85.

Chapter 8
Nutrition Assessment: Adults and Obesity

Judith A. Fulton and Alexandra W.M. Wilson

Key Points

- As patients with cystic fibrosis (CF) are living well into adulthood, nutrition-related comorbidities are becoming more common. As with children with CF, maintaining optimal nutrition status is associated with preserved lung function in adults with CF. Registered dietitians play a vital role in maintaining optimal nutrition status in adults with CF.
- An annual nutrition assessment is recommended and should include the following: assessment of dietary intake, pancreatic enzyme therapy replacement (PERT) usage, review of vitamin and mineral supplementation, and an evaluation of annual laboratory values.
- CF Foundation recommends a goal body mass index of 22 kg/m^2 or higher in adult females and 23 kg/m^2 or higher in adult males.
- A high calorie, unrestricted fat diet continues to be recommended in adults with CF with pancreatic insufficiency. Estimated protein needs are 1.5–2.0 times the recommended daily allowance. Supplemental tube feeding is recommended to adult patients with CF when other weight gain strategies have failed.
- Due to increased fat malabsorption, adults with CF are at higher risk of fat-soluble vitamin deficiency. For this reason, they are encouraged to use regular CF-specific multivitamin daily to prevent fat-soluble vitamin deficiency.
- Bone disease is common in adults with CF. Patients are encouraged to attain adequate intake of fat-soluble vitamins and calcium, participate in regular physical activity, and maintain a healthy body weight.
- CF-related diabetes is the most common co-morbidity in CF. It should be treated by a multi-disciplinary team familiar with CF and in consultation with the CF team.
- Gastroesophageal reflux is common in adults with CF. Appropriate medical, diet, and lifestyle management of reflux are encouraged.
- Overweight and obesity does occur in CF. Healthy weight, physical activity, and healthy diet are encouraged in overweight or obese patients with CF.

J.A. Fulton, M.P.H., R.D., L.D.N.
Clinical Nutrition, Children's Hospital Colorado, University of Colorado, Cystic Fibrosis Center,
13123 East 16th Avenue, B395, Aurora, CO 80045, USA
e-mail: judith.fulton@childrenscolorado.org

A.W.M. Wilson, M.S., R.D.N., C.D.E. (✉)
Food Service and Clinical Nutrition, National Jewish Health, Adult Cystic Fibrosis Program,
Colorado Cystic Fibrosis Center, 1400 Jackson Street, Room A02C, Denver, CO 80206, USA
e-mail: wilsona@njhealth.org

E.H. Yen, A.R. Leonard (eds.), *Nutrition in Cystic Fibrosis: A Guide for Clinicians*, Nutrition and Health,
DOI 10.1007/978-3-319-16387-1_8, © Springer International Publishing Switzerland 2015

Keywords Assessment • Dietitian • Nutrition • Body mass index • Pancreatic enzyme replacement therapy • Vitamin supplementation • Bone health • Cystic fibrosis related diabetes • Obesity • Overweight

Abbreviations

BMI   Body mass index
CDC   Center of disease control and prevention
CF   Cystic fibrosis
CFRD   Cystic fibrosis related diabetes
DEXA   Dual X-ray absorptiometry
FEV_1 Forced expiratory volume in 1 second
GER   Gastroesophageal reflux
PERT   Pancreatic enzyme replacement therapy

Introduction

"No achievement highlights the striking developments of the past few decades in cystic fibrosis (CF) care more clearly than the tremendous growth of the adult CF population" [1]. With the average life expectancy of an individual with CF increasing dramatically over the last three decades, we are seeing CF patients living well into adulthood and experiencing new non-respiratory illness such as diabetes, osteoporosis, and reproductive concerns. The importance of nutrition in the long-term survival of patients with CF has been well documented [2–5]. This section provides an overview of adult CF nutrition assessment and the importance of nutritional status in the long-term survival of patients with CF.

In the 1950s, CF was a childhood disease. At that time, a child diagnosed with CF would not live long enough to attend elementary school. With continual medical advancements as well as optimizing nutrition the median predicted survival age in 2013 was 40.7 (95% confidence interval: 37.7–44.1 years) [6]. In 2013 the CF Foundation Patient Registry followed 28,103 CF patients, and the number of patients greater than 18 years of age was 13,975 or 49.7% [6]. As new drug therapies and treatments continue to be developed, the number of adults living with this disease will only continue to increase. The CF Foundation Patient Registry has also reported adults with CF are living fulfilling lives [6, 7]. Throughout the phases of adult life, maintaining optimal nutrition status can be challenging.

In general, as the disease advances, adults with CF have more severe pulmonary disease than they do as children. This puts them at an increased risk for serious complications such as pneumothorax and massive hemoptysis. The majority of adult CF patients die of respiratory failure [6]. Slowing or preventing the decline in lung function is the most important challenge for a majority of patients. Although pulmonary physiotherapy and antibiotics are important to maintain lung health, good nutrition is a critical piece of this puzzle. By not accepting nutritional failure in pediatric CF patients, we can preserve their lung function as adults.

CF Nutrition Assessment: Adults

The CF Foundation recommends that a registered dietitian complete a structured nutrition assessment annually, in addition to nutrition follow-up and reinforcement visits. The CF annual visit should include the following: assessment of dietary intake, pancreatic enzyme therapy replacement (PERT) usage, and review of vitamin and mineral supplementation, and an evaluation of annual laboratory values. The assessment should also include assessment of nutrition and metabolic complications, and the appropriate screening tests [8, 9] as discussed in greater detail in this chapter. The annual nutrition assessment provides the framework for future nutrition care planning and anticipatory guidance. Refer to Table 8.1 for an adult CF nutrition assessment flow sheet.

Adult Weight/Height Assessment

Growth of a child with CF is monitored by tracking weight and height at intervals on a standard growth curve. After 20 years of age the growth chart is no longer used, but this doesn't mean the importance of weight and height diminishes when assessing nutrition. The CF Foundation Clinical Practice Guidelines Growth and Nutrition Subcommittee published data looking at the relationship between body mass index (BMI) and lung function in the CF population in 2008 [8]. As a result of this data CF Foundation recommends a goal BMI of 22 kg/m^2 or higher in females and 23 kg/m^2 or higher in males [8]. These values correlated with a forced expiratory volume in 1 second (FEV_1)>60% predicted [8]. In this adult CF group, there was no evidence of decreased FEV_1 up to a BMI of 29 and the sample of adults with a BMI over 29.9 (obesity) was too small for analyses [8]. As described in the obesity section this population is growing which may allow us to observe this trend change. It is not known whether a BMI greater than the CF Foundation goal would be associated with further increased lung function.

Pancreatic Status

Pancreatic insufficiency usually develops during infancy, and approximately 90% of adult patients with CF are pancreatic insufficient resulting in chronic nutrient malabsorption [9]. There is a correlation between genotype and phenotype in regard to the exocrine function of the pancreas [10]. Being pancreatic insufficient suggests not enough pancreatic function is available to achieve normal digestion. That is, absorption of fat and protein is compromised, resulting in symptoms of malabsorption. These symptoms include poor weight gain despite adequate calories, frequent bowel movements, abdominal pain, bulky, large and/or light colored stools, oil or grease in stool, and excessive gas. PERT adequacy is determined clinically by monitoring nutritional status, signs and symptoms of malabsorption, and excessive appetite with poor weight gain. Inadequate doses of PERT may result in malabsorption, abdominal pain, and constipation. Please refer to Chapter 7 for more detailed information on pancreatic enzyme dosing and management.

In adult patients with CF, who are pancreatic sufficient, the pancreatic function can decline with age. The result is pancreatic insufficiency [1]. Pancreatic sufficient patients should be routinely asked about their stools so that malabsorption can be addressed early. These patients are at higher risk for acute or recurrent episodes of pancreatitis as compared to the general population [11]. Treatment of pancreatitis with CF is similar to the general population and requires adequate pain management and gut rest. Recurrent episodes of pancreatitis may lead to pancreatic insufficiency requiring PERT. Please refer to Chapter 12 for more information regarding pancreatitis.

Assessing Intake

Calorie and protein requirements can sometimes be higher in adults than children with CF, despite not having to account for growth [12]. Higher calories may be needed for the increased work of breathing and frequent infections along with the progressive pancreatic insufficiency [9, 13]. A broad

Table 8.1 Adult CF nutrition assessment

Table 2:   **Adult CF Nutrition Assessment**

Name:_____   Pt's Home: _____

DOB: _____   Insurance: Private / Government

                                                        Enzyme Program: Yes / No

Medications: _____

Other Diagnoses: _____

Height: _____

	Date	Date	Date
Age			
Weight & %IBW			
BMI & IBW			
Recent weight changes			
Appetite			
Supplement			
PERT - dose & TDD			
PERT - timing			
Vitamins			
Calcium			
Other vitamins / herbals			
Food allergies or intolerances			
Nausea / Vomiting			
Diarrhea			
Constipation			
Meds for D/C			
#BMs daily			
Consistency			
Heartburn & meds			
Dysgeusia			
Early satiety			
Dry mouth			
Chewing / Dysphagia			
CFRD / IGT / Indeterminate			
Insulin / CHO ratio			
SMBG			
Exercise / Activity			
Pregnant or desiring			
FEV1 %			

_____
_____
_____
_____
_____
_____
_____
_____
_____

(continued)

Table 8.1 (continued)

Labs			
	Date	Date	Date
Vitamin A			
Vitamin D			
Vitamin E			
PTT or vitamin K			
Glucose			
Albumin			
HgbA1c			
Ferritin / Iron			
Other labs:			
OGTT: fast, 30 min, 1hr, 2hr			
Bone DEXA			
L1-L4 (t-score, z-score)			
L femur (t-score, z-score)			
R femur (t-score, z-score)			
Radius (t-score, z-score)			

recommendation for energy requirements for patients with CF is 120–150% of requirements for the general population [14, 15]. Actual caloric requirements vary from person to person, but often increase as the lung disease progresses. For example, an adult male could require between 3500 and 4500 cal which is approximately 150% more than an individual without CF. To meet these higher caloric needs the adult patient with CF needs to consume at least 3 meals and 2–3 snacks a day. Skipping a meal or snack or not taking pancreatic enzymes as prescribed will cause caloric intake or nutrient absorption to be inadequate. Monitoring weight at each CF clinic visit is important along with assessing caloric intake. Please refer to Chapter 2, Table 2.1 for a review of the 2005 Estimated Energy Requirement equations.

A high calorie, liberal fat diet is standard practice for the CF population throughout the life cycle. The tendency to restrict fat consumption in these patients should be discouraged because dietary fat is calorically dense, improves the palatability of the foods and is needed to prevent essential fatty acid deficiency. Research suggests lipid profiles of adult CF patients who have been on a high calorie, high fat diet their entire life were not elevated; therefore a high calorie, unrestricted fat diet continues to be recommended in adults with CF with pancreatic insufficiency [16].

Of note, reports of adult patients who were pancreatic sufficient did have high-normal cholesterol levels [17]. Higher serum triglyceride levels in patients with CF compared to the standard population with several incidences of hypertriglyceridemia have been observed [18, 19]. The etiology is not fully understood, but chronic inflammation, excessive carbohydrate intake, or absorption of a high fat diet has been proposed [18, 19]. There are reports of premature atrial damage compared to controls [20] and a few reports of myocardial infarction in the aging CF population [21, 22]. Due to the potential for cardiovascular disease in the adult CF population, encouraging increased intake of mono-unsaturated and poly-unsaturated fatty acids rather than saturated fatty acids may be prudent. Please refer to Chapter 2, Table 2.2 to review common food sources of unsaturated and saturated fatty acids.

Protein is an important nutrient to prevent catabolism. The recommended intake for adults with CF is 1.5–2 times the recommended daily allowance [23, 24]. A protein intake of 15–20% of total calories [23, 24] has been suggested. When recommending a protein amount to an adult patient with CF, it may be best to provide the goal in total grams of protein per day. Please refer to Chapter 2, Table 2.4 for recommended daily allowance for protein.

Some adult patients with CF are not able to consume enough calories in their diet to maintain a healthy weight and adequate BMI. For these patients, supplemental tube feedings can counter the challenge of consuming enough calories every day. This option of nutrition therapy should be discussed with each patient who continues to struggle with his or her weight and when other recommendations have failed. There is concern placing and using feeding tubes in adults with advanced lung disease and this is related to a decreased ability to achieve a productive cough and do chest physiotherapy. With this decreased mucous clearance, there is more risk of lung infections. Most feeding tube research in CF has been done in children, who usually have less lung disease. It is important to place a gastrostomy tube prior to significant decline in lung function to result in better outcome results. The option of supplemental tube feeding should be initiated as a means to maintain lung health and nutrition rather than a rescue option or a threat when all else has failed. Please refer to Chapter 8 for more detail regarding supplemental tube feedings.

Adult Nutrition Intervention

Nutrition intervention and counseling are important parts of the CF clinic visit. The medical team needs to work with the CF patient to help reach their BMI goal by using diet intervention and nutrition counseling strategies. Table 8.2 offers examples of nutrition strategies to counsel adult CF patients.

Table 8.2 Nutrition strategies to counsel adult CF patients

• Have snack foods available away from home, in office, backpack, or car.
• Use a diet phone app to track calories to help reach caloric goal.
• Avoid soda, empty calories, and try and drink milk with meals.
• Keep peanut butter readily available to eat a spoonful 1–2x/day (1 tablespoon=95 cal)
• Investigate insurance coverage of oral supplements—use a prior authorization form or letter.
• Utilize the enzyme company programs for free CF vitamins and oral supplements.
• Take the time to eat 3 meals and 2–3 snacks a day—use a phone alarm to remind you.
• Target 1 meal or snack a day to add extra calories. 100 extra calories can add up.
• Easy ways to add calories—order extra cheese on pizza, butter the bread of your sandwich.
• Have a container of heavy cream available to add when cooking.
• Use a weekly pillbox, so you don't have to open bottles all the time and can help compliance.
• Remember to take PERT with all meals and snacks to absorb all those calories.
• If you forget to take enzymes at certain times, set a phone alarm to help remember.
• Make meals on weekends for the week, or use a crockpot for a meal when you return home.
• Put meal doses of enzymes in Baggies and put them next to your cell phone and car keys.
• Take enzymes at the start of the meal or if eating >45 min spread over meal.
• When eating fatty fast food take extra enzymes for those extra calories.
• Keep enzymes in several places, backpack, office, friends and relatives, etc.
• Remember to take enzymes with all beverages including lattes, milk, oral supplements.
• Remember some foods don't require PERT (fruit, popsicles, juice, plain pretzels).
• If doing night tube feedings, take PERT as prescribed to maximize absorption.
• Remember enzymes are heat sensitive and cannot be stored in a hot place like a car.

Similar to guidelines in the United States, the European CF Society Standards of Care published guidelines in 2014 recommending adults to maintain a BMI > 20 with an ideal BMI of 22 for females and of 23 for males [25]. They also recommend nutrition intervention to be tried stepwise for a limited period of time or until nutritional status is optimized, depending on the severity of malnutrition and the age of the patient. They recommend the first step to be anticipatory guidance and include the following: reinforcement of adherence to the CF diet, enzyme recommendations, vitamin and mineral supplementation, and using behavioral modification or motivational interviewing. The second step of nutrition intervention for moderate malnutrition includes the use of oral supplements for additional calories in a time-limited trial or temporarily as meal replacement for ill patients. In addition, temporary tube feeds may be used to maintain calories during a pulmonary exacerbation to prevent weight loss. In severe malnutrition, and when these two steps fail, the third step of nutrition intervention would be enteral feeding to improve and then maintain nutrition [25].

Vitamin and Mineral Supplementation

Optimal vitamin and minerals are essential for the overall health of an individual with CF. Although a balanced diet contributes to the overall nutrient intake, there is a need for oral vitamin and mineral supplements. CF patients, especially those with pancreatic insufficiency, are at risk of fat-soluble vitamin deficiency and the importance of supplementing vitamins A, D, E, and K has been well documented [1, 9, 26, 27]. Through all stages of life, patients with CF are prescribed fat-soluble vitamins as part of their medical therapy. The doses are higher than recommended for people without

CF to prevent deficiency and keep their vitamin levels in an optimal range. Low vitamin levels occur for several reasons including inadequate adherence to recommended therapy, inadequate dietary intake, malabsorption, drug-nutrient interactions, liver disease, or bowel resection [28–30].

The introduction of CF-specific multivitamin supplements coupled with improved pancreatic enzyme replacement therapy has contributed to the reduction in the incidence and prevalence of vitamin deficiency. It is standard practice for all adult patients with CF who are followed at a CF Foundation-accredited Center to have their fat-soluble vitamin levels monitored annually. If levels are low and require repletion, they should be re-evaluated, ideally in 3 months until optimal levels are reached. Adult patients with CF are at risk of iron-deficiency and iron-deficiency anemia from chronic disease. Finally, due to malabsorption of vitamins D and K, adult CF patients are at risk of low bone mineral density, making assessment of calcium intake also important. Please review Chapter 6 on vitamins and minerals for more specific information on the research and the current recommendations.

Bone Health

The prevalence of bone disease among adult patients with CF is growing as this population ages, and is exacerbated by malnutrition and advanced lung disease [31]. As of 2012, the CF Foundation Patient Registry reports 36% of adult's ages 35 and older had CF-related bone disease (including fractures, osteopenia, and osteoporosis) [32]. Multiple factors contribute to the development of bone disease including: inadequate nutrition, suboptimal vitamin D levels, glucocorticoid therapy, physical inactivity, delayed puberty, and early hypogonadism [31, 33]. Chronic pulmonary inflammation can also increase serum cytokine levels, which may increase bone resorption and decrease bone formation [31, 33].

Although prevention therapy of bone disease is encouraged in the pediatric population, adults currently treat osteopenia to prevent progression to osteoporosis. According to the CF Foundation guidelines, starting at 18 years of age, all individuals with CF should have a baseline dual X-ray absorptiometry (DEXA) scan to determine bone mineral density. If the DEXA scan is normal, then repeat scans should be conducted every five years to monitor for disease [31]. Individuals with CF can maintain their bone health by ensuring adequate intake of fat-soluble vitamins and calcium, participating in regular physical activity, and maintaining a healthy body weight. The European CF Society Standards of Care recommend all CF Centers be familiar with the risk factors contributing to the development of reduced bone mass density. The most common risk factors include: pulmonary infections, poor nutritional status, lack of weight bearing exercise, delayed puberty, glucocorticoid treatment, hypogonadism, and vitamins D and K, as well as calcium deficiencies [32]. Please refer to Chapter 4 for specific guidelines for screening and treating bone disease in the CF population.

Cystic Fibrosis Related Diabetes

The number of patients diagnosed with CFRD is rapidly increasing, possibly reflecting better screening and improved CF survival. The annual incidence of CFRD is reported to increase with age at 5% a year in patients 10 years of age and 9.3% a year in patients 20 years of age and older [33, 34]. Data from the University of Minnesota, where they preformed annual screening oral glucose tolerance test (OGTT) starting at age 6 years, reported CFRD in 2% of children, 19% of adolescents, and 40–50% adults [34]. Patients with CFRD require medical care from a multi-disciplinary management team with experience in CFRD and in consultation with the CF team. CFRD is caused by progressive insulin deficiency secondary to progressive destruction of the pancreas in CF, specifically to the insulin-producing Beta cells [35]. CFRD shares characteristics of both type 1 and type 2 diabetes, but is clinically distinct and requires a unique management approach [34]. Treatment with systemic glucocorticoids can exacerbate hyperglycemia in CF. Declining lung function, weight loss, protein catabolism and increased mortality are all associated with the CFRD diagnosis [34, 35]. In 2010 the CF Foundation along with the American Diabetes Association and the Pediatric Endocrine Society published clinical care guidelines for the screening, diagnosis, and medical management of CFRD [35]. Refer to Chapter 10 on additional guidance for the screening, treatment, and nutritional management of CFRD.

Gastroesophageal Reflux

Approximately 80% of adults with CF have heartburn or gastroesophageal reflux (GER) [36]. Delayed gastric emptying, increased stomach acid, the altered shape of the chest, and changes in the diaphragm found in adults with CF may contribute to GER. The CF team should be aware of the signs and symptoms of GER and be able to provide appropriate diagnostic testing (impedance and pH probe, upper endoscopy) and treatment [25]. In most instances, typical GER symptoms are heartburn, regurgitation of stomach contents into the mouth, and upper abdominal pain [36, 37]. The dietitian should review the diet history and offer recommendations for avoiding foods that could be aggravating symptoms and encourage smaller more frequent meals, eating slower and avoiding lying flat after eating. The usual medication treatment for GER is acid suppression and the use of motility agents. Please refer to Chapter 12 for more details on GER in CF.

Obesity in Cystic Fibrosis

Cystic fibrosis (CF) is often associated with malnutrition primarily from pancreatic insufficiency, inadequate intake, and increased energy expenditure. Malnutrition has been associated with the rapid progression of lung disease and shortened lifespan [38]. Countering malnutrition by promoting normal growth velocity and maintaining adequate nutrition is standard CF therapy. With earlier CF diagnosis through newborn screening, aggressive nutrition therapy and regular medical follow-up, the prevalence of malnutrition has significantly decreased in patients with CF [26]. In contrast, the 2013 CF Foundation Patient Registry reports that the percentage of both overweight and obesity in this population is on the rise. The Centers for Disease Control and Prevention (CDC) has classified overweight and obesity in pediatrics and adults using BMI [39, 40]. Tables 8.3 and 8.4 summarize the metrics referenced by the CDC for overweight and obesity in the general population [39, 40].

Table 8.3   Pediatric CDC classification of overweight and obesity [3]

BMI percentile	Weight status
>85th and <95th	Overweight
>95th	Obesity

Table 8.4   Adult CDC classification of overweight and obesity [4]

BMI	Weight status
25–29.9	Overweight
30 and above	Obesity

Pediatrics

The 2013 CF Foundation Patient Registry followed 28,103 patients with CF in the United States; 15,707 were children less than 20 years of age. Approximately 3.5% (or 543 of 15,707) of children ages 2–19 years had a BMI>95th percentile were considered obese. Approximately 8% (or 1279 of 15,707) of the CF pediatric population had a BMI %>85% and <95th percentile were considered overweight [6]. Some CF Centers have reported an obesity and overweight rate as high as 23% in children and have noted 28% of their obese patients were pre-hypertensive and 6% were hypertensive [41]. The overweight and obese patients were mostly pancreatic insufficient and were not associated with better lung function [41]. The increase in the obesity rate in the CF population may be related to the increased prevalence in the general population. In addition, the earlier diagnosis through neonatal screening, combined with earlier intensive interventions could be contributing to this trend [42].

Adults

The 2013 CF Foundation Patient Registry followed 12,396 adults (non-transplant) with CF over the age of 20. Approximately 5% (or 623 of 12,396) of adults had a BMI>30 were considered obese [6]. Approximately 18% (or 2209 of 12,396) of the CF adult population reported a BMI between 25 and 29.9 were considered overweight [6]. This higher percentage of overweight and obese adult CF patients is projected to increase as the life expectancy increases for this population.

The CF Foundation Clinical Practice Guidelines Growth and Nutrition Subcommittee published the importance of BMI status as a function of optimal lung function in the CF population in 2008 [8]. They published recommended BMI percentile in children and recommended BMI in adults that were sensitive to changes on percent predicted forced expiratory volume in 1 second (FEV_1) [8]. The FEV_1 is a spirometry measurement used to evaluate lung function. In children, they reported better FEV_1 status at 80% predicted or above to be associated with a BMI at or above the 50th percentile [8]. In adults they reported an FEV_1 of 60% predicted or above to be associated with a BMI of 22 or higher in females and a BMI of 23 or higher in males. For adults, there was no evidence of decreased FEV_1 up to a BMI of 29 and the sample of adults with a BMI>29 (obesity) was too small for analyses [8]. From the 2013 CF Patient Registry Report, we can see a subgroup of patients have achieved BMIs higher than what is considered healthy for the general population. It is not known whether a BMI higher than the CF Foundation goal would be associated with further increased lung function.

Since the CF Foundation nutrition guideline publication in 2008, the many CF Centers have initiated quality improvement programs aimed at improving BMI in their CF populations. To date the majority of nutrition guidelines for individuals with CF focus on increasing BMI. There is a lack of recommendations to manage obese or overweight patients in this population. Since there are no specific guidelines for CF, recommendations similar to those for the general population, including a lower calorie, healthy diet along with increased exercise, may be some of the first step in counseling these patients. Further studies are needed to better determine optimal management of overweight and obese pediatric and adult patients with CF.

Conclusion

Although CF has long been viewed as a pediatric disease, it has now evolved into an adult disease bringing new medical advances, research breakthroughs, and interdisciplinary healthcare teams that have led to a dramatic improvement in the life expectancy and the quality of life for these individuals.

Advanced age with CF can lead to complications, but it also means individuals can develop careers, marry, and start families. Careful monitoring of nutritional status is important for early detection and correction of unfavorable trends. Patients of all ages should be aware of their weight goals for optimal nutrition. Dietitians should be a key member of the CF medical team and assist when a patient presents with malnutrition or weight loss. The primary nutrition goal of the CF medical team should be the prevention of malnutrition at all ages, including adults, and adequate management of nutrition-related comorbidities.

References

1. Yankaskas JR, Marshall BC, Sufian B, Simon RH, Rodman D. Cystic fibrosis adult care- consensus conference report. Chest. 2004;125:1S–39.
2. Kraemer R, Rudeberg A, Hadorn B. Relative underweight in cystic fibrosis and its prognostic value. Acta Paediatr Scand. 1978;67:33–7.
3. Huang NN, Schidlow DV, Szatrowski TH. Clinical features, survival rate and prognostic factors in young adults with cystic fibrosis. Am J Med. 1987;82:871–9.
4. Corey M, McLaughlin FJ, Williams M, Levison H. A comparison of survival, growth, and pulmonary function in patients with cystic fibrosis in Boston and Toronto. J Clin Epidemiol. 1988;41 suppl 6:583–91.
5. Liou TG, Adler FR, FitzSimmons SC. Predictive 5-year survivorship model of cystic fibrosis. Am J Epidemiol. 2001;153:345–52.
6. Cystic fibrosis patient registry. Bethesda, MD: Cystic Fibrosis Foundation; 2013.
7. Orenstein DM, Spahr JE, Weiner DJ. Cystic fibrosis: a guide for patient and family. 4th ed. Philadelphia, PA. Lippincott Williams & Wilkins; 2012.
8. Stallings VA, Stark LJ, Robison KA, Feranchak AP, Quinton H, The Clinical Practice Guidelines on Growth and Nutrition Subcommittee. Evidence-based practice recommendations for nutrition-related management of children and adults with cystic fibrosis and pancreatic insufficiency: results of a systemic review. J Am Diet Assoc. 2008;108 suppl 5:832–9.
9. Ramsey BW, Farrell PM, Pencharz P, Consensus Committee. Nutritional assessment and management in cystic fibrosis: a consensus report. Am J Clin Nutr. 1992;55:108–16.
10. Schibli S, Durie PR, Tullis ED. Proper usage of pancreatic enzymes. Curr Opin Pulm Med. 2002;8(6):542–6.
11. Cohn JA, Friedman KJ, Noone PG. Relation between mutations of the cystic fibrosis gene and idiopathic pancreatitis. N Engl J Med. 1998;339:653–8.
12. Bell SC, Saunders MJ, Elborn JS, Shale DJ. Resting energy expenditure and oxygen cost of breathing in patients with cystic fibrosis. Thorax. 1996;51:126–31.
13. Murphy JL, Wootton SA, Bond SA, Jackson AA. Energy content of stools in normal healthy controls and patients with cystic fibrosis. Arch Dis Child. 1991;61:495–500.
14. Dodge JA. Nutritional requirements in cystic fibrosis: a review. J Pediatr Gastroenterol Nutr. 1988;7 suppl 1:S8–11.
15. Dodge JA, Turck D. Cystic fibrosis: nutritional consequences and management. Best Pract Res Clin Gastroenterol. 2006;20 suppl 3:531–46.
16. Slesinenski MJ, Gloninger MF, Costantino JP, Orenstein DM. Lipid levels in adults with cystic fibrosis. J Am Diet Assoc. 1994;94:402–8.
17. Rhodes B, Nash EF, Tullis E, Pencharz PB, Brotherwood M, Dupuis A, Stephenson A. Prevention of dyslipidemia in adults with cystic fibrosis. J Cyst Fibros. 2010;9:24–8.
18. Figueroa V, Milla C, Parks EJ, Schwarzenberg SJ, Moran A. Abnormal lipid concentrations in cystic fibrosis. Am J Clin Nutr. 2002;75:1005–11.
19. Georgiopoulou VV, Denker A, Bishop KL, Brown JM, Hirsh B, Wolfenden L, Sperling L. Metabolic abnormalities in adults with cystic fibrosis. Respirology. 2010;15:823–9.
20. Hull JH, Garrod R, Ho TB, Knight RK, Cockcroft JR, Shale DJ, Bolton CE. Increased augmentation index in patients with cystic fibrosis. Eur Respir J. 2009;34 suppl 6:1322–8.
21. O'Nady GM, Farinet CL. An adult cystic fibrosis patient presenting with persistent dyspnea: case report. BMC Pulm Med. 2006;6:9–12.
22. Aratari MT, Venuta F, DeGiacoma T, Rendina EA, Anile M, Diso D, Francioni F, Quattrucci S, Rolla M, Pugliese F, Liparulo V, DiStasio M, Ricella C, Tsagkaropoulos S, Ferretti G, Coloni CF. Lung transplantation for cystic fibrosis: ten years of experience. Transplant Proc. 2008;40:2001–2.
23. Macdonald A, Holden C, Harris G. Nutritional strategies in cystic fibrosis: current issues. J R Soc Med. 1991; 84 suppl 18:28–35.

24. MacDonald A. Nutritional management of cystic fibrosis. Arch Dis Child. 1996;74:81–7.
25. Smyth AR, Bell SC, Bojein S, Bryon M, Duff A, Flume P, Kashirskaya N, Munck A, Ratjen F, Schwarzebberg SJ, Sermet-Gaudelus I, Southern KW, Taccetti G, Ullrich G, Wolfe S. European Cystic Fibrosis Society standards of care: best practice guidelines. J Cyst Fibros. 2014;13:23–42.
26. Sinaasappel M, Stern M, Littlewood J, Wolfe S, Steinkamp G, Harry GM, Heijerman HGN, Robberecht E, Doring G. Nutrition in patients with cystic fibrosis: a European consensus. J Cyst Fibros. 2002;1:51–75.
27. Borowitz D, Durie PR, Clarke L. Gastrointestinal outcomes and confounders in cystic fibrosis. J Pediatr Gastroenterol Nutr. 2005;41(3):273–85.
28. Hollander FM, DeRoos NM, Dopheide J, Hoekstra T, Van Berkhout FT. Self-reported use of vitamin and other nutritional supplements in adult patients with cystic fibrosis. Is daily practice in concordance with recommendations? Int J Vitam Nutr Res. 2010;80(6):408–15.
29. Palmery M, Saraceno A, Vaiarelli A, Carlomagno G. Oral contraceptives and changes in nutritional requirements. Eur Rev Med Pharmacol Sci. 2013;17:1804–13.
30. Siwamogsatham O, Dong W, Binongo JN, Chowdhury R, Alvarez JA, Feinman SJ, Enders J, Tangpricha V. Relationship between fat-soluble vitamin supplementation and blood concentrations in adolescents and adult patients with cystic fibrosis. Nutr Clin Pract. 2014;29:491–7.
31. Aris RM, Merkel PA, Bachrach LK. Guide to bone health and disease in cystic fibrosis. J Clin Endocrinol Metab. 2005;90(3):1888–96.
32. Lrgroux-Gerot I, Leroy S, Prudhomme C. Bone loss in adults with cystic fibrosis: prevalence, associated factors, and usefulness of biological markers. Joint Bone Spine. 2012;79(1):73–7.
33. Moran A, Becker D, Casella SJ. Epidemiology, pathophysiology, and prognostic implications of cystic fibrosis related diabetes: a technical review. Diabetes Care. 2010;33(12):2677–83.
34. Moran A, Dunitz J, Nathan B, Saeed A, Holme B, Thomas W. Cystic fibrosis related diabetes: current trends in prevalence, incidence and mortality. Diabetes Care. 2009;32(9):1626–31.
35. Moran A, Brunzell C, Cohen RC, Katz M, Marshal BS, Onady G. Clinical care guidelines for cystic fibrosis related diabetes: a position statement of the American Diabetes Association and a clinical practice guideline of the Cystic Fibrosis Foundation, endorsed by the Pediatric Endocrine Society. Diabetes Care. 2010;33:2697–708.
36. Ledson M, Tran J, Walshaw M. Prevalence and mechanisms of gastro-esophageal reflux in adult cystic fibrosis patients. J R Soc Med. 1998;91:7–9.
37. Orenstein S, Khan S. Gastroesophageal reflux. In: Walker W, Goulet OJ, Kleinman R, Sherman P, Shneider B, Sanderson I, editors. Pediatric gastrointestinal disease: pathophysiology, diagnosis, management. 4th ed. Ontario: BC Decker; 2003.
38. Yen EH, Quinton H, et al. Better nutritional status in early childhood is associated with improved clinical outcomes and survival in patients with cystic fibrosis. J Pediatr. 2013; 162:530–535. e 531.
39. About BMI for Children's and Teens. Centers for Disease Control and Prevention. 2015. http://www.cdc.gov/healthyweight/assessing/bmi/childrens_bmi/about_childrens_bmi.html.
40. About BMI for Adults. Centers for Disease Control and Prevention. 2015. http://www.cdc.gov/healthyweight/assessing/bmi/adult_bmi/.
41. Reem HM, Weiner DJ. Overweight and obesity in patients with cystic fibrosis: a center-based analysis. Pediatr Pulmonol. 2014. doi:10.1002/ppul.23033.
42. Farrell PM, Kosorok MR, et al. Early diagnosis of cystic fibrosis through neonatal screening prevents severe malnutrition and improves long-term growth. Wisconsin Cystic Fibrosis Neonatal Screening Study Group. Pediatrics. 2001;107:1–13.

Chapter 9
Nutrition Intervention

Ala K. Shaikhkhalil, Suzanne H. Michel, Maria R. Mascarenhas, and Virginia A. Stallings

Key Points

- Optimizing nutrition and obtaining goal body mass index is correlated with improved survival in children and adults with cystic fibrosis (CF).
- Maintaining an adequate intake of nutrients is often challenging in this patient population and nutrition interventions become necessary.
- Education, behavioral counseling, oral formulas, and calorie boosting are commonly used to increase energy intake.
- When interventions using the oral route are not sufficient to maintain weight and or growth, enteral tube feeding is used.
- Management of enteral tube feeding requires knowledge of caloric requirements, methods of administration including use of enzymes and choice of formula, effect of tube feeding on quality of life, and long-term health and pulmonary outcomes related to its use.
- Appetite stimulants can serve as an adjuvant to other interventions and have been proven to provide nutrition-related advantages with a reasonably safe side effect profile.
- There is a role for using parenteral nutrition in severely ill patients, those who have short bowel, or can't tolerate enteral nutrition
- Well-designed, large-scale clinical trials are required to provide additional evidence on what interventions are appropriate given the complexity of modern CF care.

Keywords Cystic fibrosis • Nutrition interventions • Oral supplements • Calorie boosting • Enteral tube feeding • Appetite stimulants • Parenteral nutrition

A.K. Shaikhkhalil, M.D. (✉)
Division of Gastroenterology, Hepatology and Nutrition, The Ohio State University College of Medicine, Nationwide Children's Hospital, 700 Children's Drive, Columbus, OH 43205, USA
e-mail: ala.shaikhkhalil@nationwidechildrens.org

S.H. Michel, M.P.H., R.D., L.D.N.
Pulmonary Medicine, Medical University of South Carolina, PO Box 1674, Folly Beach, SC 29439-1674, USA
e-mail: Smichelrd@aol.com

M.R. Mascarenhas, M.B.B.S. • V.A. Stallings, M.D.
Division of Gastroenterology, Hepatology and Nutrition, Children's Hospital of Philadelphia, Philadelphia, PA, USA

Perelman School of Medicine University of Pennsylvania, Philadelphia, PA, USA
e-mail: Mascarenhas@email.chop.edu; stallingsv@email.chop.edu

E.H. Yen, A.R. Leonard (eds.), *Nutrition in Cystic Fibrosis: A Guide for Clinicians*, Nutrition and Health, 129
DOI 10.1007/978-3-319-16387-1_9, © Springer International Publishing Switzerland 2015

Abbreviations

BMI   Body mass index
BMR   Basal metabolic rate
CF   Cystic fibrosis
CFF   Cystic fibrosis foundation
COA   Coefficient of fat absorption
FFM   Fat-free mass
GERD   Gastroesophageal reflux disease
PEG   Percutaneous endoscopic gastrostomy
PERT   Pancreatic enzyme replacement therapy
PI   Pancreatic insufficient
PN   Parenteral nutrition
$ppFEV_1$ Percentage of predicted forced expiratory volume in 1 second
PS   Pancreatic sufficient
RD   Registered dietitian
STF   Supplemental tube feeding
WHO   World Health Organization

Introduction

Optimal energy intake is paramount for persons who have CF. There is conflicting evidence describing energy intake by persons who have CF. Some research describes inadequate intake therefore compromising weight and linear growth, [1–5] other studies reveal adequate energy intake, with varied fat intake [6, 7]. Use of diet records may not provide data reflective of actual intake and therefore be unreliable [7, 8]. Determining appropriate energy intake for persons who have CF is challenging and impacted by a constellation of factors including: sex [9, 10], age [11], pulmonary status [12, 13], gastrointestinal status with resultant maldigestion and malabsorption [9], pubertal stage [14], pulmonary exacerbation [15], fat-free mass [10], genotype [16, 17], physical activity [18], and medical complications such as CF-related liver disease and diabetes [19].

Mathematical formulas are available to estimate patients' energy needs [19–21]. Trabulsi et al. evaluated formulas and concluded the estimated energy requirement of the Dietary Reference Intake at the active level is best for the CF population, see Table 9.1 [19, 21]. Formulas are best used as a starting point for calculating energy needs. Increases in weight and stature (length or height), velocity of increase in weight and length/height, and fat stores are best used to assess adequacy of energy intake. In clinical care, adjustment in energy estimated intake may be needed to achieve optimal weight and linear growth.

In general, energy intake of 110% or greater (up to 200%) of that for persons without CF is recommended, this needs to be individualized to reflect each patient's energy needs [22]. Little is known about energy needs specific to pancreatic sufficient patients. A diet high in fat, with 35–40% of calorie intake as fat, is necessary to meet high energy needs in patients with PI [22, 23]. Although there are no specific recommendations regarding the type of fat to be consumed, to prevent essential fatty acid deficiency a diet containing adequate energy, a balanced intake of polyunsaturated fatty acids n-6 and n-3, and antioxidants is best [23, 24]. Vegetable oils such as flax, canola, and soy, and cold-water marine fish are good sources of linolenic acid and energy [23]. Breast milk is a good source of DHA and is recommended for infants [23].

Table 9.1 Determination of energy requirements per US Cystic Fibrosis Foundation using active level

1. Calculate basal metabolic rate (BMR) using WHO equations.		
Age range in years	Females	Males
0–3	61.0 wt−51	60.9 wt−54
10–18	12.2 wt+746	17.5 wt+651
18–30	14.7 wt+496	15.3 wt+679

2. Calculate the daily energy expenditure (DEE) by multiplying the BMR by activity plus disease coefficients.		
	Activity coefficients (AC)	Disease coefficients
	Confined to bed: BMR × 1.3	FEV_1 > 80% predicted: BMR × (AC+0)
	Sedentary: BMR × 1.5	FEV_1 40–79% predicted: BMR × (AC+0.2)
	Active: BMR × 1.7	FEV_1 < 40% predicted: BMR × (AC+0.3[a])

3. Calculate total daily energy requirements (DERs) from DEE and degree of steatorrhea. If a stool collection is not available to determine the fraction of fat intake, an approximate value of 0.85 may be used in the calculation. For pancreatic sufficient patients and pancreatic insufficient patients with a coefficient of fat absorption (COA) > 93% of intake, DER = DEE. For example: a patient with a COA of 0.78 the factor is 0.93/0.78 or 1.2. If the COA is not known the factor is 1.

Example:
Ten year old boy. Weight=32 kg; AC=active; FEV_1% predicted=85%. COA not available.
12.2 × 32 + 746 = 1136
1136 × (1.7+0) = 1931
1931 × 1.1 = 2124 cal/day

[a]May range up to 0.5 with very severe lung disease

It is logical to expect that diet counseling and provision of oral energy supplements will result in increased total caloric intake and improved anthropometric measures. Yet the data from research studies are inconsistent. Early work documenting the change to high-fat diets with patients previously maintained on low-fat diets showed improved energy intake and BMI, as shown by Corey et al. in the 1988 report of better survival in patients consuming a high fat diet [1]. Recent work does not provide a clear answer regarding the success of interventions to increase energy intake through diet counseling and/or oral supplements and improvement in health parameters such as BMI. In a study by White et al. adults did not achieve recommended energy and fat intake. The sickest patients used gastrostomy tubes and although they achieved increased energy intake, BMI did not change [25]. Home visits, improved adherence to supplemental enzymes, and energy supplements promoted increased energy intake in patients less than 5 years of age [26]. Steinkamp et al. [27] randomized thirty-six CF patients to standard nutrition counseling or nutrition counseling plus an energy supplement rich in fat and linoleic acid. Those who received the energy supplement had greater energy intake, weight gain, and fat mass than those who did not. No improvement was found in a group of malnourished patients with CF provided either an oral energy supplement or diet counseling [28]. Use of an oral protein energy supplement with mildly malnourished patients did not result in improvement in BMI [29]. A Cochrane review of efficacy of oral supplements in CF care concluded that no benefit was seen for moderately malnourished patients [30]. Use of diet counseling, oral supplements, and/or tube feeding did not result in improved BMI for patients waiting for lung transplant. Weight gain was achieved after lung transplant. Groleau et al. [31] reported improved energy intake, growth status, and muscle stores in school age children with mild lung disease given a structured, easily absorbable lipid supplement, or a placebo supplement with the same energy level [32]. Supplemental energy intake was approximately 100 cal daily for both groups. This is the first randomized placebo controlled trial that showed sustained increase in energy intake and a growth response.

Studies have shown that behavioral intervention is feasible in toddlers [33], can be incorporated into clinical practice [34], and resulted in increased knowledge and self-management skills in relation to nutrition and PERT in adult subjects [35]. In a study by Stark et al. in 2009 [36], behavior modification with nutrition intervention resulted in short-term increase in energy intake and BMI when compared to nutrition intervention alone, but long-term evaluation revealed that both groups had similar outcomes.

The energy demands of the diet for CF and the resultant diet recommendations can impact parent/ child relations starting in infancy and continuing throughout life. Parents of infants newly diagnosed with CF exhibit adaptive feeding behavior [37]. Stark and Powers described parenting behaviors surrounding meals that interfered with normal feeding development in young children [38, 39]. Adolescents and young adults with CF reported poorer quality of life when prescribed oral formulas or tube-feeding [40].

To achieve an energy intake that promotes normal weight and growth yet avoids negative feeding/ eating behavior; diet education should be addressed in a step-wise fashion based in patient-centered care with behavior modification and motivational interviewing. Using benchmarking and quality improvement the Cystic Fibrosis Foundation (CFF) recommends techniques described in Table 9.2 [41]. Additionally, using quality improvement strategies may improve overall nutrition status at CF Centers [41]. Chapter 18 provides a full review of nutrition-related quality improvement experience. Incorporating methods of motivational interviewing into the design of the patient's nutrition plan and education may improve energy intake.

Maneuvers specific to increasing oral energy intake (increasing caloric density) include "boosting" usual food intake and use of proprietary energy supplements in the form of drinks and/or energy bars.

Table 9.2 Nutrition smart changes ideas and benchmarking recommendations

Nutrition smart change ideas
1. Re-educate and set goals with patient and family surrounding increasing calories and vitamins/minerals and proactive nutrition
2. Prevent malabsorption: Routine enzyme use in pancreatic insufficient patients. Review and evaluate use
3. Increase RD patient contact time and frequency
4. Provide standard screening and/or assessment of nutrition at every visit
5. Assess and address feeding behaviors
6. Form relationships with and increase referrals to gastroenterology, endocrinology, and psychology. Treat adverse pulmonary, endocrine, and/or gastrointestinal symptoms
7. Formulate individual nutrition action plan with mutual goals set by patient, family and CF care team at every visit
8. Introduce the idea of a g-tube early in CF care
9. Standardize nutrition interventions
10. Provide more frequent monitoring of "at risk" patients: clinic visits, phone calls, emails, Skype
11. Have nutrition protocols in place
12. Perform in-depth reviews of patient nutritional status at a time other than clinic visits and activate nutrition care plans
Benchmarking
1. Define nutrition status at every visit as goal is prevention not rescue
2. Involve the whole team and meet regularly with focus on patient nutrition
3. Increase RD time and frequency
4. Develop patient take-home materials
4. Develop patient take-home materials
5. Increase g-tube use earlier rather than later
6. Assure that every team member and family know the nutrition assessment
7. Develop consensus that a patient without acceptable nutrition status needs an intervention
8. Deliver message to families by all team members regarding the importance of nutrition
9. Use the services of gastroenterology

Table 9.2 (continued)

10. Increase RD time for:
a. One on one nutrition education
b. Information on increasing calories
c. Obtaining diet history
11. Take-home material examples
a. Information from PortCF
b. Growth curve
c. Written nutrition information
d. Notebook for families to keep nutrition plan and materials
e. Menus
f. Information about appropriate websites
g. Nutrition information in quarterly newsletters
12. Team to support g-tube as part of CF care
13. All team members should feel empowered to bring up the idea of a g-tube

The goal of "boosting" a meal or snack is to increase the energy content without increasing the volume of food and beverages, see Table 9.3 for an example. Concentrating formula or adding powdered formula to expressed breast milk to increase to 24 or 27 calories per ounce (cal/oz) may be used with infants. Increasing energy content to 30 cal/oz may be achieved with the addition of a high calorie additive such as: Solcarb®, Duocal®, or MCTProcal®. Energy content of infant solid foods can be increased by using homemade baby foods thinned with infant formula or breast milk and adding fat calories via butter, margarine, or vegetable oil. Parents may need direction from the CF Center RD as to how to prepare homemade high calorie infant and toddler foods. Use of soft, energy-dense foods, such as ripe avocado, contributes to overall energy intake. Directing parents toward high calorie commercially prepared baby foods, including meats, will avoid the pitfalls of an infant/toddler diet with excess amounts of lower calorie fruits and vegetables. Baby food companies provide lists of high calorie baby foods, which are helpful to parents in choosing higher calorie products (Table 9.3).

Teaching parents and patients how to increase calories without increasing food/beverage volume is central to optimizing energy intake in children. "Boosting" usual food intake introduces techniques for high calorie "additives" to the usual diet and selecting high calorie foods rather than those lower in calories. Table 9.3 provides an example of "boosting" a breakfast meal. High calorie additives and spreadable include, but are not limited to: heavy cream, cheese, mayonnaise, butter, vegetable oil, cream cheese, avocado, and thick salad dressings. Other more unusual ideas include: olives, ice cream sprinkles, chocolate chips, and chopped nuts. The child's development level must be considered when selecting the additive. Examples of higher calorie snack foods for a young child are: mini muffin vs dry cereal; cereal bar vs. puff cereal, whole milk with added cream vs. plain milk; full-fat yogurt vs. low fat yogurt. Many other ways to increase energy intake without increasing food volume can be found at the CFF website, PORTCF website, and others such as Chef4CF.com.

Some persons with CF require even more calories than easily achieved with "boosting" usual food intake. Canned or powdered supplemental nutritional products may be used. Taste fatigue and cost often determines which product and how long a patient will use this approach. Some health insurance plans pay for nutritional supplements, although in most cases they do not. Patient assistance programs available through companies that make pancreatic enzyme medications provide a small amount of supplemental nutritional products monthly. See Table 9.4 for a list of products provided through company programs. There is limited evidence documenting the benefit of the use of oral supplemental nutrition products in increasing total caloric intake and weight gain. With appropriate use of pancreatic enzyme replacement therapy (PERT), patients will digest and absorb these products as well as usual foods [42]. Patient taste preference is a factor and influences the product selection. Higher calorie

Table 9.3 Example of "Boosting" a meal

Food	Calories	Food	Calories
½ cup oatmeal	83	½ cup oatmeal	83
Made with water		Made with ½ cup "super" milk[a]	165
½ cup whole milk on oatmeal	65	½ cup "Super" milk on oatmeal	165
		1 tsp soft margarine on oatmeal	33
		1 tbsp walnuts in oatmeal	48
½ cup orange juice	61	½ cup orange juice	61
Toast 1 slice	69	Toast 1 slice	69
1 tsp jelly	18	1 tsp jelly	18
		1 tsp soft margarine	33
Total calories:	296		675

[a]Super milk: 4 oz whole milk with two tablespoons of cream

Table 9.4 Nutrition Supplements Available Through Supplemental Enzyme Company Patient Assistance Programs: October 2014

AbbVie (Creon®)
Similac®
Pediasure®
Pediasure® Peptide 1.5
Pediasure® 1.5
Ensure Complete™
Ensure Plus®
Ensure Clear™
Zone Perfect®Bars
Myoplex 30®Bars
Myoplex® Ready to Drink Shake
Forest (Ultresa®, Zenpep®)
Scandishake®
Scandical©
Boost®VHC
Boost® Kid Essential 1.5
Boost Plus®
Cliff Bar
Cliff Kid Bar
Chiesi (Pertzye®)

Patient will receive $75, up to $225 for each 3-month supply of enzyme, to use for vitamins and nutritional supplements

products may have a thicker texture. Some patients use milk-based powdered supplements mixed with whole milk and heavy cream to make a high calorie, lower cost supplement from typically available foods. Another strategy to add calories without volume is the use of high calorie commercial additives such as: Scandical®, Solcarb®, Polycose®, Duocal®, MCTProcal®, and Microlipid®. These products are slowly added to the diet with adjustment of enzymes as needed based on the fat content of the product.

Children and adults with CF need to consistently consume sufficient calories to optimize weight status and ensure childhood growth at the individual's genetic potential. Achieving calorie goals is challenging and requires the expertise and support of the CF Center dietitian and other experts who will help support improving feeding and eating behavior.

Enteral Tube Feeding

Supplemental enteral tube feeding generally involves overnight delivery of a commercially available enteral formula by the nasogastric, gastrostomy, or jejunostomy route. Below is a discussion of indications, methods of administration, in addition to advantages and complications of supplemental tube feeding (STF).

Indications of Supplemental Tube Feeding in Patients with CF

The decision to start STF should be individualized taking into consideration many factors including patient's nutrition status, success of previous nutrition interventions, comorbid conditions, in addition to psychosocial factors and, financial and time resources that will affect adherence. While evidence regarding the optimal time to initiate STF is scarce; what is available seems to point to better outcomes when STF is introduced before the patient has advanced lung disease [43, 44]. On the other hand, individuals with advanced lung disease and who are candidates for transplantation may benefit from pre-operative STF.

STF is considered when behavioral and dietary interventions to improve nutritional status have failed in patients with clinically significant weight or growth deficits. These approaches are discussed elsewhere in this chapter and in Chapter 13. Diagnosis and treatment of CF and non-CF-related co-morbidities (such as CF-related diabetes, liver disease, constipation, or bacterial overgrowth) are important to understand the etiology and treatment of suboptimal nutritional and growth status in patients of all ages.

In 2008 the CFF updated the definition and approach to nutritional status monitoring using weight for stature [22] to employ age appropriate BMI criteria that are based on CDC growth charts [45]. Use of the percentage of ideal body weight method is no longer recommended [23]. The monitoring approach, guidelines, and definitions are summarized in Table 9.5.

The STF literature in CF includes patients with different degrees of malnutrition. Many studies [44, 46–49] were conducted before the 2008 changes in approach to weight for stature assessment [22] (see Table 9.5). Some studies evaluated STF in patients with a weight z score of < -1.0 [46, 50–52], while others intervened in participants with more significant malnutrition and weight z score < -2.0 [44, 48, 49].

Bradley et al. [50] is one of the few studies that used an outcome benchmark of BMI >50th percentile [22] for their intervention in 20 children with an average age of 9 years and included a one year follow-up. The authors found that children who received STF were ten times more likely to attain the BMI goal than control subjects with similar baseline characteristics. Control subjects received standard nutrition management including dietitian evaluation, counseling, and in some oral nutritional supplements and/or appetite stimulants. The observed BMI gain in STF-treated children was sustained up to 12 months. White et al. [53], in the UK, retrospectively studied a cohort of adults with CF. Patients were eligible for STF with a BMI <19, or with a history of a minimum 5% weight loss over 2 months and failure of oral nutrition supplements. This study design was generally based on European consensus recommendations [24] for care of patients with CF. The study included 23 adults, 17 of whom agreed to STF and the remainder declined and served as a comparison group. The authors found that those who were treated with STF had a significant increase in weight (average 19.5%), the BMI moved into the recommended range, and lung function was stable over the three-year follow-up. Patients who did not accept STF had a decline in lung function and no weight gain over the three years.

Table 9.5 CFF recommendations on the appropriate method of weight for stature assessment by age group (and gender in adults) modified from [22]

Age group	Recommended method for weight for stature assessment, goal
<2 years	Weight for length percentile, ≥50th percentile
2–20 years	BMI percentile, BMI ≥ 50th percentile
≥20 years- women	BMI ≥ 22
≥20 years- men	BMI ≥ 23

The variation in the timing of introduction of STF in research studies highlights the need of large-scale prospective studies in children and adults to provide the evidence needed to establish the ideal time to introduce STF across the range of ages and clinical status encountered in the care of patients with CF.

Using its modified and more clinically applicable definitions [22]; the Consensus Committee recommends the use of nutritional supplements (oral or enteral) in addition to dietary counseling to help restore an ideal weight; a measure that has long been linked to improved pulmonary outcomes. The CFF recommends starting with intensive behavioral intervention and counseling for children aged 1–12 years but reported having insufficient evidence to support similar interventions in children older than 13 years or adults.

Effects of Supplemental Tube Feeding on Pulmonary Function, Nutritional Status, and Quality of Life

STF is used to achieve an increase in energy intake with the purpose to improve weight, BMI, and linear growth (in children). Improved nutritional status is associated with better lung function expressed as percentage of predicted FEV_1 ($ppFEV_1$), and most importantly longer survival. The literature evaluating STF in CF contains no randomized controlled trials directly evaluating these goals [54]. The ethical implications of randomizing malnourished subjects to a placebo/usual care treatment arm represent an important barrier to conducting such trials.

Many studies assessed the effect of STF on lung function and frequency of pulmonary exacerbations. There is no strong evidence that STF resulted in a reduction in pulmonary exacerbations or hospital days [44, 49, 50, 53]. The effect of STF on $ppFEV_1$, however, varied among studies. Some showed stable $ppFEV_1$ over study duration [49, 50], others showed improvement or decrease in the rate of decline of $ppFEV_1$ [47, 52, 53]. One study [44] reported a small initial reduction in $ppFEV_1$ in the first year of STF and was followed by stabilization during the second year. Oliver et al. [43] found that individuals who had $ppFEV_1$ less than 50% at time of gastrostomy tube placement had higher mortality over one year follow-up than those who had a greater than 50% at baseline. This may highlight the importance of early intervention with STF and not waiting to offer it as a "last resort" [23].

There is variability in nutrition outcomes reported in studies of STF in CF. Only two studies reported absolute changes in weight in addition to changes in BMI percentile [50, 53]. Studies usually reported changes in BMI z score [44, 48, 49], BMI percentile [44, 46], or weight z score [43, 47]. Only a few studies evaluated the impact on height [44, 46, 48]. Several studies found significant improvement in weight variables with STF that were sustained from one year [49, 50], two years [43, 44, 47, 48], three years [46, 53], and up to four years [52]. One group [50] found that the degree of improvement in BMI z score was greater at 6- than at 12-months and speculated that changes in adherence may play a role in this observation. Other STF studies also showed faster or greater gains of weight in the first 6–12 months [53, 55]. In a subgroup analysis of 46 subjects, Best et al. [52] found that women had a negative BMI response following STF and speculated that body image issues may increase reluctance to use STF in women with CF; this likely will apply to teenage girls.

As for the STF effect on height, Rosenfeld et al. [46] showed that, as expected, height improvement temporally lagged behind weight improvements and increased from an average of 5th percentile to 10th percentile after 18–20 months of STF. Efrati et al. [44] reported that height Z score showed a trend toward improvement in the second year of STF. Those who started STF in infancy had the greatest benefit. Finally, Van Biervliet et al. [48] showed significant improvements in catch-up linear growth after 12 months of STF. Improvements were, however, incomplete especially in peri-pubertal children.

Most of these studies were retrospective and all but one [50] did not include a control or comparison group. Generally, the patients were used as their own control when comparing outcomes before and after STF. The cohorts included in these studies also had variable degrees of baseline malnutrition, lung disease, energy intake, and enzyme administration; all of which might impact nutrition outcomes. A systematic Cochrane Review reported that there were no well-designed multicenter randomized controlled trials of STF in subjects with CF [54]. As mentioned above, the ethical implications represent a barrier to designing and conducting randomized trials in malnourished participants. There is, however, great need for prospective multicenter evaluations of feasibility and tolerance of STF, optimal timing to start STF, choice of formula and method of administration, dose and administration of PERT, and finally the effect of STF on short- and long-term outcomes that include nutrition status, lung function, quality of life, and survival.

There is little published on quality of life in patients with CF who receive STF. Gunnel et al. evaluated the attitudes toward percutaneous endoscopic gastrostomy (PEG) placement by survey with patients and their families with and without a PEG. Most with PEG, who responded ($n = 29$), thought that it helped them gain weight, grow taller, be healthier, and have more energy. They did not perceive the PEG as painful, embarrassing, or limiting to their abilities to play sports. Those without a PEG were more likely to perceive it to be painful, to look bad or embarrassing, and were less likely to think that a PEG would result in improved weight gain or pulmonary function. Van Biervliet et al. [48] found that parents had more difficulty accepting tube feeding than children themselves. Parents also felt that although they had seen the tube on a doll, they were surprised by the degree of disturbance of the body image of their child. They also reported that they forgot some of the information provided in the initial teaching sessions. In a different study of only adults [53], the median time from first discussion of STF to initiation of treatment was five months (range 0.2–36). A study in adults to evaluate prevalence of disordered eating, self-image, and quality of life among patients with CF with variable nutrition interventions (oral supplement, enteral feeds) and CF and healthy controls [40] reported that those who receive STF were more likely to have a negative body image and a poorer quality of life compared to the other groups. It is important to note, however, that the subjects on STF (in this cohort) had the lowest ppFEV$_1$ and it is possible that their worse disease course (and not the tube feeds alone) played a role in their perception of self and quality of life.

This literature suggests that while patients with CF on STF may have favorable views of their quality of life and health outcomes; patients and families can experience significant difficulties when considering and accepting STF. It is important that healthcare professionals introduce the discussion of STF early, provide guidance and repeated education, and quite possibly the opportunity to meet with patients and families who have gone through the experience. The Consensus Committee [23] recommended that STF be discussed as supplemental therapy with positive outcomes as opposed to a threat, sign of failure, or poor outcome. More research should focus on prospectively assessing attitudes, quality of life, and barriers experienced by individuals who receive STF and their families.

Supplemental Tube Feeding Methods

There is no evidence that one type of enteral access is superior to others for patients with CF. The Consensus Committee recommended that the choice of tube and technique of placement should be based on expertise at the CF Center [23]. Options include nasogastric, orogastric, gastrostomy, or jejunostomy tubes. Gastrostomy feeding was the STF access of choice in patients with CF in the published literature [43, 44, 46, 47, 49, 50, 52, 53, 56, 57] and likely reflects their common use and low risk of complications. All of the cited studies used continuous nocturnal feeding; this is consistent with the Consensus Committee recommendations [23] and promotes a more normal eating pattern during the day.

Nasogastric tubes can be considered for administration of STF when the expected duration of treatment is short, prior to insertion of gastrostomy tube, or in teenagers who fear significant changes to their body image. Jejunostomy feeding was less commonly used and can be delivered through a surgically created jejunostomy or by extending a gastrostomy catheter to the jejunum. Jejunostomy feeding may be used in patients with severe gastroesophageal reflux (as an alternative or adjuvant to a surgical anti-reflux procedure), those with short bowel syndrome, or more severe feeding intolerance.

Gastroesophageal reflux disease (GERD) is common in patients with CF (see Chapter 12). Gastrostomy (and nasogastric) tube feeding can worsen underlying GERD, but is not a contraindication to STF. The Consensus Committee [23] stated that many clinicians advocate for assessing the presence and severity of GERD before initiation of STF so that an anti-reflux procedure (fundoplication) can be considered at the time of gastrostomy tube placement in patients with severe GERD. There is little information on the outcomes of fundoplication in patients with CF. One study [58] retrospectively evaluated nutrition and pulmonary outcomes in children with CF who underwent fundoplication (with or without gastrostomy tube placement). A higher incidence of recurrence of symptoms following fundoplication was reported compared to children with neurological impairment and severe GERD treated with fundoplication. Over the course of the follow-up period (average 33 months), the authors reported that there was no increase in BMI, BMI percentile, or change in the slope of ppFEV$_1$. In a subgroup analysis, however, children with ppFEV$_1$ greater than 60% at fundoplication showed an improvement in the slope of ppFEV$_1$. Another study that included adult and pediatric patients [59] retrospectively evaluated 48 patients with CF who underwent fundoplication, 60% of whom also had gastrostomy tube placement. This cohort showed significant reductions in pulmonary exacerbations, slower rate of decline of ppFEV$_1$, and increased weight gain over the two-year follow-up. Patients who had milder lung disease and those who received gastrostomy tube feeding exhibited the greatest benefits from fundoplication.

Formula Choice and Calorie Goals

Many studies used intact polymeric formulas for tube feeds in patients with CF [46–48, 53] and reported good tolerance. One author gave all patients with PI semi-elemental formula [49], while others used elemental or semi-elemental formula in children who developed nausea or diarrhea (not responsive to change in PERT dose) [43, 49]. Some authors used a mix of intact and elemental or semi-elemental formula but did not explain why different formula choices were made [44, 50]. Many studies provided about 50% of estimated energy requirements through STF [43, 46, 48–50], while some delivered a range of 40–60% or 20–60% [53].The caloric density of the study formulas also varied. Two groups used 1.0 kcal/mL [43, 44], while the remainder used more calorically dense formulas with a range of 1.5–2.0 kcal/mL [46–49, 53].

The Consensus Committee report [23] stated that intact polymeric formula with high caloric density (1.5–2.0 kcal/mL) appeared to be tolerated and delivered adequate calories while minimizing the volume. The Committee also recommended providing 30–50% of estimated energy requirements with a continuous nocturnal infusion. Calories delivered are titrated based on feeding tolerance and the patient's weight gain and growth response. Clinical experience of some practitioners, in accordance with the experience of Williams et al. [49], supports using a semi-elemental or elemental formula in patients who develop nausea, bloating, morning anorexia, or diarrhea with standard formula.

Pancreatic Enzymes and Supplemental Tube Feeding

Data on appropriate dosing and timing of pancreatic enzymes with overnight tube feeds are lacking. STF studies in children and adults with CF reported variable practices of enzyme administration. The majority reported giving enzymes orally before overnight feeds and again at the end of the infusion [43, 44, 48, 50], with one group recommending an additional dose mid-way through the infusion [48]. Some authors provided enzymes only before the start of feeds [47]. Those who reported the dose of PERT chose doses similar to a mealtime dose [50], calculated the dose based on the formula's fat content [43], or gave 2500 lipase units per kg of body weight [47].

The CF Consensus Committee [23] recommended that pancreatic enzymes be given orally in a mealtime dose just before overnight tube feeding was started and suggested that additional doses may be needed mid-way or at the end of the feeding. In patients who receive elemental or low fat formula, pancreatic enzymes administration may not be necessary. More research is needed to determine ideal methods to administer pancreatic enzymes with STF.

There is no consensus among CF healthcare professionals on method of administration of pancreatic enzymes to patients who are unable to take them by mouth. Variable practices have been reported including suspending the capsule contents in a thicker fluid and giving as a bolus through the feeding tube, crushing the capsule contents, and adding them to the feeding bag, or mixing the contents with sodium bicarbonate then adding them to the feeding bag or giving them directly through the feeding tube [60]. These practices can increase the risk of clogging the feeding tube. Nicolo et al. [61] reported success in eliminating clogging of feeding tubes by diluting the contents of the capsule with sodium bicarbonate before directly administering pancreatic enzymes through the feeding tube.

Complications of Supplemental Tube Feeding

Nasogastric tubes can cause discomfort (especially in patients with nasal polyps) and when dislodged can increase the risk of aspiration. Studies of gastrostomy tube feeding in CF reported no major complications such as gastric perforation or wall separation. Granulation tissue [46, 50], redness and tenderness at the site [48, 56], leakage [43, 46, 48], tube malfunction or displacement [50, 56] were seen. One study also documented bedwetting and night sweats in some patients [48]. Nausea and vomiting were also reported and in some cases and responded to treatment with prokinetic agents [46, 56]. STF associated diarrhea improved with elemental or semi-elemental formula [43, 46]. Enzyme dosing adjustments and obtaining stool for infectious studies (including *Clostridium Difficile*) are appropriate in patients who develop diarrhea while on STF.

CF-related diabetes can occur following the initiation of STF [43, 44]. It is possible that the increase in calories can unmask already existing carbohydrate intolerance. The Consensus Committee [23] recommended screening for glucose intolerance with measurement two to three hours after initiation and at the end of the feeding cycle on two separate nights after caloric goal is reached. Blood glucose should also be monitored when patients are ill, receiving steroids, or if they are unable to gain weight with additional calories.

Other potential complications related to enteral feeding include worsening of existing GERD, micro-aspiration, or bronchospasm. Assessment for and treatment of GERD is an important component of considering STF (discussed in the previous section).

Summary

While there are many gaps in the current literature, it appears that delivery of STF can improve nutritional status and possibly pulmonary health in patients with CF who have weight or growth deficits. The process requires a great deal of education and support from healthcare providers and commitment on the part of patients and families. STF must be monitored closely and tailored to the individual needs of the patient with adjustments made in response to changes in nutrition status.

Appetite Stimulants

The use of appetite stimulants is common practice in treating anorexia and promoting weight gain in children and adults with CF. These agents are not licensed for this indication and controversy regarding their efficacy and side effect profile continues. As we have outlined so far in this chapter, effective treatment of weight loss, inadequate weight gain, or growth faltering in CF can be challenging.

Anorexia can be an important contributor to reduced energy intake in CF. The exact mechanism of anorexia remains uncertain and objective tools for assessment of appetite are lacking. There are multiple factors contributing to poor appetite and reduced energy intake in CF [62]. Many of these are unique to CF and some are not. CF-related factors include pulmonary exacerbations, anorectic effect of increased cytokines, GERD, poor gastric emptying, distal intestinal obstruction syndrome, and constipation. Nasal polyps and sinus disease alter the patient's ability to smell and taste food and to eat while breathing comfortably. Factors that are not unique to CF, but carry great importance, include depression, anxiety, stress, eating disorder, medication use (i.e., ADHD medications and possibly antibiotics), economic issues, impact of medical therapies on time and energy to prepare and eat food, endocrine issues, and finally abnormalities in appetite neuro-transmitters (ghrelin, peptide Y, leptin, and insulin) [62, 63].The above-mentioned factors are considered when evaluating reduced energy intake in patients with CF, as successfully treating underlying issues can provide an effective and safe treatment of malnutrition. If problems with appetite or food intake persist despite treating underlying issues, then appetite stimulants can be considered based on the individual's needs.

Appetite Stimulants and Mechanisms

There is a variety of medications that have been used for appetite stimulation in CF, these agents have a range of pharmacological characteristics and include hormones, antihistamines, steroids, cannabinoids, antidepressants, and antipsychotics. Some of the most studied agents include megestrol acetate, cyproheptadine hydrochloride, dronabinol, and mirtazapine.

Megestrol Acetate (MA) or Megace® is a synthetic, orally active form of progesterone. It is used in treatment of advanced breast cancer and also in uterine and prostate cancers. It has been used as appetite stimulant in patients with AIDS and cancer where it was found to increase appetite, weight gain, and promote a sense of well-being [62, 64]. The mechanism of how MA affects appetite has not been well established. Some of the postulated mechanisms include inhibition of action of tumor necrosis factor, altering serum cytokine profile, inducing adipocyte differentiation, and stimulating synthesis and release of neuropeptide Y, a potent appetite stimulant [62, 65, 66]. Given its glucocorticoid base, it is possible that a portion of the weight gain observed with MA treatment is due to water retention.

Cyproheptadine Hydrochloride (CH) or Periactin® is a first generation anti-histamine which is both a histamine and serotonin antagonist with the secondary effect of appetite stimulation [67, 68]. It has been used as an appetite stimulant in anorexia nervosa [69], tuberculosis [70], and in underweight adults [71]. The mechanism of action of CH is not fully understood and does not appear to be related to hypoglycemic-induced hyperphagia or changes in growth hormone secretion [62, 68, 72].

Dronabinol or Marinol® is an orally active synthetic cannabinoid with central sympathomimetic activity. It has reversible effects on appetite, mood, cognition, memory, and perception. It has been studied in patients with cancer and HIV with noted improvements in appetite and weight gain. In a comparison trial with MA, it was not as effective but the study was criticized because a low dose of dronabinol was used [73, 74]. Studies in patients with CF are limited [62, 75].

Mirtazapine or Remeron® is a non-adrenergic and specific serotonergic antidepressant and is used primarily in the treatment of depression. Other uses include appetite stimulation, control of emesis, anxiolysis, and hypnosis. Sudden cessation will cause withdrawal symptoms. Data regarding use in patients with CF are limited [62, 76, 77].

Efficacy of Appetite Stimulants in CF

The literature examining appetite stimulants in CF includes case reports and case series [78, 79]. The number of randomized controlled studies [65, 72, 80] is limited and the ones that exist have relatively small sample size and heterogeneous study design.

In 2007 Chinuck et al. [66] published a systematic review that evaluated the results of fifteen studies of appetite stimulation in CF (6 peer reviewed papers, 8 abstracts, and 1 letter to the editor). Out of these fifteen reports, ten used MA, one used dronabinol, two used mirtazapine, and one used CH, and included a total of 139 subjects. Only three studies were randomized and placebo-controlled, two were double-blinded. Studies evaluating use of MA demonstrated significant gains in weight in subjects who received the drug. Two randomized controlled trials used MA as the appetite stimulant in CF [65, 80]. Both studies found significant improvements in weight and lung function. The two studies that evaluated the use of CH showed beneficial effects on weight gain and variable results on lung function [72, 81].

Homnick et al. in 2004 [72] randomized 16 children and adults to receive placebo or CH (4 mg four times daily) in a double-blinded fashion for 12 weeks. The CH group had more significant weight gain, (3.45 kg vs. 1.1 kg), increased weight-for-age Z score, and ideal body weight. Side effects included transient drowsiness in a few subjects. To evaluate the long-term outcomes of the use of CH in a more "real-life" treatment program, the authors asked the subjects to continue the trial in an open-label design for an additional nine months and started all placebo subjects on CH [81]. Twelve of the original sixteen completed the subsequent nine months of the study. Subjects who changed from placebo to CH gained weight significantly over 3–6 months and those who continued on CH generally maintained previously gained weight over the duration of the study. There was no difference in pulmonary outcomes. Important observations in this study include a fairly significant variability in the degree of weight gain among subjects who were switched from placebo to CH (ranged from +1.8 to +6.3 kg). In the group who continued CH, two subjects lost weight while the remainder maintained their weight. The authors speculated that this variability was caused by changes in adherence after long-term therapy especially with four-times per day dosing. Decreasing drug effect or intrinsic individual variations may be factors too.

The authors concluded that after one year of therapy, CH appeared to be safe and well tolerated, with a small weight gain in most subjects and most of weight gain occurring in the first few months of therapy. They, therefore, recommended the use of appetite stimulants as an intermediate step in a program of CF nutritional interventions.

Marchand et al. [65] published a randomized double-blinded, placebo-controlled study with a cross-over design. Twelve children with CF were randomized to receive placebo or MA (10 mg/kg/ dose) for 12 weeks, followed by a 12-week wash-out period, and 12 weeks of alternate treatment. The study outcomes included weight, appetite, caloric intake, and ppFEV$_1$. Importantly half of the study sample (6 of 12) did not complete the study (three unrelated to the study, two children developed diabetes while on MA and one developed glucose intolerance while on placebo). Treatment group had significant increases in weight gain and weight-for-age- Z score. There was a slight increase in height in the treatment group. The authors also demonstrated gains in fat mass, fat-free mass (FFM), and ppFEV$_1$. Many subjects lost weight after the medication was stopped or when the dose was reduced.

In another randomized, double-blinded, placebo-controlled study of MA, Eubanks et al. [80] included 17 participants who all had PI and met criteria for growth failure for preceding six months. Subjects were randomized to receiving placebo or MA at 10 mg/kg/day (with adjustment at subsequent visits as discussed below in the dosing section). The treatment group had significant increases in weight, weight-for-age Z score, and ppFEV$_1$ compared with the placebo group. The authors speculated that the anti-inflammatory properties of MA could be playing a role in the improvement of pulmonary outcomes. When they evaluated the quality of weight gain, Eubanks et al. showed, by use of DXA, that both fat mass and FFM increased among MA users at 3- and 6-month intervals. In a subgroup analysis, peri-pubertal children had the most increase in FFM which constituted up to 50% of their weight gain.

Homnick et al. [81] showed that, in the short term, CH appears to induce more fat mass gain than FFM. It can be argued, however, that restoration of fat mass and energy stores is of value in malnourished patients with CF [66] and it is possible that long-term use can result in improvements in FFM, an outcome linked to ppFEV$_1$. Some studies reported trends toward improvement in quality of life [65, 80]. Only one study reported an increase in dietary energy and protein intake [80].

A recently published Cochrane Review [82] on the use of appetite stimulants in CF concluded that both MA and CH, despite many limitations to the studies included, have demonstrated efficacy in short-term (up to six months) treatment of anorexia in CF patients. It could not be concluded that one therapy was more effective than the other. The available evidence did not provide enough data to recommend optimal dosing, duration, or timing of treatment. The authors added that given the limitations in the available evidence, clinicians should be aware of and monitor for potential side effects (discussed below) and continuously weigh those against clinical benefits in an individualized fashion. Further, the authors of the Cochrane Review called for future prospective, multi-centered, adequately powered, randomized trials of appetite stimulation in CF to address some of the many gaps in our current knowledge.

An important consideration in evaluating the literature pertaining to appetite stimulation in CF is that the mechanisms of anorexia are not fully understood and there is no validated measure to assess appetite; it is difficult to study the relationship among appetite, dietary intake, and subsequent weight gain. The quality and sustainability of weight gain has not been well studied in the literature. Finally, although many individuals gained weight, it is unclear how many achieved weight gain goals or reached optimal weight and BMI. Other clinical questions include the optimal dose and duration of use of appetite stimulants among different age groups, and whether patients awaiting lung transplants should receive a different therapeutic approach, for example, including timing of the intervention and possibly avoiding MA due to the speculative risk of osteoporosis.

Dosing and Duration of Appetite Stimulants

In a systematic literature review, Chinuck et al. [66] reported variable daily doses of MA ranging from 1.27 to 10 mg/kg or 15 to 800 mg. The doses were often divided in four daily doses. The duration of use was also highly variable and ranged from 2 to 28 months. Eubanks et al. [80] used MA with a starting dose of 10 mg/kg/day and increased by 2.5 mg/kg/day for weight gain <2% above baseline at 30 days and decreased the dose for weight gain >5% at 30 days or >10% at day 60 or 90. The mean dose of MA was 7.5 mg/kg/day. Marchand et al. [65] commented that when doses of MA were dropped to 5 mg/kg/day (for irritability and insomnia), weight loss was observed. In their randomized controlled trial of CH, Homnick et al. [72] used a dose of 4 mg four times daily for three months.

Side Effects of Appetite Stimulants in CF

Use of MA was associated with abnormalities in glucose tolerance [65, 80], development of diabetes [65], and reversible adrenal suppression [65, 80]. Testicular failure and impotence have been reported with the use of MA in a patient with CF [79]. Of note, diabetes and impaired glycemic control was reported with the use of higher MA doses (10 mg/kg/day). Hyperglycemia was reversible in only one study [80]. Glycaemia should be monitored closely after initiation of MA therapy. Although this has not been reported in CF population, MA has been speculated to be a risk factor for osteoporosis [66, 83]. Osteoporosis can be a contraindication for CF-related lung transplant. CH side effects were relatively minor and included sedation, mood changes, and perceived excessive weight gain. Adherence to appetite stimulants can be a problem given the need for two to four times daily doses.

In summary, appetite stimulants appear to be effective in the short-term to induce weight gain in patients with CF and anorexia. It is important to evaluate and manage any treatable conditions that contribute to anorexia. While there are more studies on the use of MA, its side effect profile makes it a less attractive option and leads to more use of CH in the CF clinical setting. It is important to individualize therapeutic decisions and discuss the risk-benefit ratio with the patient and family.

Our knowledge of appetite regulation has expanded with the understanding of the roles of peptides and CFTR in appetite regulation which may expand future therapeutic options. Adequately powered, randomized-controlled trials of various appetite stimulants are needed in CF. Future studies should incorporate objective methods of assessment of appetite and energy intake, changes in weight including fat and FFM, sustainability of weight gain in the long-term, side effects, in addition to potential changes in lung function and quality of life.

Parenteral Nutrition

Studies on the use of parenteral nutrition (PN) in patients with CF are limited. In general PN is used as a supportive measure when enteral plus oral nutrition cannot be used or fail to maintain or improve patients' nutritional status. In 1980, Shepherd et al. [84] studied 12 subjects with CF for 6 months before and after 21 days of hyper-caloric PN while hospitalized. They noted catch-up weight and height gain by 1 month and 3 months, respectively and this continued for 6 months. They also noted decreased rate of lung infections, improvements in pulmonary function, well-being, and oral intake. The PN regimen (protein 20%, carbohydrate 20% and fat 40% of calories) used, provided 90–100% RDA for calories and consisted of crystalline amino acids, dextrose, and Intralipid® administered via a peripheral IV. Eight of twelve participants also received IV antibiotics for pulmonary infections.

Goal for caloric intake from oral and PN routes was 130% RDA. Some improvement may have been due to successful treatment of pulmonary infections and treatment of essential fatty acid deficiency.

PN tends to be used primarily in the inpatient setting when a patient is critically ill, during a pulmonary exacerbation, or with severe feeding intolerance. When a patient is NPO, PN is used to provide full nutrition support. It can also be used to treat essential fatty acid deficiency in patients, in whom enteral supplementation failed (personal experience). Typically, PN is administered via a central venous line since these patients often have central access for administration of antibiotics. This allows the provision of a more concentrated PN solution which has a high osmolality. Some patients may exhibit hyperglycemia, especially when PN is cycled and/or if a patient is on concomitant corticosteroids.

There is experience with Home PN in CF. Allen et al. [85] treated 25 subjects with CF with declining nutritional and pulmonary status at home over a four-year period. Participants ranged in age from 4 to 27 years with an average age of 16 and had previously failed a focused enteral approach to improve nutritional status or linear growth. They had moderate to severe lung disease (mean ppFEV$_1$ 40.9%). PN regimens were started in the hospital and advanced to provide 50–100% of total daily needs over several days. Patients were discharged home on stable regimens and some needed insulin. Weight loss returned within six months after PN was stopped. No change in lung function was noted. Increased complications were noted while on PN: increased days needed for IV antibiotics, sepsis, major vessel thrombosis, and mechanical problems. A subset of four subjects accounted for the majority of the sepsis episodes. More than 50% of patients reported increased energy, better appearance, weight gain, and less pressure to eat. Negative outcomes included nausea, activity limitations with infusions, and more nighttime urinary frequency. Skeie et al. [86] followed two people with severe lung disease and malnutrition on home PN and showed weight gain, improved exercise tolerance, and increased participation in daily activities. Currently in the USA, the use of omega-3 fatty acid is popular in patients with chronic inflammation. At this time, intravenous fish oil products are not FDA approved, however their use in CF has been explored. Katz et al. [87] compared intravenous fish oil (Omegaven 10%®) to traditional IV fat emulsion containing soybean and safflower oils (Liposyn III® 10%) for 1 month (dose of 150 mg/day) in 18 adult patients with CF at home. During the study period patients were given standard PN (glucose, Novamine® amino acid solution 11.4%, Liposyn® 20%, mineral, vitamins, electrolytes, and trace elements). Caloric intake from PN was set at 115% of measured REE with 14% calories derived from protein. No changes were noted in pulmonary function or with fatty acid panels other than an increase in levels of omega-3 fatty acids. The authors concluded that the short-term use of IV fish oil products was safe in patients with CF.

Conclusion

The information presented here describes the many approaches to be considered to provide an effective nutrition intervention for an individual patient within his/her clinical and social environment. Clearly, more well-designed clinical research is needed to provide additional evidence of what strategies are best suited to the different degrees of malnutrition, ages, and other clinical and psychosocial variables in the modern CF care setting.

References

1. Corey M, McLaughlin FJ, Williams M, Levison H. A comparison of survival, growth, and pulmonary function in patients with cystic fibrosis in Boston and Toronto. J Clin Epidemiol. 1988;41(6):583–91.
2. Powers SW, Patton SR, Byars KC, Mitchell MJ, Jelalian E, Mulvihill MM, et al. Caloric intake and eating behavior in infants and toddlers with cystic fibrosis. Pediatrics. 2002;109(5):E75–5.

3. Schall JI, Bentley T, Stallings VA. Meal patterns, dietary fat intake and pancreatic enzyme use in preadolescent children with cystic fibrosis. J Pediatr Gastroenterol Nutr. 2006;43(5):651–9.

4. Kawchak DA, Zhao H, Scanlin TF, Tomezsko JL, Cnaan A, Stallings VA. Longitudinal, prospective analysis of dietary intake in children with cystic fibrosis. J Pediatr. 1996;129(1):119–29.

5. Moen IE, Nilsson K, Andersson A, Fagerland MW, Fluge G, Hollsing A, et al. Dietary intake and nutritional status in a Scandinavian adult cystic fibrosis-population compared with recommendations. Food Nutr Res. 2011;55.

6. Maqbool A, Dougherty KA, Rovner AJ, Michel SH, Stallings VA. Nutrition. In: Alan J, Panitch H, Rubenstein R, editors. Cystic Fibrosis, vol 242. New York, New York: Informa Healthcare; 2010. p. 308–27.

7. Woestenenk JW, Castelijns SJ, van der Ent CK, Houwen RH. Dietary intake in children and adolescents with cystic fibrosis. Clin Nutr. 2014;33(3):528–32.

8. Trabulsi J, Schall JI, Ittenbach RF, Olsen IE, Yudkoff M, Daikhin Y, et al. Energy balance and the accuracy of reported energy intake in preadolescent children with cystic fibrosis. Am J Clin Nutr. 2006;84(3):523–30.

9. Allen JR, McCauley JC, Selby AM, Waters DL, Gruca MA, Baur LA, et al. Differences in resting energy expenditure between male and female children with cystic fibrosis. J Pediatr. 2003;142(1):15–9.

10. Stallings VA, Tomezsko JL, Schall JI, Mascarenhas MR, Stettler N, Scanlin TF, et al. Adolescent development and energy expenditure in females with cystic fibrosis. Clin Nutr. 2005;24(5):737–45.

11. Bines JE, Truby HD, Armstrong DS, Phelan PD, Grimwood K. Energy metabolism in infants with cystic fibrosis. J Pediatr. 2002;140(5):527–33.

12. Fried MD, Durie PR, Tsui LC, Corey M, Levison H, Pencharz PB. The cystic fibrosis gene and resting energy expenditure. J Pediatr. 1991;119(6):913–6.

13. Kalnins D, Pencharz PB, Grasemann H, Solomon M. Energy expenditure and nutritional status in pediatric patients before and after lung transplantation. J Pediatr. 2013;163(5):1500–2.

14. Barclay A, Allen JR, Blyler E, Yap J, Gruca MA, Asperen PV, et al. Resting energy expenditure in females with cystic fibrosis: is it affected by puberty? Eur J Clin Nutr. 2007;61(10):1207–12.

15. Reilly JJ, Ralston JM, Paton JY, Edwards CA, Weaver LT, Wilkinson J, et al. Energy balance during acute respiratory exacerbations in children with cystic fibrosis. Eur Respir J. 1999;13(4):804–9.

16. Magoffin A, Allen JR, McCauley J, Gruca MA, Peat J, Van Asperen P, et al. Longitudinal analysis of resting energy expenditure in patients with cystic fibrosis. J Pediatr. 2008;152(5):703–8.

17. Bradley GM, Blackman SM, Watson CP, Doshi VK, Cutting GR. Genetic modifiers of nutritional status in cystic fibrosis. Am J Clin Nutr. 2012;96(6):1299–308.

18. Johnson MR, Ferkol TW, Shepherd RW. Energy cost of activity and exercise in children and adolescents with cystic fibrosis. J Cyst Fibros. 2006;5(1):53–8.

19. Michel SH, Maqbool A, Hanna MD, Mascarenhas M. Nutrition management of pediatric patients who have cystic fibrosis. Pediatr Clin North Am. 2009;56(5):1123–41.

20. Ramsey BW, Farrell PM, Pencharz P. Nutritional assessment and management in cystic fibrosis: a consensus report. The Consensus Committee. Am J Clin Nutr. 1992;55(1):108–16.

21. Trabulsi J, Ittenbach RF, Schall JI, Olsen IE, Yudkoff M, Daikhin Y, et al. Evaluation of formulas for calculating total energy requirements of preadolescent children with cystic fibrosis. Am J Clin Nutr. 2007;85(1):144–51.

22. Stallings VA, Stark LJ, Robinson KA, Feranchak AP, Quinton H, Clinical Practice Guidelines on Growth, et al. Evidence-based practice recommendations for nutrition-related management of children and adults with cystic fibrosis and pancreatic insufficiency: results of a systematic review. J Am Diet Assoc. 2008;108(5):832–9.

23. Borowitz D, Baker RD, Stallings V. Consensus report on nutrition for pediatric patients with cystic fibrosis. J Pediatr Gastroenterol Nutr. 2002;35(3):246–59.

24. Sinaasappel M, Stern M, Littlewood J, Wolfe S, Steinkamp G, Heijerman HG, et al. Nutrition in patients with cystic fibrosis: a European Consensus. J Cyst Fibros. 2002;1(2):51–75.

25. White H, Morton AM, Peckham DG, Conway SP. Dietary intakes in adult patients with cystic fibrosis–do they achieve guidelines? J Cyst Fibros. 2004;3(1):1–7.

26. Adde FV, Rodrigues JC, Cardoso AL. Nutritional follow-up of cystic fibrosis patients: the role of nutrition education. J Pediatr (Rio J). 2004;80(6):475–82.

27. Steinkamp G, Demmelmair H, Ruhl-Bagheri I, von der Hardt H, Koletzko B. Energy supplements rich in linoleic acid improve body weight and essential fatty acid status of cystic fibrosis patients. J Pediatr Gastroenterol Nutr. 2000;31(4):418–23.

28. Kalnins D, Corey M, Ellis L, Pencharz PB, Tullis E, Durie PR. Failure of conventional strategies to improve nutritional status in malnourished adolescents and adults with cystic fibrosis. J Pediatr. 2005;147(3):399–401.

29. Poustie VJ, Russell JE, Watling RM, Ashby D, Smyth RL, Group CTC. Oral protein energy supplements for children with cystic fibrosis: CALICO multicentre randomised controlled trial. BMJ. 2006;332(7542):632–6.

30. Smyth RL, Walters S. Oral calorie supplements for cystic fibrosis. Cochrane Database Syst Rev. 2012; 10, CD000406.

31. Hollander FM, van Pierre DD, de Roos NM, van de Graaf EA, Iestra JA. Effects of nutritional status and dietetic interventions on survival in Cystic Fibrosis patients before and after lung transplantation. J Cyst Fibros. 2014;13(2):212–8.

32. Groleau V, Schall JI, Dougherty KA, Latham NE, Maqbool A, Mascarenhas MR, et al. Effect of a dietary intervention on growth and energy expenditure in children with cystic fibrosis. Journal of Cyst Fibros. 2014;13(5):572–8.

33. Powers SW, Byars KC, Mitchell MJ, Patton SR, Schindler T, Zeller MH. A randomized pilot study of behavioral treatment to increase calorie intake in toddlers with cystic fibrosis. Child Health Care. 2003;32:297–311.

34. Stark LJ, Opipari-Arrigan L, Quittner AL, Bean J, Powers SW. The effects of an intensive behavior and nutrition intervention compared to standard of care on weight outcomes in CF. Pediatr Pulmonol. 2011;46(1):31–5.

35. Watson H, Bilton D, Truby H. A randomized controlled trial of a new behavioral home-based nutrition education program, "Eat Well with CF," in adults with cystic fibrosis. J Am Diet Assoc. 2008;108(5):847–52.

36. Stark LJ, Quittner AL, Powers SW, Opipari-Arrigan L, Bean JA, Duggan C, et al. Randomized clinical trial of behavioral intervention and nutrition education to improve caloric intake and weight in children with cystic fibrosis. Arch Pediatr Adolesc Med. 2009;163(10):915–21.

37. Tluczek A, Clark R, McKechnie AC, Orland KM, Brown RL. Task-oriented and bottle feeding adversely affect the quality of mother-infant interactions after abnormal newborn screens. J Dev Behav Pediatr. 2010;31(5):414–26.

38. Janicke DM, Mitchell MJ, Stark LJ. Family functioning in school-age children with cystic fibrosis: an observational assessment of family interactions in the mealtime environment. J Pediatr Psychol. 2005;30(2):179–86.

39. Powers SW, Paton SR, Henry R, Heidemann M, Stark LJ. A tool to individualize nutritional care for children with cystic fibrosis: Reliability, validity and utility of the CF Indiviualized NuTritional Assessment of Kids Eating (CF INTAKE). Child Health Care. 2005;34:113–31.

40. Abbott J, Morton AM, Musson H, Conway SP, Etherington C, Gee L, et al. Nutritional status, perceived body image and eating behaviours in adults with cystic fibrosis. Clin Nutr. 2007;26(1):91–9.

41. Savant AP, Britton LJ, Petren K, McColley SA, Gutierrez HH. Sustained improvement in nutritional outcomes at two paediatric cystic fibrosis centres after quality improvement collaboratives. BMJ Qual Saf. 2014;23 Suppl 1:i81–9.

42. Erskine JM, Lingard CD, Sontag MK, Accurso FJ. Enteral nutrition for patients with cystic fibrosis: comparison of a semi-elemental and nonelemental formula. J Pediatr. 1998;132(2):265–9.

43. Oliver MR, Heine RG, Ng CH, Volders E, Olinsky A. Factors affecting clinical outcome in gastrostomy-fed children with cystic fibrosis. Pediatr Pulmonol. 2004;37(4):324–9.

44. Efrati O, Mei-Zahav M, Rivlin J, Kerem E, Blau H, Barak A, et al. Long term nutritional rehabilitation by gastrostomy in Israeli patients with cystic fibrosis: clinical outcome in advanced pulmonary disease. J Pediatr Gastroenterol Nutr. 2006;42(2):222–8.

45. Kuczmarski RJ, Ogden CL, Guo SS, Grummer-Strawn LM, Flegal KM, Mei Z, et al. 2000 CDC growth charts for the United States: methods and development. Vital and health statistics Series 11, Data from the national health survey. Vital Health Stat 11. 2002;246:1–190.

46. Rosenfeld M, Casey S, Pepe M, Ramsey BW. Nutritional effects of long-term gastrostomy feedings in children with cystic fibrosis. J Am Diet Assoc. 1999;99(2):191–4.

47. Walker SA, Gozal D. Pulmonary function correlates in the prediction of long-term weight gain in cystic fibrosis patients with gastrostomy tube feedings. J Pediatr Gastroenterol Nutr. 1998;27(1):53–6.

48. Van Biervliet S, De Waele K, Van Winckel M, Robberecht E. Percutaneous endoscopic gastrostomy in cystic fibrosis: patient acceptance and effect of overnight tube feeding on nutritional status. Acta gastro-enterologica Belgica. 2004;67(3):241–4.

49. Williams SG, Ashworth F, McAlweenie A, Poole S, Hodson ME, Westaby D. Percutaneous endoscopic gastrostomy feeding in patients with cystic fibrosis. Gut. 1999;44(1):87–90.

50. Bradley GM, Carson KA, Leonard AR, Mogayzel Jr PJ, Oliva-Hemker M. Nutritional outcomes following gastrostomy in children with cystic fibrosis. Pediatr Pulmonol. 2012;47(8):743–8.

51. Truby H, Cowlishaw P, O'Neil C, Wainwright C. The long term efficacy of gastrostomy feeding in children with cystic fibrosis on anthropometric markers of nutritional status and pulmonary function. Open Respir Med J. 2009;3:112–5.

52. Best C, Brearley A, Gaillard P, Regelmann W, Billings J, Dunitz J, et al. A pre-post retrospective study of patients with cystic fibrosis and gastrostomy tubes. J Pediatr Gastroenterol Nutr. 2011;53(4):453–8.

53. White H, Morton AM, Conway SP, Peckham DG. Enteral tube feeding in adults with cystic fibrosis; patient choice and impact on long term outcomes. J Cyst Fibros. 2013;12(6):616–22.

54. Conway S, Morton A, Wolfe S. Enteral tube feeding for cystic fibrosis. Cochrane Database Syst Rev. 2012;12, CD001198:1–14.

55. Steinkamp G, Rodeck B, Seidenberg J, Ruhl I, von der Hardt H. Stabilization of lung function in cystic fibrosis during long-term tube feeding via a percutaneous endoscopic gastrostomy. Pneumologie. 1990;44(10):1151–3.

56. Steinkamp G, von der Hardt H. Improvement of nutritional status and lung function after long-term nocturnal gastrostomy feedings in cystic fibrosis. J Pediatr. 1994;124(2):244–9.

57. Gunnell S, Christensen NK, McDonald C, Jackson D. Attitudes toward percutaneous endoscopic gastrostomy placement in cystic fibrosis patients. J Pediatr Gastroenterol Nutr. 2005;40(3):334–8.

58. Boesch RP, Acton JD. Outcomes of fundoplication in children with cystic fibrosis. J Pediatr Surg. 2007;42(8): 1341–4.
59. Sheikh SI, Ryan-Wenger NA, McCoy KS. Outcomes of surgical management of severe GERD in patients with cystic fibrosis. Pediatr Pulmonol. 2013;48(6):556–62.
60. O'Brien CE, Harden H, Com G. A survey of nutrition practices for patients with cystic fibrosis. Nutr Clin Pract. 2013;28(2):237–41.
61. Nicolo M, Stratton KW, Rooney W, Boullata J. Pancreatic enzyme replacement therapy for enterally fed patients with cystic fibrosis. Nutr Clin Pract. 2013;28(4):485–9.
62. Nasr SZ, Drury D. Appetite stimulants use in cystic fibrosis. Pediatr Pulmonol. 2008;43(3):209–19.
63. Strang P. The effect of megestrol acetate on anorexia, weight loss and cachexia in cancer and AIDS patients (review). Anticancer Res. 1997;17(1B):657–62.
64. Alexieva-Figusch J, van Gilse HA, Hop WC, Phoa CH, Blonk-van der Wijst J, Treurniet RE. Progestin therapy in advanced breast cancer: megestrol acetate--an evaluation of 160 treated cases. Cancer. 1980;46(11):2369–72.
65. Marchand V, Baker SS, Stark TJ, Baker RD. Randomized, double-blind, placebo-controlled pilot trial of megestrol acetate in malnourished children with cystic fibrosis. J Pediatr Gastroenterol Nutr. 2000;31(3):264–9.
66. Chinuck RS, Fortnum H, Baldwin DR. Appetite stimulants in cystic fibrosis: a systematic review. J Hum Nutr Diet. 2007;20(6):526–37.
67. Bergen Jr SS. Appetite Stimulating Properties of Cyproheptadine. Am J Dis Child. 1964;108:270–3.
68. Stiel JN, Liddle GW, Lacy WW. Studies on mechanism of cyproheptadine-induced weight gain in human subjects. Metabolism. 1970;19(3):192–200.
69. Goldberg SC, Halmi KA, Eckert ED, Casper RC, Davis JM. Cyproheptadine in Anorexia-Nervosa. Br J Psychiatry. 1979;134(Jan):67–70.
70. Rahman KM. Appetite stimulation and weight gain with cyproheptadine (periactin) in tuberculosis patients (double-blind clinical study). Med J Malaysia. 1975;29(4):270–4.
71. Noble RE. Effect of cyproheptadine on appetite and weight gain in adults. J Am Med Assoc. 1969;209(13): 2054–5.
72. Homnick DN, Homnick BD, Reeves AJ, Marks JH, Pimentel RS, Bonnema SK. Cyproheptadine is an effective appetite stimulant in cystic fibrosis. Pediatr Pulmonol. 2004;38(2):129–34.
73. Amar MB. Cannabinoids in medicine: a review of their therapeutic potential. J Ethno-Pharmacol. 2006;105:1–25.
74. Beal JE, Olson R, Laubenstein L, Morales JO, Bellman P, Yangco B, et al. Dronabinol as a treatment for anorexia associated with weight loss in patients with AIDS. J Pain Symptom Manage. 1995;10(2):89–97.
75. Anstead MI, Kuhn RJ, Martyn D, Craigmyle L, Kanga JF. Dronabinol, an effective and safe appetite stimulant in cystic fibrosis. Pediatr Pulmonol Suppl. 2003;25:343.
76. Young J, Danduran MJ, McColley SA, Boas SR. The role of mirtazapine as an appetite stimulant in malnourished individuals with cystic fibrosis. Pediatr Pulmonol Suppl. 2000;20S:325.
77. Sykes R, Kittel F, Marcus M, Tarter E, Schroth M. Mirtazapine for appetite stimulation in children with cystic fibrosis. Pediatr Pulmonol Suppl. 2006;506:389.
78. Nasr SZ, Hurwitz ME, Brown RW, Elghoroury M, Rosen D. Treatment of anorexia and weight loss with megestrol acetate in patients with cystic fibrosis. Pediatr Pulmonol. 1999;28(5):380–2.
79. McKone EF, Tonelli MR, Aitken ML. Adrenal insufficiency and testicular failure secondary to megestrol acetate therapy in a patient with cystic fibrosis. Pediatr Pulmonol. 2002;34(5):381–3.
80. Eubanks V, Koppersmith N, Wooldridge N, Clancy JP, Lyrene R, Arani RB, et al. Effects of megestrol acetate on weight gain, body composition, and pulmonary function in patients with cystic fibrosis. J Pediatr. 2002; 140(4):439–44.
81. Homnick DN, Marks JH, Hare KL, Bonnema SK. Long-term trial of cyproheptadine as an appetite stimulant in cystic fibrosis. Pediatr Pulmonol. 2005;40(3):251–6.
82. Chinuck R, Dewar J, Baldwin DR, Hendron E. Appetite stimulants for people with cystic fibrosis. Cochrane Database Syst Rev. 2014;7, CD008190:1–48.
83. Wermers RA, Hurley DL, Kearns AE. Osteoporosis associated with megestrol acetate. Mayo Clin Proc. 2004;79(12):1557–61.
84. Shepherd R, Cooksley WG, Cooke WD. Improved growth and clinical, nutritional, and respiratory changes in response to nutritional therapy in cystic fibrosis. J Pediatr. 1980;97(3):351–7.
85. Allen ED, Mick AB, Nicol J, McCoy KS. Prolonged parenteral nutrition for cystic fibrosis patients. Nutr Clin Pract. 1995;10(2):73–9.
86. Skeie B, Askanazi J, Rothkopf MM, Rosenbaum SH, Kvetan V, Ross E. Improved exercise tolerance with long-term parenteral nutrition in cystic fibrosis. Crit Care Med. 1987;15(10):960–2.
87. Katz DP, Manner T, Furst P, Askanazi J. The use of an intravenous fish oil emulsion enriched with omega-3 fatty acids in patients with cystic fibrosis. Nutrition. 1996;12(5):334–9.

Chapter 10
Pancreatic Insufficiency

Elissa Downs and Sarah Jane Schwarzenberg

Key Points

- Pancreatic sufficiency (PS) occurs in approximately 11–15% of patients diagnosed with cystic fibrosis.
- Most infants diagnosed with CF PS will progress to pancreatic insufficiency in the first 2 years of life, although a more gradual decline in pancreatic function is possible.
- Testing for pancreatic exocrine status may be conducted annually using the fecal elastase-1 (FE-1) immunoabsorbent assay to monitor for progression to pancreatic insufficiency status.
- Although PS generally is associated with milder CFTR phenotypes and better nutritional status, patients with CF and PS may experience clinically significant nutritional and gastrointestinal problems.
- Nutritional standards determined by the Cystic Fibrosis Foundation for growth during infancy, childhood and adolescence, maintenance of appropriate BMI during adult life, and nutrient adequacy apply to all CF patients regardless of pancreatic status. However, caloric and nutrient requirements may differ for the CF PS patient and should be evaluated on an individual basis.
- Acute pancreatitis may occur in CF PS patients. Testing for pancreatitis is indicated for the CF PS patient if clinical symptoms are present.

Keywords Pancreatic insufficiency • Pancreatic sufficiency • Pancreatic enzyme therapy • Coefficient of fat absorption • Immunoreactive trypsinogen • Fecal elastase • Malabsorption • Cholecystokinin

Abbreviations

CCK   Cholecystokinin
CF   Cystic fibrosis
CFA   Coefficient of fat absorption
CFF   Cystic Fibrosis Foundation

E. Downs, M.D., M.P.H. • S.J. Schwarzenberg, M.D. (✉)
Department of Pediatrics, Division of Pediatric Gastroenterology, Hepatology, and Nutrition, University of Minnesota, East Building, 6th Floor, 2450 Riverside Avenue, Minneapolis, MN 55454, USA
e-mail: down0015@umn.edu; schwa005@umn.edu

E.H. Yen, A.R. Leonard (eds.), *Nutrition in Cystic Fibrosis: A Guide for Clinicians*, Nutrition and Health, DOI 10.1007/978-3-319-16387-1_10, © Springer International Publishing Switzerland 2015

CFRD   Cystic fibrosis-related diabetes
CFTR   Cystic fibrosis transmembrane receptor
FDA   Food and Drug Administration
FE-1   Fecal elastase
IRT   Immunoreactive trypsinogen
PERT   Pancreatic enzyme replacement therapy
PI   Pancreatic insufficiency
PS   Pancreatic sufficiency

The Clinical Manifestations of Pancreatic Insufficiency in CF

Since the publication in 1938 by Andersen [1], cystic fibrosis (CF) has been a disease characterized by pancreatic insufficiency (PI). Careful measurement of pancreatic function and study of the multiple mutations in the CFTR gene led to recognition of both PI and pancreatic sufficient (PS) CF. The development of pancreatic enzyme replacement therapy (PERT) and its application to children with CF dramatically altered the outcomes of this disease. Microencapsulated pancreatic enzyme products made provision of adequate enzyme therapy achievable. Further improvements in the detection and management of PI in CF include the development of the fecal elastase test (FE-1), newborn screening, and FDA regulations requiring testing of pancreatic enzymes.

The pancreas has both exocrine and endocrine functions [2]. Exocrine pancreatic functions include synthesis and secretion into the duodenum of bicarbonate and a group of digestive enzymes, including amylase, lipase, and trypsin. Loss of exocrine function leads to maldigestion and subsequent malabsorption of many macronutrients (starches, proteins, and long-chain fats) and many micronutrients (including vitamins B12, A, E, D, and K). Nutrients not specifically requiring pancreatic secretions for digestion may be malabsorbed as a result of "intestinal hurry," the rapid movement of the small bowel as undigested fat reaches the colon and creates irritant diarrhea. Fatty stools increase absorption of dietary oxalates from the fecal stream, creating a risk for oxalate kidney stones.

Today, most North American children with CF are diagnosed at birth and rarely manifest the full clinical picture of exocrine PI prior to diagnosis and treatment. Clinicians should be aware of the clinical presentation of exocrine PI (Table 10.1). Children with PI may manifest poor growth, and adults may have weight loss. Patients with poorly controlled PI may experience severe abdominal pain, bloating, excessive flatus passage, and/or steatorrhea. Some patients are asymptomatic. Absence or denial of symptoms should not be considered evidence of PS nor should diarrhea and abdominal pain be assumed to represent inadequate pancreatic enzyme therapy.

The primary endocrine functions are the synthesis and secretion into the bloodstream of insulin (β-cell) and glucagon (α-cell) to regulate blood glucose levels. Loss of endocrine function, which occurs gradually in many CF patients, leads to glucose dysregulation, and, ultimately, cystic fibrosis-related diabetes (CFRD; see Chapter 10). Aggressive screening programs now detect CFRD ahead of serious clinical problems [3]. If not detected early, CFRD may present with weight loss, or be

Table 10.1 Symptoms of exocrine pancreatic insufficiency in cystic fibrosis

Failure to thrive	Meconium ileus
Short stature	Rectal prolapse
Poor weight gain; weight loss	Clinical deficiency of vitamin A, E, D, K
Hypoproteinemia; edema	
Steatorrhea	

Derived from [104]

asymptomatic until the individual experiences an infection. During illness or infection, individuals who until then have been glucose tolerant may develop glucose intolerance or diabetes. This condition may last several weeks after recovery from the illness that precipitated it.

The Pancreas in CF

CFTR protein is expressed in the ductal epithelium of the pancreas, where it allows water and anions access to the ductal lumen. It is also important in pancreatic bicarbonate transport. In the absence of functional CFTR, there is diminished ductal fluid, increased concentration of proteins in the fluid, and consequent precipitation of solutes in the ducts. The resulting ductal obstruction leads to acinar damage and fibrosis [4, 5]. The injury begins in utero, and at birth the pancreas is often severely damaged. Although some exocrine pancreatic tissue may be present at birth, and endocrine function appears unimpaired, most individuals homozygous for two severe CFTR mutations are functionally PI early in the first year of life [6].

Exocrine PI is the gastrointestinal complication of CF that is most predictable from genotype [7, 8]. Patients homozygous for severe CFTR mutations (class I, II, III, and VI) are generally PI, while individuals homozygous for mild CFTR mutations (class IV or V), or heterozygous for a mild and a severe mutation, are generally born PS. This is not to suggest that genotype alone should be used to make a clinical diagnosis of PI or PS. Investigation of pancreatic function is discussed below.

CFRD occurs in approximately 19% of adolescents and 40–50% of adults [9]. The development of CFRD is complex, involving reduced insulin secretion, genetic factors, insulin resistance, and other factors [3]. Damage to the α- and β-cells results from the gradual pancreatic destruction associated with obstruction of the ductal system.

The pancreas in the patient who is PS is generally not completely normal [10]. Some PS patients may have diminished bicarbonate secretion or reduced pancreatic enzyme secretion. Because the PI state requires loss of >85% of pancreatic function [11], PS individuals may have significant pancreatic functional impairment and still be clinically PS. Individuals born PS may become PI as they age. In one study, about 25% of PS patients became PI over a 5-year period. This change may occur very rapidly in some patients slowly in others [12].

Measuring Pancreatic Insufficiency

Choice of Tests and When to Use Them

PI can be measured by several different methods. Direct measurement, long considered the "gold standard" due to high levels of sensitivity and specificity, can be used for research purposes or when the indirect testing methods are inconclusive. Indirect testing methods, assaying serum or fecal enzymes or enzymatic activity, are usually low cost, noninvasive, straightforward to perform, and can largely be done on an outpatient basis. A number of different indirect tests exist with varying sensitivities and specificities. No test accurately identifies mild pancreatic insufficiency. In CF patients with compromised lung function, intubation or procedures that require additional sedation may aggravate respiratory insufficiency [13], and therefore, an indirect test may be preferable. In pediatric patients, indirect tests may also be preferable as they are less invasive and better tolerated [14].

Tests may also be categorized as useful for diagnosing PI status, for the purposes of initiating PERT, or tests useful for monitoring adequacy of PERT. The use of indirect tests to monitor adequacy of PERT has not been standardized and no test thus far has proven completely accurate for this purpose.

Direct Measurement Methods

Direct measurement methods are often referred to as invasive "tube" tests, as they use an enteric tube to collect stimulated pancreatic secretions from administration of secretin, cholecystokinin (CCK), combined secretin-CCK, or a meal (Lundh test meal) [15]. Secretin stimulation provokes bicarbonate production from the ductal cells, while CCK stimulation provokes enzyme secretion from the acinar cells. Although perhaps easier to perform, the Lundh test meal is no longer widely used as secretin testing has slightly improved sensitivity to detect mild PI [16].

The secretin stimulation test was modified by Dreiling [17] in 1948 and became the primary methodology to directly measure pancreatic secretion. As described by Lieb and Draganov [18], a large bore enteric tube is placed with gastric and duodenal ports and baseline measurements of pH are taken from both ports. A bolus dose or continuous infusion of secretin is then given; duodenal fluid over the next hour, at 15-min increments, is collected and analyzed for volume, pH, and bicarbonate concentration. Peak bicarbonate less than the reference range (80–130 mEq/L) [18] correlates with PI.

The stimulation test can also be performed with CCK or cerulein, a CCK analogue. In this test, two double-lumen enteric tubes are placed and again, baseline measurements from gastric and duodenal ports are obtained [19]. A constant infusion of mannitol and polyethylene glycol is administered duodenally, while IV CCK or cerulein is administered as a bolus or continuous infusion. Duodenal fluid over the next 80 min is collected in 20-min increments and analyzed for enzymatic output as well as bicarbonate concentration. Enzymatic activity or concentration should rapidly increase in response to CCK administration; peak concentration is significantly decreased in those with pancreatic disease [20].

More recently, variations on the direct stimulation test that are more feasible and better tolerated by patients were published. One such test is the secretin-stimulated endoscopic test [21], comparable in performance to the Dreiling test, measuring peak bicarbonate secretion, but at less cost, decreased procedure time, less radiation exposure, and with greater overall availability [22]. A secretin-enhanced MRI may allow even mild PI to be detected [23], but would require sedation in younger patients.

While these direct measurement methods are considered the "gold standard" for diagnosing pancreatic dysfunction, they are expensive, time consuming, and only performed at specialized centers [24]. Studies that have compared these direct methods with indirect methods [13] found that some indirect tests give comparable results with less cost, time commitment, and discomfort to the patient.

Indirect Methods

Currently, the three most commonly used indirect methods of assessing pancreatic insufficiency are coefficient of fat absorption (CFA), FE-1, and serum trypsinogen assays. Other tests will be described, but have limited use.

Coefficient of Fat Absorption

A quantitative fecal fat measurement can be obtained by the van de Kamer method [25]. This entails a 72-h stool collection on a diet with a fixed amount of fat (80–100 g/day in older patients). Normal fecal fat excretion on this fixed-fat diet should be <7 g/day for those aged 10 years and older, or <4–5 g/day for those aged 2–10 years [14].

CFA can then be calculated from this 72-h stool collection comparing exact intake versus excretion ([fat intake − fat excretion]/intake × 100). CFA values differ by age, with a CFA >85% normal for infants less than 6 months old [26, 27], and a CFA >93% normal for older infants, children, and adults [26, 28]. Steatorrhea would then be defined as >15% malabsorption in infants or >7% in adults.

CFA values have been found to vary widely in PI CF patients, reflective of the multifactorial etiology of malabsorption in CF [29]; despite the wide range, these values are still markedly abnormal with CFA values in untreated patients around 40% [29].

Disadvantages of quantifying fecal fat and calculating a CFA include low specificity as steatorrhea can be caused by conditions such as celiac disease, Crohn's disease, or small intestinal bacterial overgrowth [24]. Thus, the CFA can be abnormal even in pancreatic sufficient patients with confounding factors. Other disadvantages are that it requires 72 h collection on a fixed-fat diet and the patient must be off pancreatic enzymes if they have already been started [24]. Many patients find this test unpleasant. A single stool sample measurement of fecal fat is not recommended as fat content will vary significantly based on dietary intake [30].

In a study of CF patients with PI, the percentage fat in multiple single stool samples over several days had a strong correlation with the CFA and could be used instead of the 72-h stool collection for total fat measurement or for CFA calculation [31].

Fecal Elastase

The level of FE-1 is the predominately used indirect test. Elastase is an enzyme produced by the pancreas, is not degraded during intestinal transit, and becomes concentrated in stool [32]. Testing is via ELISA assay [32, 33], with a normal value defined as >200 micrograms of elastase per gram stool (μg/g). Assays using a monoclonal antibody may have higher sensitivity than those using a polyclonal antibody [34]. This test is specific for the human enzyme, and will not detect exogenous enzyme replacement [35]. It has defined sensitivity that detects severe PI more accurately: the sensitivity is approximately 100% in severe, 77–100% in moderate, and 0–63% in mild PI [36–38]. In a study of infants with cystic fibrosis, FE-1 was abnormal even at an initial visit around 3–4 months of age; by 6 months of age, all infants in the study had values <100 μg/g [6], leading the authors to conclude this test should be used early for the monitoring of pancreatic insufficiency development. The specificity of the test is also high (approximately 90%), but this may be decreased in those with type 1 diabetes or small bowel disease [38].

FE-1 is an attractive test as it is easy to perform, can be done with a single stool sample, and patients can continue PERT [24]. In some algorithms of diagnosing PI, it is one of the first steps in the process [14, 15]. Disadvantages include results that are unreliable on loose stool [39] and in newborn infants under 2 weeks of age [40]; it also has decreased sensitivity in mild pancreatic insufficiency. FE-1 does not distinguish between primary and secondary causes of PI [39]. False positives can be due to mucosal villous atrophy from celiac disease, or infectious or allergic enteropathy [41]. Researchers have also identified both within stool and day-to-day mild variation in levels of FE-1. Thus if results are uncertain (in the borderline area as defined by Hamwi et al. [42] of ±25% of the normal 200 μg/g), this assay should be repeated on a different stool sample [38].

Studies comparing CFA, serum immunoreactive trypsinogen (IRT), and FE-1 have shown poor correlation of these three assays in PS CF patients [43]. FE-1 also has a lower sensitivity and high false positive rate compared to direct measurement of pancreatic function by secretin-stimulated endoscopic method [44]. However, for most purposes, the convenience of the FE-1 will outweigh its limitations.

Immunoreactive Trypsinogen

Levels of plasma IRT are elevated in infants with CF [45–47]; this test forms the basis of the newborn screen for CF. However, IRT levels are significantly elevated in CF infants under 1 year old regardless of PS or PI status [48]; thus this test would not be appropriate to use in infants to diagnose pancreatic status. When CF infants become PI, IRT levels fall rapidly and a large proportion of patients will have subnormal values by 6 years old [45], with >95% subnormal by 7 years old [46]. No corresponding age-related declines have been found in CF patients who remain PS [45, 46]. After 7 years of age, the difference in IRT levels between the PS and PI patients became statistically significant [45] and was an accurate predictor of pancreatic function. Lower IRT levels in older age groups were also significantly associated with steatorrhea [47]. The trends in IRT levels could be used to monitor for the development of PI [46], but only after 7 years of age.

Other Fecal Tests

A stool steatocrit is a rough estimation of stool fat concentration and thus, malabsorption. Values decline over the first 3 months of life [49]. It is proposed as a means to monitor fat absorption and sufficiency of PERT in infants [50]. It should not be used to diagnose PI. Acidification of the stool improves sensitivity of the test [51]. In CF, some groups find good correlation of acid steatocrit and CFA [51] and others find the correlation to be poor [52]. Its advantages are that it can be done on a small volume of stool (0.5 g) [53]. This test is less accurate in older children as fat is not distributed evenly throughout stool as it is in younger children [54].

Chymotrypsin, a pancreatic protease, is not degraded in the stool and can be used to assess pancreatic enzyme secretion. Activity is calculated by units per gram of stool (U/g); values <3 U/g are abnormal [38]; an abnormal value of <6 U/g may increase the sensitivity of the test [55]. An advantage to this test is that is can be performed off a single stool sample. It had 100% sensitivity and specificity in one study in identifying CF patients with total PI [56], but in patients with mild PI, the sensitivity drops significantly [55]. Chymotrypsin is altered by exogenous enzyme supplementation, thus the test may be useful to monitor compliance to therapy [14, 57]. A disadvantage of this test is an increased rate of false positives in diarrhea stool due to diluted activity [18]. To assay PI, patients need to be off pancreatic enzymes for several days prior. In comparison to FE-1, chymotrypsin was less sensitive in detecting mild, moderate, and severe PI [55].

Breath Tests

The breath test is unique in that rather than measuring enzyme levels or enzymatic activity, it measures triglyceride digestion. Patients are given a meal with labeled triglyceride substrates; the substrates are then hydrolyzed, absorbed, and waste products are released across the pulmonary epithelium as labeled CO_2 [24]. This can then be measured via breath test at 6 h postingestion of the meal. In healthy subjects, recovered labeled CO_2 has ranged between 20 and 40%, with lower values for younger children [58, 59]. Studies have demonstrated a sensitivity of 89–90% and specificity of 81–91% [60, 61]. Examples of different substrates that have been used include 13C-triolein [62, 63], 13C-tripalmitin [64], and 13C-mixed triglyceride [65, 66].

Other Tests

The serum lipase can be measured in response to a meal challenge (Lundh test meal). A baseline lipase is measured prior to the meal, and then a peak around 30 min after the meal. Consistently low levels in response to the Lundh test meal correlated with known severe PI in CF patients [67].

So-called "tube-less" tests of pancreatic function, including the NBT-PABA test and pancreolauryl or fluorescein dilaurate test are no long used. Studies of newer assays, such as a nonabsorbable lipid marker (behenic acid) have not shown good enough correlation with CFA to justify use [68].

The malabsorption blood test (MBT) is a novel approach to quantifying digestion and absorption of fat [69]. Simultaneous oral doses of pentadecanoic acid (a free fatty acid) and triheptadecanoic acid (a triglyceride with three saturated fatty acids) are given. These are naturally occurring but uncommon lipids. The triheptadecanoic acid must undergo hydrolysis by pancreatic lipase before absorption. On initial testing, the differential between the absorption of these substrates reflected pancreatic digestion. Ultimately, this may prove to be a useful tool to assess lipase-deficient fat malabsorption.

Pancreatic Enzyme Replacement Therapy

Description of Enzyme Therapy

PERT has long been available in the USA for patients with cystic fibrosis or other causes of pancreatic insufficiency. These formulations are of bovine or porcine origin. Most of them had been in place prior to 1938 and the enactment of the Federal Food, Drug, and Cosmetic Act, which required new drugs to obtain government approval. In 1991, the FDA required that pancreatic enzyme replacement products be provided by prescription only and in 2004, current products required new drug application approval to assure safety, effectiveness, and product quality [70] by a deadline extended to 2010. Products have evolved over time with the advent of micro-drug development and enteric coating to protect the enzymes against gastric acid inactivation. The majority of enzymes currently available in the USA are formulated in this manner; only one product is not enteric coated.

A non-porcine-derived pancreatic enzyme preparation is desirable for several reasons, including the batch-to-batch variability associated with an animal-derived product and some religious objections to animal-derived or porcine products [71, 72]. A synthetic non-porcine enzyme product is in development and has undergone a phase III trial with outcomes of improved fat and nitrogen absorption. This formulation contains only biotechnology-derived amylase, lipase, and trypsin engineered to be stable at acidic pH; it does not require enteric coating. Further clinical trials will be needed to determine if this approach can replace porcine-derived enzymes.

Dosing Pancreatic Enzymes

PERT should be started in the following situations: (1) based on presence of two CFTR mutations associated with PI [73], (2) evidence of PI by testing methods as described above, or (3) frank malabsorption symptoms [74].

Most PERT is provided via enteric-coated formulations to avoid gastric acid inactivation of unprotected lipase; this coating will dissolve at alkaline pH in the small intestine. The enteric-coated formulations should not be crushed or chewed [75]. However, the capsules can be opened and mixed with food such as applesauce or another non-alkaline food to avoid premature dissolution of the coating and thus enzyme activation [75].

A single pancreatic enzyme preparation is available that is not micro-encapsulated (Viokase). Some providers use it during enteral feedings, as it can be crushed and added to the formula. It should be noted that there is no evidence to support this practice. Viokase is also used by some providers to treat or prevent the pain of chronic pancreatitis by reducing CCK and pancreas secretion [76].

While it is more physiologic to dose enzymes based on the grams of fat per meal, it is more practical and convenient to use a weight-based dose or standard dose per meal or snack [28, 75].

Meal Method

Meal method dosing varies by age. In infants and children, doses per kilogram of body weight are targeted. In adults, a standard dose is chosen independent of body weight. However regardless of age, doses should not exceed 10,000 lipase units per kilogram per day [74, 77]. Doses higher than 10,000 lipase units/kg/day may be associated with side effects (see below) [77, 78]. Some authors have questioned this limit, particularly for young infants, but as yet the optimal dose of enzymes in this group is unknown [79]. Care should be taken in exceeding the recommended doses without further evidence.

For infants, enzymes should be given for all types of formula and breast milk feedings [26]. The capsules should be opened and mixed with an acidic baby food (like applesauce) or cereal. If uncoated enzyme preparations are used, the infant's mouth and gums should be cleaned with sterile water after administration to prevent mucosal injury [80]. If coated preparations are used, the infant's mouth should be examined for residual microspheres.

The Cystic Fibrosis Foundation (CFF) recommends starting at a standard dose of 2000–5000 lipase units per feeding (defined as 120 mL of formula or each breast feeding occurrence) for infants and those under 12 months of age [26, 74]. For children from 12 months to 4 years of age, an initial dose of 1000 lipase units per kilogram per meal is recommended. A dose of 500 lipase units per kilogram per meal is a recommended starting point for older children, adolescents and adults [28, 75]. For all ages the maximum recommended meal dose is 2,500 lipase units/kg [75]. In a study of Pancrease MT, a dose of 500 lipase units per kilogram per meal was also well tolerated in infants and toddlers; higher doses did not increase CFA significantly [81]. For those consuming snacks, one-half the meal dose should be given as coverage. Frequent reassessment of dosing is necessary at each visit to ensure proper growth and weight gain. Doses should be adjusted as needed based on weight and on presence of symptoms indicative of malabsorption [75].

To avoid excessive dosing for overweight/obese adults another recommendation is to provide 25,000–40,000 (up to 75,000) units of lipase per meal, and 5000–25,000 units of lipase per snack, as long as doses do not exceed 10,000 units per kilogram per day [24, 77]. Total doses of more than 75,000 units per meal are not recommended [77]. Half of the dose should be taken at the start of the meal, with the remainder half-way through the meal [57, 82].

Fat Gram Method

Dosing enzymes by amount of fat per meal is more physiologic, but less convenient overall; however it does take into account that fat intake is relatively higher in infancy and decreases over time [75]. Daily dosing by this method ranges from 500 to 4000 lipase units per gram of fat ingested per day. In a study of delayed release pancrelipase (Creon), target doses of 4000 lipase units per gram of dietary fat were well tolerated compared to placebo in those aged 7–11 years [83] and in those aged >12 years [84]. In one study, matching enzyme dose to grams of fat per meal led to improvement in symptoms of abdominal pain and diarrhea [85]. Patients took over twice as many capsules per day on this routine versus a fixed meal dose routine (5–11.5). If patients or their families are motivated, this regimen is recommended to optimize absorption.

Enteral Feeds

Individuals who receive nocturnal enteral feeds should divide their doses throughout the feeding, with a dose at the beginning of the feeding, midway, and at the end administered via the enteral tube [77]. Non-enteric-coated enzymes (Viokase) tablets can also be crushed and mixed directly into the formula itself to start predigesting the formula [86]. If enteric-coated formulations are used, these should be mixed with applesauce and delivered through a larger bore feeding tube [77]. Alternatively, some institutions will dissolve the capsule contents in sodium bicarbonate solution and then administer via the enteral tube [87, 88]. There are no randomized controlled trials to assess the comparative efficacy of these techniques.

Other Issues

PI may lead to malabsorption of fat-soluble vitamins, including vitamins A, E, D, and K [89]. As pancreatic enzymes are necessary for the release of vitamin B12 from proteins binding it prior to complexing with intrinsic factor, deficiency of B12 is possible in PI, but with appropriate care it is not a clinical problem [90]. The CFF recommends supplementation of PI individuals with vitamin preparations containing both fat-soluble and water-soluble vitamins. Yearly monitoring of vitamins A, E, and D is recommended [89]. Serum levels of vitamin K are not recommended, as it reflects recent intake.

Complications of Excessive Doses of PERT

In the early 1990s, case reports detailing the development of fibrosing colonopathy in young children and adolescents appeared in the UK [91, 92]. During examination of the National Cystic Fibrosis Patient Registry, a total of 31 cases were identified in the USA between 1990 and 1994 [78] with a strong dose-dependent response. In their analysis models, a dose between 24,000 and 50,000 lipase units per kilogram per day had a relative risk of fibrosing colonopathy of 10.9; higher than 50,000 lipase units per kilogram per day had a relative risk of fibrosing colonopathy of 199.5. In 1995, a CFF Consensus statement was published with recommendations to not exceed 10,000 units per kilogram per day based on this risk [75]. This equates to <2500 lipase units per kilogram per meal or <4000 lipase units per gram of fat per day [89].

Monitoring Effectiveness of Enzymes

Efficacy of therapy is usually monitored clinically on the basis of improvement in symptoms of steatorrhea and weight gain [57, 89]. If it is unclear whether poor weight gain or diarrhea is the result of inadequate enzyme administration, some of the methods discussed above, such as the CFA, would be appropriate measures to assess this [89].

Detecting Failure and Its Causes

Failure of PERT occurs due to numerous factors and analysis should be undertaken on a patient-by-patient basis; a good history should detect a number of these factors and underscores the importance of working with a registered dietitian well trained in the management of cystic fibrosis. A common cause of failure is poor adherence to medication dosing and administration. Rates of adherence have been problematic in children [93], adolescents, and teenagers [94]. In studies of adolescents and adults [95, 96], those with more severe disease were found to be more adherent, suggesting the converse is also true.

Dietary factors—such as excessive juice intake causing toddler's diarrhea or a periodic extremely high-fat meal that a standard dose of enzymes may not cover [75]—all can lead to perceived failure, and should be assessed with a good diet history before pursuing other interventions.

In addition, other lifestyle factors, such as a perception that enzymes do not need to be given with all meals or snacks or difficulty dosing enzymes for children and adults who "graze" or snack all day long [75], should be assessed. Clinicians should query the timing of enzyme administration as well; enzymes should be taken no more than 30 min before or after a meal [86].

Underdosing may occur based on overall fat intake or when a patient "outgrows" their body weight-based dosing. In this sense, underdosing is likely more common with meal method versus the fat gram method [85]. Dosing may also be sufficient to decrease symptoms of steatorrhea, but may not be sufficient enough to correct nutritional deficiencies [97].

Failure can also be caused by an inappropriate intestinal pH milieu. Uncoated enzymes can be inactivated by prolonged exposure to gastric acid [98]. Cystic fibrosis leads to impairment of bicarbonate secretion [99]; this leads to a relatively acidic duodenal environment that may decrease dissolution of the coating on micro-encapsulated enzyme replacement therapy [75, 100]. Enzymes may then be activated in the distal jejunum or ileum, bypassing important areas of nutrient absorption. Some providers administer proton pump inhibitor therapy in an attempt to reduce gastric acid secretion and improve intestinal pH.

For enzyme therapy to be maximally effective, the enzymes need to reach the proximal duodenum in conjunction with food substrate. With delayed gastric emptying, enzymes may exit the stomach prior to the food bolus; in these patients, PERT is not as successful [101]. If delayed gastric emptying is suspected, the timing of enzyme administration could be adjusted to midway through or at the end of a meal [101], which has been shown to optimize efficacy [102]. The addition of non-coated enzyme could be considered if rapid gastric emptying [86, 101], as this will empty from the stomach earlier with the liquid portion of the meal.

PERT is costly; some insurance providers do not pay for PERT or pay only part of the costs. This may lead patients to use fewer enzymes than prescribed. They may also try over-the-counter "enzymes," often sold in health food stores. These do not contain functional pancreatic enzymes and cannot be substituted for PERT.

Patients with CF may develop confounding gastrointestinal disorders that may cause poor weight gain or growth failure; this may also lead to perceived failure of PERT. Examples of these conditions include lactose intolerance, gastroenteritis, small intestinal bacterial overgrowth, celiac disease, Crohn's disease, or *Clostridium difficile* colitis [75]. Comorbid conditions of CF, including CFRD and CF liver disease, or pulmonary infections, may lead to poor growth and perceived failure of PERT.

Diagnosis of Persistent Malabsorption

Persistent failure of weight gain or growth when using adequate pancreatic enzyme doses should be investigated carefully. If adherence and appropriate dosing is known, causes of poor appetite and/or malabsorption other than PI should be suspected. Increasing enzyme doses above 10,000 lipase units/kg/day without performing CFA or other tests of malabsorption should not be done. In addition, even when fat malabsorption is demonstrated at appropriate doses of PERT, other causes should be considered (see Chapter 11).

Fieker et al. [57] outline a systematic approach to detect causes of failure, starting with assessment of compliance. If noncompliance is suspected, a fecal chymotrypsin level can be obtained and if low, then education can be provided on adherence [14, 57]. If the patient is compliant, the lipase dose can be increased, the diet can be modified, and/or acid suppression can be added. If these interventions fail to reveal an etiology of the failure, further evaluation can be undertaken to look for alternate etiologies of steatorrhea such as bacterial overgrowth, giardiasis, and blind loop among others, such as celiac disease [24].

Monitoring PS CF for Developing PI (10%)

Individuals with CF who are PS at birth do not have completely normal pancreas function [4]. They may remain PS throughout their life, or may become PI at any time during their life [12]. Development of pancreatitis, which occurs in about 25% of PS CF patients, and most commonly in those with the best preserved pancreatic function [103], may increase the risk for development of PI as a result of injury to the pancreas. The CFF recommends that individuals with CF who are PS be evaluated yearly for possible development of PI [74]. This may be done clinically or by using established tests of pancreatic function, including CFA, direct pancreatic function, or FE-1 testing. Clinical evaluation may miss early development of PI.

Conclusion

In summary, PI is a critical complication of cystic fibrosis, affecting 80–90% of patients over the life-span. Left untreated or undertreated, it can lead to malnutrition, vitamin and mineral deficiencies, and abdominal pain. Fecal elastase provides a simple measure of PI allowing recognition of individuals transitioning from PS to PI and appropriate use of PERT. Meticulous attention to providing appropriate doses of PERT, managing malabsorption related to non-PI medical complications, and promoting adherence to PERT will improve the lives of individuals with CF.

References

1. Andersen DH. Cystic fibrosis of the pancreas and its relation to celiac disease: a clinical and pathological study. Am J Dis Child. 1938;56:344–99.
2. Owyang C, Williams J. Pancreatic secretion. In: Yamada T, Alpers DH, Kalloo AN, Kaplowitz N, Owyang C, Powell DW, editors. Textbook of gastroenterology. 5th ed. Oxford: Wiley-Blackwell; 2008. p. 368–400.
3. Kelly A, Moran A. Update on cystic fibrosis-related diabetes. J Cyst Fibros. 2013;12(4):318–31.
4. Wilschanski M. Novel therapeutic approaches for cystic fibrosis. Discov Med. 2013;15(81):127–33.
5. Durie PR, Forstner GG. Pathophysiology of the exocrine pancreas in cystic fibrosis. J R Soc Med. 1989;82 Suppl 16:2–10.
6. Walkowiak J, Sands D, Nowakowska A, Piotrowski R, Zybert K, Herzig KH, et al. Early decline of pancreatic function in cystic fibrosis patients with class 1 or 2 CFTR mutations. J Pediatr Gastroenterol Nutr. 2005;40(2): 199–201.
7. Kristidis P, Bozon D, Corey M, Markiewicz D, Rommens J, Tsui LC, et al. Genetic determination of exocrine pancreatic function in cystic fibrosis. Am J Hum Genet. 1992;50(6):1178–84.
8. Kerem E, Corey M, Kerem BS, Rommens J, Markiewicz D, Levison H, et al. The relation between genotype and phenotype in cystic fibrosis—analysis of the most common mutation (delta F508). N Engl J Med. 1990; 323(22):1517–22.
9. Moran A, Dunitz J, Nathan B, Saeed A, Holme B, Thomas W. Cystic fibrosis-related diabetes: current trends in prevalence, incidence, and mortality. Diabetes Care. 2009;32(9):1626–31.
10. Wilschanski M, Novak I. The cystic fibrosis of exocrine pancreas. Cold Spring Harb Perspect Med. 2013;3(5): a009746.
11. DiMagno EP, Go VL, Summerskill WH. Relations between pancreatic enzyme outputs and malabsorption in severe pancreatic insufficiency. N Engl J Med. 1973;288(16):813–5.

12. Walkowiak J, Nousia-Arvanitakis S, Agguridaki C, Fotoulaki M, Strzykala K, Balassopoulou A, et al. Longitudinal follow-up of exocrine pancreatic function in pancreatic sufficient cystic fibrosis patients using the fecal elastase-1 test. J Pediatr Gastroenterol Nutr. 2003;36(4):474–8.

13. Walkowiak J, Cichy WK, Herzig KH. Comparison of fecal elastase-1 determination with the secretin-cholecystokinin test in patients with cystic fibrosis. Scand J Gastroenterol. 1999;34(2):202–7.

14. Walkowiak J, Nousia-Arvanitakis S, Henker J, Stern M, Sinaasappel M, Dodge JA. Indirect pancreatic function tests in children. J Pediatr Gastroenterol Nutr. 2005;40(2):107–14.

15. Lindkvist B. Diagnosis and treatment of pancreatic exocrine insufficiency. World J Gastroenterol. 2013;19(42):7258–66.

16. Gyr K, Agrawal NM, Felsenfeld O, Font RG. Comparative study of secretin and Lundh tests. Am J Dig Dis. 1975;20(6):506–12.

17. Dreiling DA, Hollander F. Studies in pancreatic function; preliminary series of clinical studies with the secretin test. Gastroenterology. 1948;11(5):714–29.

18. Lieb 2nd JG, Draganov PV. Pancreatic function testing: here to stay for the 21st century. World J Gastroenterol. 2008;14(20):3149–58.

19. Go VL, Hofmann AF, Summerskill WH. Simultaneous measurements of total pancreatic, biliary, and gastric outputs in man using a perfusion technique. Gastroenterology. 1970;58(3):321–8.

20. Conwell DL, Zuccaro G, Morrow JB, Van Lente F, Obuchowski N, Vargo JJ, et al. Cholecystokinin-stimulated peak lipase concentration in duodenal drainage fluid: a new pancreatic function test. Am J Gastroenterol. 2002;97(6):1392–7.

21. Stevens T, Conwell DL, Zuccaro Jr G, Van Lente F, Purich E, Khandwala F, et al. A randomized crossover study of secretin-stimulated endoscopic and dreiling tube pancreatic function test methods in healthy subjects. Am J Gastroenterol. 2006;101(2):351–5.

22. Conwell DL, Zuccaro Jr G, Vargo JJ, Morrow JB, Obuchowski N, Dumot JA, et al. An endoscopic pancreatic function test with cholecystokinin-octapeptide for the diagnosis of chronic pancreatitis. Clin Gastroenterol Hepatol. 2003;1(3):189–94.

23. Czako L. Diagnosis of early-stage chronic pancreatitis by secretin-enhanced magnetic resonance cholangiopancreatography. J Gastroenterol. 2007;42 Suppl 17:113–7.

24. Sikkens EC, Cahen DL, Kuipers EJ, Bruno MJ. Pancreatic enzyme replacement therapy in chronic pancreatitis. Best Pract Res Clin Gastroenterol. 2010;24(3):337–47.

25. Van De Kamer JH, Ten Bokkel Huinink H, Weyers HA. Rapid method for the determination of fat in feces. J Biol Chem. 1949;177(1):347–55.

26. Ramsey BW, Farrell PM, Pencharz P. Nutritional assessment and management in cystic fibrosis: a consensus report. The Consensus Committee. Am J Clin Nutr. 1992;55(1):108–16.

27. Fomon SJ, Ziegler EE, Thomas LN, Jensen RL, Filer Jr LJ. Excretion of fat by normal full-term infants fed various milks and formulas. Am J Clin Nutr. 1970;23(10):1299–313.

28. Yankaskas JR, Marshall BC, Sufian B, Simon RH, Rodman D. Cystic fibrosis adult care: consensus conference report. Chest. 2004;125(1 Suppl):1S–39.

29. Borowitz D, Konstan MW, O'Rourke A, Cohen M, Hendeles L, Murray FT. Coefficients of fat and nitrogen absorption in healthy subjects and individuals with cystic fibrosis. J Pediatr Pharmacol Ther. 2007;12(1):47–52.

30. Taylor JR, Gardner TB, Waljee AK, Dimagno MJ, Schoenfeld PS. Systematic review: efficacy and safety of pancreatic enzyme supplements for exocrine pancreatic insufficiency. Aliment Pharmacol Ther. 2010;31(1):57–72.

31. Caras S, Boyd D, Zipfel L, Sander-Struckmeier S. Evaluation of stool collections to measure efficacy of PERT in subjects with exocrine pancreatic insufficiency. J Pediatr Gastroenterol Nutr. 2011;53(6):634–40.

32. Sziegoleit A, Krause E, Klor HU, Kanacher L, Linder D. Elastase 1 and chymotrypsin B in pancreatic juice and feces. Clin Biochem. 1989;22(2):85–9.

33. Sziegoleit A, Knapler H, Peters B. ELISA for human pancreatic elastase 1. Clin Biochem. 1989;22(2):79–83.

34. Borowitz D, Lin R, Baker SS. Comparison of monoclonal and polyclonal ELISAs for fecal elastase in patients with cystic fibrosis and pancreatic insufficiency. J Pediatr Gastroenterol Nutr. 2007;44(2):219–23.

35. Dominici R, Franzini C. Fecal elastase-1 as a test for pancreatic function: a review. Clin Chem Lab Med. 2002;40(4):325–32.

36. Dominguez-Munoz JE. Pancreatic enzyme therapy for pancreatic exocrine insufficiency. Curr Gastroenterol Rep. 2007;9(2):116–22.

37. Beharry S, Ellis L, Corey M, Marcon M, Durie P. How useful is fecal pancreatic elastase 1 as a marker of exocrine pancreatic disease? J Pediatr. 2002;141(1):84–90.

38. Loser C, Mollgaard A, Folsch UR. Faecal elastase 1: a novel, highly sensitive, and specific tubeless pancreatic function test. Gut. 1996;39(4):580–6.

39. Daftary A, Acton J, Heubi J, Amin R. Fecal elastase-1: utility in pancreatic function in cystic fibrosis. J Cyst Fibros. 2006;5(2):71–6.

40. Nissler K, Von Katte I, Huebner A, Henker J. Pancreatic elastase 1 in feces of preterm and term infants. J Pediatr Gastroenterol Nutr. 2001;33(1):28–31.

41. Walkowiak J, Herzig KH. Fecal elastase-1 is decreased in villous atrophy regardless of the underlying disease. Eur J Clin Invest. 2001;31(5):425–30.

42. Hamwi A, Veitl M, Maenner G, Vogelsang H, Szekeres T. Pancreatic elastase 1 in stool: variations within one stool passage and individual changes from day to day. Wien Klin Wochenschr. 2000;112(1):32–5.

43. Weintraub A, Blau H, Mussaffi H, Picard E, Bentur L, Kerem E, et al. Exocrine pancreatic function testing in patients with cystic fibrosis and pancreatic sufficiency: a correlation study. J Pediatr Gastroenterol Nutr. 2009;48(3):306–10.

44. Wali PD, Loveridge-Lenza B, He Z, Horvath K. Comparison of fecal elastase-1 and pancreatic function testing in children. J Pediatr Gastroenterol Nutr. 2012;54(2):277–80.

45. Durie PR, Forstner GG, Gaskin KJ, Moore DJ, Cleghorn GJ, Wong SS, et al. Age-related alterations of immunoreactive pancreatic cationic trypsinogen in sera from cystic fibrosis patients with and without pancreatic insufficiency. Pediatr Res. 1986;20(3):209–13.

46. Couper RT, Corey M, Durie PR, Forstner GG, Moore DJ. Longitudinal evaluation of serum trypsinogen measurement in pancreatic-insufficient and pancreatic-sufficient patients with cystic fibrosis. J Pediatr. 1995;127(3):408–13.

47. Bollbach R, Becker M, Rotthauwe HW. Serum immunoreactive trypsin and pancreatic lipase in cystic fibrosis. Eur J Pediatr. 1985;144(2):167–70.

48. Cleghorn G, Benjamin L, Corey M, Forstner G, Dati F, Durie P. Age-related alterations in immunoreactive pancreatic lipase and cationic trypsinogen in young children with cystic fibrosis. J Pediatr. 1985;107(3):377–81.

49. de Mello ED, da Silveira TR. The Steatocrit Test: a semiquantitative method to evaluate the fecal fat excretion—method standardization. J Pediatr (Rio J). 1995;71(5):273–8.

50. Colombo C, Maiavacca R, Ronchi M, Consalvo E, Amoretti M, Giunta A. The steatocrit: a simple method for monitoring fat malabsorption in patients with cystic fibrosis. J Pediatr Gastroenterol Nutr. 1987;6(6):926–30.

51. Tran M, Forget P, Van den Neucker A, Strik J, van Kreel B, Kuijten R. The acid steatocrit: a much improved method. J Pediatr Gastroenterol Nutr. 1994;19(3):299–303.

52. Wagner MH, Bowser EK, Sherman JM, Francisco MP, Theriaque D, Novak DA. Comparison of steatocrit and fat absorption in persons with cystic fibrosis. J Pediatr Gastroenterol Nutr. 2002;35(2):202–5.

53. Phuapradit P, Narang A, Mendonca P, Harris DA, Baum JD. The steatocrit: a simple method for estimating stool fat content in newborn infants. Arch Dis Child. 1981;56(9):725–7.

54. Tardelli AC, Camargos PA, Penna FJ, Sarkis PF, Guimaraes EV. Comparison of diagnostic methods for pancreatic insufficiency in infants with cystic fibrosis. J Pediatr Gastroenterol Nutr. 2013;56(2):178–81.

55. Walkowiak J, Herzig KH, Strzykala K, Przyslawski J, Krawczynski M. Fecal elastase-1 is superior to fecal chymotrypsin in the assessment of pancreatic involvement in cystic fibrosis. Pediatrics. 2002;110(1 Pt 1), e7.

56. Girella E, Faggionato P, Benetazzo D, Mastella G. The assay of chymotrypsin in stool as a simple and effective test of exocrine pancreatic activity in cystic fibrosis. Pancreas. 1988;3(3):254–62.

57. Fieker A, Philpott J, Armand M. Enzyme replacement therapy for pancreatic insufficiency: present and future. Clin Exp Gastroenterol. 2011;4:55–73.

58. Weaver LT, Amarri S, Swart GR. 13C mixed triglyceride breath test. Gut. 1998;43 Suppl 3:S13–9.

59. van Dijk-van Aalst K, Van Den Driessche M, van Der Schoor S, Schiffelers S, van't Westeinde T, Ghoos Y, et al. 13C mixed triglyceride breath test: a noninvasive method to assess lipase activity in children. J Pediatr Gastroenterol Nutr. 2001;32(5):579–85.

60. Vantrappen GR, Rutgeerts PJ, Ghoos YF, Hiele MI. Mixed triglyceride breath test: a noninvasive test of pancreatic lipase activity in the duodenum. Gastroenterology. 1989;96(4):1126–34.

61. Iglesias-Garcia J, Vilarino M, Iglesias-Rey M, Lourido V, Dominguez-Munoz E. Accuracy of the optimized 13c-mixed triglyceride breath test for the diagnosis of steatorrhea in clinical practice. Gastroenterology. 2003;124(Suppl1):A631.

62. O'Keefe SJ, Stevens S, Lee R, Zhou W, Zfass A. Physiological evaluation of the severity of pancreatic exocrine dysfunction during endoscopy. Pancreas. 2007;35(1):30–6.

63. Ritz MA, Fraser RJ, Di Matteo AC, Greville H, Butler R, Cmielewski P, et al. Evaluation of the 13C-triolein breath test for fat malabsorption in adult patients with cystic fibrosis. J Gastroenterol Hepatol. 2004;19(4):448–53.

64. Laiho KM, Gavin J, Murphy JL, Connett GJ, Wootton SA. Maldigestion and malabsorption of 13C labelled tripalmitin in gastrostomy-fed patients with cystic fibrosis. Clin Nutr. 2004;23(3):347–53.

65. Dominguez-Munoz JE, Iglesias-Garcia J, Vilarino-Insua M, Iglesias-Rey M. 13C-mixed triglyceride breath test to assess oral enzyme substitution therapy in patients with chronic pancreatitis. Clin Gastroenterol Hepatol. 2007;5(4):484–8.

66. Herzog DC, Delvin EE, Albert C, Marcotte JE, Pelletier VA, Seidman EG. 13C-labeled mixed triglyceride breath test (13C MTG-BT) in healthy children and children with cystic fibrosis (CF) under pancreatic enzyme replacement therapy (PERT): a pilot study. Clin Biochem. 2008;41(18):1489–92.

67. Augarten A, Katznelson D, Dubenbaum L, Doolman R, Sela BA, Lusky A, et al. Serum lipase levels pre and post Lundh meal: evaluation of exocrine pancreatic status in cystic fibrosis. Int J Clin Lab Res. 1998;28(4):226–9.

68. Dorsey J, Buckley D, Summer S, Jandacek RJ, Rider T, Tso P, et al. Fat malabsorption in cystic fibrosis: comparison of quantitative fat assay and a novel assay using fecal lauric/behenic acid. J Pediatr Gastroenterol Nutr. 2010;50(4):441–6.
69. Stallings VA, Mondick JT, Schall JI, Barrett JS, Wilson M, Mascarenhas MR. Diagnosing malabsorption with systemic lipid profiling: pharmacokinetics of pentadecanoic acid and triheptadecanoic acid following oral administration in healthy subjects and subjects with cystic fibrosis. Int J Clin Pharmacol Ther. 2013;51(4):263–73.
70. U.S. Department of Health and Human Services FaDA. Guidance for industry. Exocrine pancreatic insufficiency drug products—submitting NDAs.
71. Borowitz D, Stevens C, Brettman LR, Campion M, Chatfield B, Cipolli M, et al. International phase III trial of liprotamase efficacy and safety in pancreatic-insufficient cystic fibrosis patients. J Cyst Fibros. 2011;10(6):443–52.
72. Borowitz D, Stevens C, Brettman LR, Campion M, Wilschanski M, Thompson H, et al. Liprotamase long-term safety and support of nutritional status in pancreatic-insufficient cystic fibrosis. J Pediatr Gastroenterol Nutr. 2012;54(2):248–57.
73. Castellani C, Cuppens H, Macek Jr M, Cassiman JJ, Kerem E, Durie P, et al. Consensus on the use and interpretation of cystic fibrosis mutation analysis in clinical practice. J Cyst Fibros. 2008;7(3):179–96.
74. Cystic Fibrosis F, Borowitz D, Robinson KA, Rosenfeld M, Davis SD, Sabadosa KA, et al. Cystic Fibrosis Foundation evidence-based guidelines for management of infants with cystic fibrosis. J Pediatr. 2009;155(6 Suppl):S73–93.
75. Borowitz DS, Grand RJ, Durie PR. Use of pancreatic enzyme supplements for patients with cystic fibrosis in the context of fibrosing colonopathy. Consensus Committee. J Pediatr. 1995;127(5):681–4.
76. Chauhan S, Forsmark CE. Pain management in chronic pancreatitis: a treatment algorithm. Best Pract Res Clin Gastroenterol. 2010;24(3):323–35.
77. Ferrone M, Raimondo M, Scolapio JS. Pancreatic enzyme pharmacotherapy. Pharmacotherapy. 2007;27(6):910–20.
78. FitzSimmons SC, Burkhart GA, Borowitz D, Grand RJ, Hammerstrom T, Durie PR, et al. High-dose pancreatic-enzyme supplements and fibrosing colonopathy in children with cystic fibrosis. N Engl J Med. 1997;336(18):1283–9.
79. Borowitz D, Gelfond D, Maguiness K, Heubi JE, Ramsey B. Maximal daily dose of pancreatic enzyme replacement therapy in infants with cystic fibrosis: a reconsideration. J Cyst Fibros. 2013;12(6):784–5.
80. Kalnins D, Wilschanski M. Maintenance of nutritional status in patients with cystic fibrosis: new and emerging therapies. Drug Des Devel Ther. 2012;6:151–61.
81. Van de Vijver E, Desager K, Mulberg AE, Staelens S, Verkade HJ, Bodewes FA, et al. Treatment of infants and toddlers with cystic fibrosis-related pancreatic insufficiency and fat malabsorption with pancrelipase MT. J Pediatr Gastroenterol Nutr. 2011;53(1):61–4.
82. Bruno MJ, Haverkort EB, Tytgat GN, van Leeuwen DJ. Maldigestion associated with exocrine pancreatic insufficiency: implications of gastrointestinal physiology and properties of enzyme preparations for a cause-related and patient-tailored treatment. Am J Gastroenterol. 1995;90(9):1383–93.
83. Graff GR, Maguiness K, McNamara J, Morton R, Boyd D, Beckmann K, et al. Efficacy and tolerability of a new formulation of pancrelipase delayed-release capsules in children aged 7 to 11 years with exocrine pancreatic insufficiency and cystic fibrosis: a multicenter, randomized, double-blind, placebo-controlled, two-period crossover, superiority study. Clin Ther. 2010;32(1):89–103.
84. Trapnell BC, Maguiness K, Graff GR, Boyd D, Beckmann K, Caras S. Efficacy and safety of Creon 24,000 in subjects with exocrine pancreatic insufficiency due to cystic fibrosis. J Cyst Fibros. 2009;8(6):370–7.
85. Ramo OJ, Puolakkainen PA, Seppala K, Schroder TM. Self-administration of enzyme substitution in the treatment of exocrine pancreatic insufficiency. Scand J Gastroenterol. 1989;24(6):688–92.
86. Goodin B. Nutrition issues in cystic fibrosis. Pract Gastroenterol. 2005;27(5):76–94.
87. Nicolo M, Stratton KW, Rooney W, Boullata J. Pancreatic enzyme replacement therapy for enterally fed patients with cystic fibrosis. Nutr Clin Pract. 2013;28(4):485–9.
88. Ferrie S, Graham C, Hoyle M. Pancreatic enzyme supplementation for patients receiving enteral feeds. Nutr Clin Pract. 2011;26(3):349–51.
89. Borowitz D, Baker RD, Stallings V. Consensus report on nutrition for pediatric patients with cystic fibrosis. J Pediatr Gastroenterol Nutr. 2002;35(3):246–59.
90. Maqbool A, Schall JI, Mascarenhas MR, Dougherty KA, Stallings VA. Vitamin B(12) status in children with cystic fibrosis and pancreatic insufficiency. J Pediatr Gastroenterol Nutr. 2014;58(6):733–8.
91. Smyth RL, Ashby D, O'Hea U, Burrows E, Lewis P, van Velzen D, et al. Fibrosing colonopathy in cystic fibrosis: results of a case-control study. Lancet. 1995;346(8985):1247–51.
92. Smyth RL, van Velzen D, Smyth AR, Lloyd DA, Heaf DP. Strictures of ascending colon in cystic fibrosis and high-strength pancreatic enzymes. Lancet. 1994;343(8889):85–6.
93. Schall JI, Bentley T, Stallings VA. Meal patterns, dietary fat intake and pancreatic enzyme use in preadolescent children with cystic fibrosis. J Pediatr Gastroenterol Nutr. 2006;43(5):651–9.

94. Faulkner C, Taper LJ, Scott M. Adherence to pancreatic enzyme supplementation in adolescents with cystic fibrosis. Can J Diet Pract Res. 2012;73(4):196–9.
95. DeLambo KE, Ievers-Landis CE, Drotar D, Quittner AL. Association of observed family relationship quality and problem-solving skills with treatment adherence in older children and adolescents with cystic fibrosis. J Pediatr Psychol. 2004;29(5):343–53.
96. Conway SP, Pond MN, Hamnett T, Watson A. Compliance with treatment in adult patients with cystic fibrosis. Thorax. 1996;51(1):29–33.
97. Dominguez-Munoz JE, Iglesias-Garcia J. Oral pancreatic enzyme substitution therapy in chronic pancreatitis: is clinical response an appropriate marker for evaluation of therapeutic efficacy? JOP. 2010;11(2):158–62.
98. Kalnins D, Ellis L, Corey M, Pencharz PB, Stewart C, Tullis E, et al. Enteric-coated pancreatic enzyme with bicarbonate is equal to standard enteric-coated enzyme in treating malabsorption in cystic fibrosis. J Pediatr Gastroenterol Nutr. 2006;42(3):256–61.
99. Quinton PM. Cystic fibrosis: impaired bicarbonate secretion and mucoviscidosis. Lancet. 2008;372(9636):415–7.
100. Gelfond D, Ma C, Semler J, Borowitz D. Intestinal pH and gastrointestinal transit profiles in cystic fibrosis patients measured by wireless motility capsule. Dig Dis Sci. 2013;58(8):2275–81.
101. Symonds EL, Omari TI, Webster JM, Davidson GP, Butler RN. Relation between pancreatic lipase activity and gastric emptying rate in children with cystic fibrosis. J Pediatr. 2003;143(6):772–5.
102. Dominguez-Munoz JE, Iglesias-Garcia J, Iglesias-Rey M, Figueiras A, Vilarino-Insua M. Effect of the administration schedule on the therapeutic efficacy of oral pancreatic enzyme supplements in patients with exocrine pancreatic insufficiency: a randomized, three-way crossover study. Aliment Pharmacol Ther. 2005;21(8):993–1000.
103. Ooi CY, Dorfman R, Cipolli M, Gonska T, Castellani C, Keenan K, et al. Type of CFTR mutation determines risk of pancreatitis in patients with cystic fibrosis. Gastroenterology. 2011;140(1):153–61.
104. Rosenstein BJ, Cutting GR. The diagnosis of cystic fibrosis: a consensus statement. Cystic Fibrosis Foundation Consensus Panel. J Pediatr. 1998;132(4):589–95.

Chapter 11
Nutrition and Cystic Fibrosis Related Liver Disease

Kristin J. Brown, Cathy Lingard, and Michael R. Narkewicz

Key Points

- Liver involvement is common in CF, but only certain types of liver disease result in unique nutritional needs.
- Neonatal cholestasis is rare in CF, but results in increased needs for fat-soluble vitamins, energy, and fat
- Cirrhosis leads to increased basal metabolic rate and energy requirements.
- Protein restriction is generally not indicated in cirrhosis in CF
- Hepatic steatosis merits investigation for malnutrition and essential fatty acid deficiency

Keywords Cirrhosis • Hepatic steatosis • Cholestasis

Abbreviations

BMI   Body mass index (weight kg)/(height in meters)^2
CF   Cystic fibrosis
NAFLD   Nonalcoholic fatty liver disease
PIVKA   Protein induced in vitamin K absence
RBP   Retinol binding protein
TPGS   Alpha tocopherol polyethylene glycol succinate

K.J. Brown, M.S., R.D., C.N.S.C. • C. Lingard, R.D.
Children's Hospital Colorado, 13123 East 16th Avenue, B290, Aurora, CO 80045, USA
e-mail: kristin.brown@childrenscolorado.org; Catherine.Lingard@childrenscolorado.org

M.R. Narkewicz, M.D. (✉)
Children's Hospital Colorado, 13123 East 16th Avenue, B290, Aurora, CO 80045, USA

Section of Pediatric Gastroenterology, Hepatology and Nutrition, Department of Pediatrics, University of Colorado School of Medicine, Aurora, CO, USA
e-mail: michael.narkewicz@childrenscolorado.org

E.H. Yen, A.R. Leonard (eds.), *Nutrition in Cystic Fibrosis: A Guide for Clinicians*, Nutrition and Health,
DOI 10.1007/978-3-319-16387-1_11, © Springer International Publishing Switzerland 2015

Introduction

The liver is commonly affected in CF. While most individuals will have some liver involvement, significant liver disease affects 5–10% of all CF patients [1]. Despite this, liver disease is the third leading cause of death in CF and accounts for 2.5% of the overall annual mortality [2]. In this chapter, we will provide an overview of liver involvement in CF, address the disorders that occur in the liver as a result of nutritional deficiencies, and address the nutritional evaluation and management of the two liver diseases in CF that directly affect nutritional status: cholestasis and cirrhosis.

There are many forms of liver involvement in CF. A recently recommended classification of liver disease in CF is shown in Table 11.1 [1].

The two liver diseases that have a significant impact on the nutritional status of individuals with CF are neonatal cholestasis and cirrhosis with or without portal hypertension. In addition, hepatic steatosis (fatty liver) can occur as a result of malnutrition, over nutrition (obesity associated nonalcoholic fatty liver disease NAFLD), and nutritional deficiencies such as essential fatty acid (EFA) deficiency. The other disorders involving the liver do not have a significant impact on nutritional status and will not be discussed.

Neonatal Cholestasis

Neonatal cholestasis is defined as liver disease with an elevation of direct bilirubin to >2 mg/dl or >20% of the total bilirubin [3]. This is the earliest manifestation of liver involvement in CF and may mimic biliary atresia. Only 1% of infants with CF who do not have meconium ileus present with neonatal cholestasis [4]. Meconium ileus is a known risk factor for the development of cholestasis and up to 25% of infants with meconium ileus will develop cholestasis [4–7]. While cholestasis generally resolves by 9 months of age with no long-term sequelae, some studies have suggested an increased risk for cirrhosis in children with meconium ileus [8–10]. The major impact of cholestasis in infants with CF is a dramatic increase in fat malabsorption. In cholestasis, the total bile acid content and concentration of bile is reduced. As bile acids are required for efficient lipase function, whatever endogenous lipase secretion remains in infants with CF is further impaired in the face of cholestasis. A key role of bile acids is to form mixed micelles, which is the final step in the absorption of long chain fat. Thus fat malabsorption is much more severe in the infant with CF and cholestasis.

The infant with CF and cholestasis presents a unique nutritional management problem. Attention to adequate weight gain alone can underestimate the nutritional status of the infant. Anthropometric assessment should be determined at least a monthly while the child is cholestatic [11]. Breast milk should be the initial nutritional management for cholestatic infants. If infants fall off their expected

Table 11.1 Simplified classification of liver involvement in cystic fibrosis

1. CF related liver disease with cirrhosis with or without portal hypertension (based on clinical exam/ imaging, histology, laparoscopy)
2. Liver involvement without cirrhosis/portal hypertension consisting of at least one of the following:
    (a) Persistent elevation of AST, ALT or GGT >2 times upper limit of normal
    (b) Intermittent elevations of the above laboratory values
    (c) Steatosis (histologic determination)
    (d) Fibrosis (histologic determination)
    (e) Cholangiopathy (based on ultrasound, MRI, CT, ERCP)
    (f) Ultrasound abnormalities not consistent with cirrhosis
    (g) Neonatal cholestasis

Table 11.2 Options for fortification of breast milk for cholestatic infants

Brand name	Manufacturer	Percent of fat as MCT oil
Breast milk fortification		
Similac human milk fortifier	Abbott	100%
Enfamil human milk fortifier	Mead Johnson	70%
Formula supplement		
Similac special care	Abbott	50%
Enfamil premature[a]	Mead Johnson	40%
Gerber good start premature	Nestle	40%
Pregestimil	Mead Johnson	55%
Alimentum	Abbott	33%
Modulars		
Liquigen	Nutricia	96.4%
MCT oil	Nestle	100%
MCT procal	Vitaflo	99%

[a]Available for institutional use only

Table 11.3 Nutrient adjustments to parenteral nutrition in neonatal cholestasis

Nutrient	Adjustment in cholestasis
Copper: excreted in the bile, reduced excretion in cholestasis leads to elevated copper blood levels	Reduce copper to 10 mcg/kg/day (50% of recommended dose)
Manganese: similar to copper, excreted in the bile, reduced excretion in cholestasis leads to elevated manganese blood levels	Remove manganese if possible (trace amounts of manganese are found in other trace elements)
Zinc: enhanced zinc losses in cholestasis [62, 89]	Double the amount of zinc to 200 mcg/kg/day
Soy based lipids Intralipid®: evidence for worsening cholestasis with high dose lipids [90]	If possible, reduce lipids to 1 g/kg/day

optimum growth, fortification of breast milk with products higher in medium chain triglycerides is recommended. Options for supplementation are shown in Table 11.2.

Medium chain triglycerides are preferred as they are absorbed directly in the portal venous system without the need to form mixed micelles. In cholestatic infants who are not breast-fed or who fail to achieve optimum growth on fortified breast milk, a formula with at least 40–50% of fat as medium chain triglycerides is preferred. Additional supplementation may be necessary.

In cholestatic infants who fail oral intake, nasogastric supplementation can improve growth [12]. In addition, these infants are at risk for hypoglycemia due to impairment of liver glycogen storage capacity, decreased capacity for gluconeogenesis and smaller glycogen stores. In this case, it is optimal to feed every 4 hours. Older children are better able to utilize fat and protein as energy sources when fasting [13].

Rarely, parenteral nutrition is required [14]. This is more common in infants with complicated meconium ileus repair with delayed intestinal function. In the setting of cholestasis and the need for parenteral nutrition, there are several specific adjustments to the parenteral nutrition formulation that should be considered (Table 11.3). In most cases, the need for parenteral nutrition lasts for less than 1–3 months and enteral nutrition can be reestablished quickly. For children who require long-term TPN and who have cholestasis, refer to reviews from Guglielmi [15] and Feranchak [16].

Another important aspect of the evaluation and management of children with CF and cholestasis is the assessment of their fat-soluble vitamin status. Deficiencies of the fat-soluble vitamins A, D, E and K are common in cholestasis and can be much more profound than deficiencies seen in noncholestatic individuals with CF. These vitamins were discussed in Chapter 6. The importance of fat-soluble

Table 11.4 Fat-soluble vitamin assessment and supplementation in cholestasis

Vitamin	Suggested monitoring	Recommended ranges	Dosing recommendations
Vitamin A	Retinol	<20 mcg/dl (deficiency) >140 mcg/dl (toxicity)	1. 5000 IU orally daily 2. 25,000–50,000 IU orally daily for 1–4 weeks
	Retinol to RBP molar ratio	Deficiency <0.8 mol/mol	
Vitamin D	25-hydroxy-Vitamin D	<10 ng/ml: severe deficiency 10–20 ng/ml: insufficiency 20–30 ng/ml: At risk 30–40 ng/ml: Goal >150 ng/ml: Toxicity	Vitamin D3 1) 1200–4000 IU orally daily 2) 4000–8000 IU orally daily 3) Consider co-administering vitamin D3 with 5–10 ml of TPGS to enhance absorption in cholestatic children. 1, 25 dihydroxy-Vitamin D3 (calcitriol) 1) 0.05–0.2 mcg/kg/day orally *consider supplemental calcium with this transition*
Vitamin E	Alpha-tocopherol to total lipids[a] mg/g ratio	Goal: >0.8 mg/g Deficiency: <0.6 mg/g for infants <0.8 mg/g for children >1 year	TPGS 1) 25 IU/kg/day orally 2) 50 IU/kg/day orally 3) 100 IU/kg/day (orally divided 2–3 times per day)
Vitamin K	INR PIVKA	>1.2–1.4 (deficiency) >3 mcg/l (deficiency)	1) INR > 1.4 and <1.8: 2 mg orally daily 2) INR > 1.8 give 2 mg IM then oral daily dosing max 5 mg

[a]Total lipids assay has limited availability

TPGS alpha tocopherol polyethylene glycol succinate, *PIVKA* protein induced in vitamin K absence

vitamin supplementation is well understood and accepted within the nutritional management plan for both CF and cholestatic liver disease populations. When dealing with the combined malabsorption related to insufficient native pancreatic enzyme and cholestasis, fat-soluble vitamin absorption suffers. The progression of cholestasis often requires fat-soluble vitamin dosing at 2–4 times the baseline CF recommended doses for age. Levels should be monitored within the first month of cholestasis and about every 2 months while infants remain cholestatic to assure adequate intake. When deficiencies are identified, supplementation should be increased as shown in Table 11.4 [13, 17–19].

There is a unique aspect of monitoring vitamin E status in cholestasis. Vitamin E is contained in the lipid fraction and much of the vitamin E in the lipid component is not available. In cholestasis, hyperlipidemia is common due to the poor bile flow. As a result infants with cholestasis can have normal vitamin E levels but are functionally deficient. Thus in cholestasis, assessment of vitamin E status is best determined by the ratio of vitamin E (mg) to total lipids (g) with an optimal lower limit of 0.8 [20].

Cirrhosis With or Without Portal Hypertension

Multilobular Cirrhosis: Multilobular cirrhosis differs from the classical pathognomonic liver lesion in CF of focal biliary cirrhosis in that there are multiple regenerative nodules and diffuse involvement of the liver. Clinically, multilobular cirrhosis is detected by a hard nodular liver that may or may not be enlarged. On imaging, there is an irregular nodular liver edge and coarse heterogeneous parenchyma. Prior to the development of portal hypertension, there are often no other clinical features. Once portal hypertension is present, splenomegaly, esophageal or gastric varices, or ascites may be the first suggestion of previously unsuspected cirrhosis. Liver biopsy can show features consistent with cirrhosis but may not be sensitive due to the patchy nature of the nodular involvement and the large regenerative nodules that can be mistaken for normal hepatic parenchyma. Multilobular cirrhosis in CF is a pediatric disorder. The median age of discovery is 10 years with very few new cases identified after 20 years of age, and no increased prevalence with increased life span [21]. There is an average prevalence of multilobular cirrhosis of 5.6%, portal hypertension 4.2%, and varices 2.4% [8–10, 22–30]. Diabetes also seems to be more common in individuals with cystic fibrosis related liver disease [31, 32].

Nutritional consequences of Cirrhosis: Although most of the nutritional complications of cirrhosis are commonly felt to be related to portal hypertension, the presence of cirrhosis without portal hypertension does have significant physiologic effects.

First, in cirrhosis, there is an increase in cardiac output by up to twofold, related to peripheral vasodilation [33]. This increase in cardiac output leads to a significant increase in metabolic demand manifesting as increased resting energy expenditure. Second, cirrhosis is also associated with peripheral insulin resistance via mechanisms that are not clear [31]. This leads to less efficient use of carbohydrates as energy sources and can increase glucose intolerance and its associated complications.

However, the most vexing nutritional issues are faced in individuals with CF cirrhosis and obvious portal hypertension.

Complications or Portal Hypertension: The primary complications of portal hypertension include hypersplenism, esophageal or gastric variceal hemorrhage, ascites, and rarely synthetic liver failure with coagulopathy [34]. While liver disease is the third leading cause of death among CF patients, some studies report no increase in mortality among patients with CF cirrhosis [8, 26, 27]. Two recent studies report a trend towards younger age of death in those with cirrhosis [30, 35]. In a large 18-year retrospective review of 1108 patients with CF, 53 developed cirrhosis, 23 with portal hypertension, 14 with varices, 8 with coagulopathy, 6 with overt liver failure resulting in 3 liver transplants, but only one reported liver related death [23]. The incidence rate of major complications of cirrhosis (bleeding, ascites, and encephalopathy) among a cohort of 177 CF patients (17 who developed cirrhosis) followed longitudinally was 0.4%, with an all-cause mortality rate of 1.6% among cirrhotic patients [8]. This is in contrast to older reports that showed 11–19% mortality from variceal bleeding or liver failure in CF cirrhosis [36].

Once portal hypertension develops in CF, some studies report an increased risk of malnutrition, osteoporosis/hepatic osteodystrophy, and decline in lung function. The decline in lung function secondary to portal hypertension has been variously attributed to intrapulmonary vascular shunting, diaphragmatic splinting due to organomegaly and ascites, and potentially increased infections [37–40]. However, a recent retrospective study of 59 CF patients with cirrhosis and portal hypertension found no decline in lung function associated with portal hypertension as compared to age and gender matched CF specific reference values for lung function [41].

Malnutrition associated with portal hypertension is likely multifactorial due in part to decreased nutrient absorption, increased resting energy expenditure, anorexia and decreased caloric intake. A single center retrospective case–control study showed an odds ratio of 4.8 (95% CI, 2.49, 9.17) for CF-related diabetes in those with cirrhosis and portal hypertension, using a surrogate marker (thrombocytopenia) for cirrhosis with portal hypertension [32]. A case-control study of CF patients with and without advanced CF liver disease found lower weight, height, and mid-upper arm circumference z score and lower FEV_1 percent predicted in patients with advanced CF liver disease [42].

Osteoporosis is the most common form of bone disease associated with cirrhosis [43]. In one study of adults with cirrhosis awaiting liver transplantation, the individuals with cystic fibrosis had the most severe osteopenia compared to all other causes with average T and z scores at the lumbar spine of -4 and -3 [43]. The mechanism of this dramatic osteopenia is unclear, but again points to the nutritional impact of the combination of chronic liver disease with cystic fibrosis.

Portal hypertension can also have a direct effect on small bowel function via small bowel edema and decreased absorptive function. Finally, portal hypertension can lead to intrapulmonary shunting with resultant hypoxia or pulmonary hypertension and further increases in energy demand [44].

Liver Synthetic Failure: Only about 10% of individuals with CF and cirrhosis and portal hypertension progress to liver synthetic failure characterized by a high bilirubin and vitamin K-resistant coagulopathy [35]. This is in contrast to other causes of cirrhosis where the rate of progression is seemingly much higher.

Management of nutrition in Cirrhosis with and without portal hypertension: Individuals with CF and advanced liver disease require careful assessment of growth and nutritional status combining objective measures and physical exam. In addition to traditional measures of height and weight tracked on established growth curves, measurement of mid-arm circumference, triceps skinfold, subscapular skinfold, and calculated mid-arm muscle area are useful tools. Methods for obtaining these measurements and reference data have been previously reported [45, 46]. Weight is not a reliable indicator of nutritional status and is often falsely elevated related to organomegaly and/or the presence of ascitic fluid in advanced liver disease. Additionally this alteration in body composition may be due to a greater proportion of body mass contributed by a metabolically active body compartment with reduced body fat and an expansion in extracellular water [47]. Decreasing height velocity is a late indicator of chronic under-nutrition and may be difficult to assess in older children. Mid-arm circumference, triceps skinfold, and subscapular skinfold measures are indicators of the fat stores. These measures should be obtained by a skilled practitioner to assure accuracy. When tracked over time these additional measures indicate when nutritional goals are being met or when additional nutritional support strategies are required. Goals for these indicators of fat mass and fat-free mass should be within the range of a z score of 0 to +1 [11, 13, 17].

Energy Needs: For children with CF greater than 2 years of age, the general recommendation for energy is greater than that of the general healthy population [48]. Prospective and retrospective studies have found improved weight gain with intakes ranging from 110 to 200% of the recommended intakes for the general population. In addition, there are many healthy CF patients who can gain weight with a standard energy intake. For infants and children during the first 2 years of life, the CFF evidenced-based guidelines for weight gain and intake are based on term well-nourished infants and between 100 and 130 kcals/kg [49]. Data for energy expenditure in cystic fibrosis patients with cirrhosis are not available. However, children with advanced liver disease without cystic fibrosis can have an elevated energy expenditure of 27% higher REE/body weight than controls [47, 50]. It is reasonable to assume that CF patients with liver disease are also in a hypermetabolic state of the same degree or higher. An energy intake 120–150% of standard is suggested by a several sources [51–53].

Macronutrient Needs in Patients with CF and Advanced Liver Disease

Protein: Individuals with liver disease have increased protein turnover. This population benefits from a protein intake of 3 g/kg/day [53]. Note that this guideline typically provides approximately 10–15% of calories from protein. Children undergoing nutritional rehabilitation with enteral feedings to reverse malnutrition can tolerate a protein intake of 3–4 g/kg without precipitating hepatic encephalopathy [54]. Protein restriction is not necessary unless the patient has encephalopathy, and in these cases protein should not be restricted below 2 g/kg/day to prevent endogenous protein consumption [13]. It is good practice to distribute food over the course of the day to avoid undue stress to the liver at any one time [55].

Fat: Individuals with CF benefit from a high fat diet to more easily meet their increased energy needs. For children with CF without liver disease the CF Foundation recommends a fat intake of 35–40% of calories [56]. When patients have liver disease in addition to CF a higher fat intake of 40–50% is suggested [53]. The increased amount of dietary fat attempts to overcome the increased losses due to less efficient fat digestion in the setting of decreased bile acid pool and pancreatic insufficiency. The topic of fat in CF is thoroughly covered in Chapter 5.

Carbohydrates: Carbohydrates are an energy source that is easily digested in patients with fat malabsorption. After the provision of an adequate fat and protein intake for patients with CFLD, the remaining 45–50% of calories is provided through carbohydrate. In patients with cirrhosis, carbohydrates may not be optimally utilized due to peripheral insulin resistance and associated glucose intolerance. Since there is an increased incidence of CF related diabetes in patients with cirrhosis, it is also important for these patients to receive diabetes screening [32]. Continuous glucose monitoring may be helpful to detect fluctuations in serum glucose and assist in formulating a supplemental insulin regimen. In addition, a more favorable glucose control may be achieved with several small meals and snacks throughout the day rather than two or three larger meals. Refer to Chapter 10 for nutritional management of CF-related diabetes.

When malnutrition is present with cirrhosis and portal hypertension, the initial approach is oral enteral supplementation. When that is not successful, nasogastric (NG) supplementation can be successful [12]. While many centers avoid gastrostomy tube placement in the setting of portal hypertension due to the risk of gastrostomy stomal varices, one study did find that this was safe in CF patients with cirrhosis and led to improvement in pulmonary and nutritional status [57]. Specific nutritional support recommendations from a European CF group were published in 2012 [53]. Their recommendations included:

1. Providing 150% of estimated RDA for energy requirements
2. Provide 40–50% of calories as fat
3. Provide a minimum of 3 g/kg/day of protein unless liver failure is present
4. Provide fat-soluble vitamin supplementation and monitor for deficiency

Fat-soluble vitamins: Most individuals with CF and cirrhosis are not cholestatic. As such standard CF vitamin supplementation is appropriate. There are two exceptions: Vitamin K: While vitamin K deficiency is very common in CF, vitamin K deficiency as determined by PIVKA was more significant in those with liver disease compared to those without liver disease [58]. Thus individuals with CF and cirrhosis should receive an additional 5 mg orally daily of vitamin K.

Vitamin A deficiency may be difficult to assess in the setting of cirrhosis. Vitamin A in the circulation is bound to retinol binding protein (RBP). In the setting of cirrhosis, RBP is low even in the absence of hypoalbuminemia, resulting in low measured retinol (Vitamin A) levels. Individuals with retinol <20 mcg/dl should receive Vitamin A supplementation [59]. The best indicator of vitamin A status may be the molar ratio of Vitamin A to RBP [59], However, this may not be accurate in cirrhosis. Since the main toxicity of vitamin A is hepatic toxicity, care must be exercised with supplementation in the setting of cirrhosis. Close monitoring (monthly or every other month) of vitamin A status during high dose supplementation is recommended. If despite high dose supplementation vitamin A levels, or the molar ratio of vitamin A to RBP, do not improve, periodic assessment of eye complications (xerophthalmia or night blindness) should be performed to guide the need for higher dose supplementation.

Zinc: Zinc deficiency has been described in CF [60]. Zinc deficiency has also been reported in patients with cirrhosis [61]. The mechanism of zinc deficiency in cirrhosis is uncertain, but likely includes inadequate intake, increased urinary zinc losses [62], impaired intestinal transport, and hepatic sequestration. No study has investigated the zinc status of individuals with CF and cirrhosis. Zinc deficiency may contribute to dermatitis, impaired immune function, and exacerbate the effects of vitamin A deficiency [60, 61] There are no controlled trials of zinc supplementation, but 50 mg of elemental zinc given orally every day is often used in adults, while one study in infants and children with CF (but not with liver disease) used 5 mg/kg/day orally of elemental zinc [63].

Sodium Chloride: The diet of individuals with CF is generally unrestricted for added salt. In times of increased exercise or increased ambient temperatures supplemental sodium is encouraged to replace excess losses [64]. This practice is encouraged until physical and biochemical assessments in light of progressive liver disease determine that renal sodium retention has increased, leading to accumulation of abdominal ascites. In the setting of cirrhosis with portal hypertension, the associated low systemic blood volume triggers activation of the renin angiotensin system and sodium retention. This is primarily related to the peripheral vasodilation and resultant arteriolar hypotension at the level of the glomerulus. The resultant sodium retention can lead to ascites. In this setting, dietary/parenteral sodium restriction should cautiously be limited to 2000 mg/day or 2–3 mEq/kg in conjunction with diuretics to increase renal output [65]. The traditional measurement of urinary sodium and potassium to assess activation of this system is complicated in CF. Typically, urinary sodium is low and potassium high with renin angiotensin activation. However this pattern can also be seen in sodium depletion. Since individuals with CF can have increased sodium losses, restriction of sodium should be reserved for those individuals with cirrhosis, portal hypertension, and ascites.

Ursodeoxycholic acid is a hydrophilic bile acid that increases bile acid independent bile flow that is frequently used in liver disease in CF. When present at high concentrations in bile critical micellar concentrations cannot be reached. Thus patients on ursodeoxycholic acid may be at increased risk for fat-soluble vitamin deficiency and merit close monitoring [66].

Hepatic Steatosis

Steatosis (fat in the liver) is likely the most common hepatic finding in CF with a prevalence of 23–75% of CF patients in all age categories [7]. Steatosis was present in 70% of children undergoing liver biopsy for suspected liver disease [26, 67]. Hepatic steatosis has been associated with malnutrition, and deficiencies of EFA, carnitine, and choline. However, steatosis is also found in CF patients with adequate nutritional status [5]. Hepatic steatosis can also be seen with obesity. In this setting it is known as nonalcoholic fatty liver disease (NAFLD). This obesity related disorder is the leading cause of liver disease in the general population and obesity has been recently recognized as increasing in CF [68]. Independent of the cause, hepatic steatosis presents as smooth mild hepatomegaly without signs of portal hypertension. There may be elevated AST and ALT and typically, the ALT is greater than the AST. The appearance of the liver on ultrasound is usually one of uniform hyperechogenicity, but it may also have a heterogeneous appearance on ultrasound or as one or several "pseudomasses," which are lobulated fatty structures 1–2 cm in size [6, 69]. In one study, 57% of cases of steatosis detected on ultrasound were associated with elevations in aminotransferases [70]. A note of caution is warranted in regard to this finding as the ultrasound findings may not be specific for steatosis and can be seen in periportal fibrosis [17]. Thus histology is still the gold standard for the diagnosis of hepatic steatosis.

The finding of steatosis in a patient with CF should trigger an evaluation for cause. The vast majority of the causes of hepatic steatosis in CF are nutritional. In the past, the most common cause of hepatic steatosis in CF was malnutrition. In malnutrition, hepatic steatosis is common. Protein malnutrition leads to decreased apolipoprotein synthesis with subsequent decreased VLDL production and transport, leading to lipid accumulation in the liver [71]. Children or adults with protein calorie malnutrition should have their malnutrition addressed first. Correction of nutritional status is associated with an improvement in hepatic steatosis, but the improvement may lag several months after the correction of the nutritional status.

Obesity (BMI ≥ 95th percentile) is strongly associated with hepatic steatosis and NAFLD. In the USA, obesity is now the leading cause of liver disease [72, 73]. The prevalence of obesity varies between 25 and 45% with differences in prevalence associated with age, gender, race, ethnicity, and socioeconomic status. Obesity is less common in CF, with a reported prevalence of 7.5% [74]. The approach to the CF patient with obesity induced hepatic steatosis or NAFLD should focus on diet and lifestyle modification as it would for any other obese patient [75].

EFA deficiency has been reported to cause hepatic steatosis [76]. Biochemical EFA deficiency is common in patients with CF without steatosis. The predominant deficiency is linoleic acid. The etiology is multifactorial and may include an inadequate calorie and fat intake and residual fat malabsorption of 10–20% despite treatment with pancreatic enzymes [77, 78]. Deficiency has been traditionally assessed by determination of a triene to tetraene ratio of plasma fatty acids. Serum linoleic acid (LA) status has been positively associated with growth and pulmonary outcomes and may be a more clinically relevant biomarker of EFA status in children with CF and pancreatic insufficiency than the triene:tetraene ratio [79].

CF patients who also have steatosis may have additional fat malabsorption due to functional bile acid deficiency that varies depending upon the severity of the disease. These patients may require a higher amount of linoleic acid supplementation than CF patients without steatosis. They should be treated with vegetable oils or margarine containing high amounts of linoleic acid.

Table 11.5 describes the linoleic acid content of some common vegetable oils that contain a significant amount of linoleic acid. These oils can be mixed into soft foods such as strained or pureed foods, mashed potatoes, and pudding or added to pastas or toast. If the oil is not palatable for the child, corn oil margarine can be used [80]; however, a greater quantity may be required. As with all fat-containing meals, it is important to remind the families that the CF patient needs to take the prescribed pancreatic enzyme dose with the EFA supplement.

The exact amount of linoleic acid needed in CF patients is not known. The DRI for acceptable macronutrient distribution for linoleic acid intake ranges between 5 and 10% of calories for healthy children [81]. The guidelines for pre-transplant pediatric liver patients are >10% of total calories [82]. In contrast, linoleic acid repletion trials in CF patients have reported that a much higher intake of calories from linoleic acid fat is required to reverse a deficiency state, ranging from 7 to 22% [83–86]. It is possible that malnourished patients require a higher percent of calories from EFA to reverse the deficiency. Since an exact recommendation is lacking, it is reasonable to aim for an EFA intake greater than 10% of calories. Additionally, an adequate total caloric intake needs to be provided when supplementing with EFA so that the fat supplement is not metabolized for caloric utilization rather than the repletion of fatty acid stores.

While EFA deficiency should be evaluated in children with CF and hepatic steatosis, other nutritional deficiencies can cause hepatic steatosis, and these are shown in Table 11.6.

Table 11.5 Options for oral supplementation of essential fatty acids

Selected vegetable oils	Linoleic acid of oil content by weight (%)	ml/day of oil to provide 6% of kcals in a 1000 kcal diet
Corn	50.9	13
Peanut	53.8	12.5
Soybean	53.8	12.5
Safflower	76.8	9.0

Adapted from Foman [91]

Table 11.6 Causes of hepatic steatosis

Disorders of lipid metabolism	
Abetalipoproteinemia	Hypobetalipoproteinemia
Familial combined hyperlipidemia	Lipodystrophy
Acid lipase deficiency	Wolman disease
Glycogen storage disease	Disorders of fatty acid oxidation
Mitochondrial disorders	
Micronutrient deficiency	
Carnitine (primary or secondary)	Essential fatty acids
Choline	
Medications	
Corticosteroids	Parenteral nutrition
Tamoxifen	Amiodarone
HAART	Methotrexate
Others	
Surgical weight loss	Celiac disease
Obesity	Malnutrition
Wilson disease	Weber–Christian disease

Adapted in part from Kneeman et al. [92]

Children with CF who have malnutrition and/or a low carnitine intake can develop a secondary carnitine deficiency that may play a role in the development of hepatic steatosis. Carnitine deficiency causes a defect in fatty acid oxidation that can contribute at least in part to hepatic steatosis seen in cystic fibrosis patients [87]. The primary role of carnitine is to transport long chain fatty acids across the mitochondrial membrane where they undergo β-oxidation to produce energy from stored fat reserves. Carnitine is available in the food supply through meats, dairy, most enteral formulas, and human milk (although the human milk concentration is dependent on the mother's carnitine status). Carnitine is not present in parenteral nutrition unless it is added. Most infant formulas including soy formulas are now supplemented with carnitine to be comparable to or higher than that found in human milk [88]. The majority of people are able to synthesize carnitine endogenously from methionine and lysine in the liver and kidney. Infants, however, have decreased biosynthetic capacity and are at risk for developing carnitine deficiency when receiving a low carnitine diet. Children with CF and hepatic steatosis without evidence of EFA deficiency should have carnitine status assessed by plasma carnitine levels. If they are found to be deficient, it is reasonable to provide a month of supplementation of levocarnitine (50–100 mg/kg/day orally divided three to four times a day with meals) in addition to a carnitine-rich diet to reverse the deficiency.

Conclusion

Liver involvement is common in CF, but nutritional consequences related to disease are primarily seen in cholestasis and cirrhosis. Cholestasis is generally transient, but leads to increased energy, fat, and fat-soluble vitamin requirements. Cirrhosis is rare, but when present results in increased energy requirements and malnutrition in this setting can be challenging to manage. Nutritional assessment and management of cirrhosis should focus on macro- and micro-nutrient needs and aggressive intervention when standard therapies fail.

References

1. Flass T, Narkewicz MR. Cirrhosis and other liver disease in cystic fibrosis. J Cyst Fibros. 2013;12:116–24.
2. Foundation CF. 2011 Annual Data Report to the Center Directors. Bethesda, MD; 2012.
3. Moyer V, Freese DK, Whitington PF, Olson AD, Brewer F, Colletti RB, et al. Guideline for the evaluation of cholestatic jaundice in infants: recommendations of the North American Society for Pediatric Gastroenterology, Hepatology and Nutrition. J Pediatr Gastroenterol Nutr. 2004;39(2):115–28.
4. Leeuwen L, Magoffin AK, Fitzgerald DA, Cipolli M, Gaskin KJ. Cholestasis and meconium ileus in infants with cystic fibrosis and their clinical outcomes. Arch Dis Child. 2014;99(5):443–7.
5. Colombo C. Liver disease in cystic fibrosis. Curr Opin Pulm Med. 2007;13(6):529–36.
6. Diwakar V, Pearson L, Beath S. Liver disease in children with cystic fibrosis. Paediatr Respir Rev. 2001;2(4):340–9.
7. Herrmann U, Dockter G, Lammert F. Cystic fibrosis-associated liver disease. Best Pract Res Clin Gastroenterol. 2010;24(5):585–92.
8. Colombo C, Battezzati PM, Crosignani A, Morabito A, Costantini D, Padoan R, et al. Liver disease in cystic fibrosis: a prospective study on incidence, risk factors, and outcome. Hepatology. 2002;36(6):1374–82.
9. Efrati O, Barak A, Modan-Moses D, Augarten A, Vilozni D, Katznelson D, et al. Liver cirrhosis and portal hypertension in cystic fibrosis. Eur J Gastroenterol Hepatol. 2003;15(10):1073–8.
10. Lamireau T, Monnereau S, Martin S, Marcotte JE, Winnock M, Alvarez F. Epidemiology of liver disease in cystic fibrosis: a longitudinal study. J Hepatol. 2004;41(6):920–5.
11. Sokol RJ, Stall C. Anthropometric evaluation of children with chronic liver disease. Am J Clin Nutr. 1990;52(2):203–8.
12. Chin SE, Shepherd RW, Cleghorn GJ, Patrick M, Ong TH, Wilcox J, et al. Pre-operative nutritional support in children with end-stage liver disease accepted for liver transplantation: an approach to management. J Gastroenterol Hepatol. 1990;5(5):566–72.
13. Young S, Kwarta E, Azzam R, Sentongo T. Nutrition assessment and support in children with end-stage liver disease. Nutr Clin Pract. 2013;28(3):317–29.
14. Sullivan JS, Sundaram SS, Pan Z, Sokol RJ. Parenteral nutrition supplementation in biliary atresia patients listed for liver transplantation. Liver Transpl. 2012;18(1):120–8.
15. Guglielmi FW, Regano N, Mazzuoli S, Fregnan S, Leogrande G, Guglielmi A, et al. Cholestasis induced by total parenteral nutrition. Clin Liver Dis. 2008;12(1):97–110.
16. Feranchak AP, Suchy FJ, Sokol RJ. Medical and nutritional management of cholestasis in infants and children. In: Suchy FJ, Sokol RJ, Balistreri WF, editors. Liver disease in children. Cambridge: Cambridge University Press; 2014. p. 111–39.
17. Sokol RJ, Durie PR. Recommendations for management of liver and biliary tract disease in cystic fibrosis. Cystic Fibrosis Foundation Hepatobiliary Disease Consensus Group. J Pediatr Gastroenterol Nutr. 1999;28(1 Suppl):S1–13.
18. Matel JL. Nutritional management of cystic fibrosis. J Parenter Enteral Nutr. 2012;36(1 Suppl):60S–7.
19. Tangpricha V, Kelly A, Stephenson A, Maguiness K, Enders J, Robinson KA, et al. An update on the screening, diagnosis, management, and treatment of vitamin D deficiency in individuals with cystic fibrosis: evidence-based recommendations from the Cystic Fibrosis Foundation. J Clin Endocrinol Metab. 2012;97(4):1082–93.
20. Sokol RJ, Heubi JE, Iannaccone ST, Bove KE, Balistreri WF. Vitamin E deficiency with normal serum vitamin E concentrations in children with chronic cholestasis. N Engl J Med. 1984;310(19):1209–12.
21. Bartlett JR, Friedman KJ, Ling SC, Pace RG, Bell SC, Bourke B, et al. Genetic modifiers of liver disease in cystic fibrosis. JAMA. 2009;302(10):1076–83.
22. Scott-Jupp R, Lama M, Tanner MS. Prevalence of liver disease in cystic fibrosis. Arch Dis Child. 1991;66(6):698–701.
23. Bhattacharjee R, Schibli S, Rose J, Tullis E, Durie P, Ellis L, et al. The natural history of liver disease in cystic fibrosis. J Cyst Fibros. 2006;5:S61.
24. Williams SM, Goodman R, Thomson A, McHugh K, Lindsell DR. Ultrasound evaluation of liver disease in cystic fibrosis as part of an annual assessment clinic: a 9-year review. Clin Radiol. 2002;57(5):365–70.
25. Lenaerts C, Lapierre C, Patriquin H, Bureau N, Lepage G, Harel F, et al. Surveillance for cystic fibrosis-associated hepatobiliary disease: early ultrasound changes and predisposing factors. J Pediatr. 2003;143(3):343–50.
26. Lindblad A, Glaumann H, Strandvik B. Natural history of liver disease in cystic fibrosis. Hepatology. 1999;30(5):1151–8.
27. Desmond CP, Wilson J, Bailey M, Clark D, Roberts SK. The benign course of liver disease in adults with cystic fibrosis and the effect of ursodeoxycholic acid. Liver Int. 2007;27(10):1402–8.
28. Lewindon PJ, Ramm GA. Cystic fibrosis-cirrhosis, portal hypertension, and liver biopsy: reply. Hepatology. 2011;53(3):1065–6.

29. Feigelson J, Anagnostopoulos C, Poquet M, Pecau Y, Munck A, Navarro J. Liver cirrhosis in cystic fibrosis—therapeutic implications and long term follow up. Arch Dis Child. 1993;68(5):653–7.

30. Chryssostalis A, Hubert D, Coste J, Kanaan R, Burgel PR, Desmazes-Dufeu N, et al. Liver disease in adult patients with cystic fibrosis: a frequent and independent prognostic factor associated with death or lung transplantation. J Hepatol. 2011;55:1377–82.

31. Minicucci L, Lorini R, Giannattasio A, Colombo C, Iapichino L, Reali MF, et al. Liver disease as risk factor for cystic fibrosis-related diabetes development. Acta Paediatr. 2007;96(5):736–9.

32. Sullivan KM, Moran A, Schwarzenberg S. Cystic fibrosis related diabetes in CF patients with cirrhosis. Pediatr Pulmonol. 2009;44:414.

33. Hsu EK, Murray KF. Cirrhosis and chronic liver failure. In: Suchy FJ, Sokol RJ, Balistreri WF, editors. Liver disease in children. 4th ed. Cambridge: Cambridge University Press; 2014. p. 51–67.

34. Shneider BL. Portal hypertension. In: Suchy FJ, Sokol RJ, Balistreri WF, editors. Liver disease in children. 4th ed. Cambridge: Cambridge University Press; 2014. p. 68–87.

35. Rowland M, Gallagher CG, O'Laoide R, Canny G, Broderick A, Hayes R, et al. Outcome in cystic fibrosis liver disease. Am J Gastroenterol. 2011;106(1):104–9.

36. Debray D, Lykavieris P, Gauthier F, Dousset B, Sardet A, Munck A, et al. Outcome of cystic fibrosis-associated liver cirrhosis: management of portal hypertension. J Hepatol. 1999;31(1):77–83.

37. Milkiewicz P, Skiba G, Kelly D, Weller P, Bonser R, Gur U, et al. Transplantation for cystic fibrosis: outcome following early liver transplantation. J Gastroenterol Hepatol. 2002;17(2):208–13.

38. Colombo C, Russo MC, Zazzeron L, Romano G. Liver disease in cystic fibrosis. J Pediatr Gastroenterol Nutr. 2006;43 Suppl 1:S49–55.

39. Westaby D. Cystic fibrosis: liver disease. Prog Respir Res. 2006;34:251–61.

40. Linnane B, Oliver MR, Robinson PJ. Does splenectomy in cystic fibrosis related liver disease improve lung function and nutritional status? A case series. Arch Dis Child. 2006;91(9):771–3.

41. Polineni D, et al. Pulmonary function (FEV1) in cystic fibrosis patients with and without severe liver disease with portal hypertension (CFLD). Am J Respir Crit Care Med. 2009;179.

42. Corbett K, Kelleher S, Rowland M, Daly L, Drumm B, Canny G, et al. Cystic fibrosis-associated liver disease: a population-based study. J Pediatr. 2004;145(3):327–32.

43. Bonkovsky HL, Hawkins M, Steinberg K, Hersh T, Galambos JT, Henderson JM, et al. Prevalence and prediction of osteopenia in chronic liver disease. Hepatology. 1990;12(2):273–80.

44. Rodriguez-Roisin R, Krowka MJ, Herve P, Fallon MB, Committee ERSTFP-HVDS. Pulmonary-hepatic vascular disorders (PHD). Eur Respir J. 2004;24(5):861–80.

45. Frisancho AR. New norms of upper limb fat and muscle areas for assessment of nutritional status. Am J Clin Nutr. 1981;34(11):2540–5.

46. Ryan AS, Martinez GA. Physical growth of infants 7 to 13 months of age: results from a national survey. Am J Phys Anthropol. 1987;73(4):449–57.

47. Greer R, Lehnert M, Lewindon P, Cleghorn GJ, Shepherd RW. Body composition and components of energy expenditure in children with end-stage liver disease. J Pediatr Gastroenterol Nutr. 2003;36(3):358–63.

48. Stallings VA, Stark LJ, Robinson KA, Feranchak AP, Quinton H, Clinical Practice Guidelines on Growth and Nutrition Subcommittee; Ad Hoc Working Group. Evidence-based practice recommendations for nutrition-related management of children and adults with cystic fibrosis and pancreatic insufficiency: results of a systematic review. J Am Diet Assoc. 2008;108(5):832–9.

49. Borowitz D, Robinson KA, Rosenfeld M, Davis SD, Sabadosa KA, Spear SL, et al. Cystic Fibrosis Foundation evidence-based guidelines for management of infants with cystic fibrosis. J Pediatr. 2009;155(6 Suppl):S73–93.

50. Pierro A, Koletzko B, Carnielli V, Superina RA, Roberts EA, Filler RM, et al. Resting energy expenditure is increased in infants and children with extrahepatic biliary atresia. J Pediatr Surg. 1989;24(6):534–8.

51. Cleghorn G. The role of basic nutritional research in pediatric liver disease: an historical perspective. J Gastroenterol Hepatol. 2009;24 Suppl 3:S93–6.

52. Kocoshis SA, Wleman RE. Hepatic disease. In: Corkins MR, Ballant J, Bobo E, Plogsted S, Yaworski JA, Seebeck ND, editors. A.S.P.E.N pediatric nutrition support core curriculum. Silver Spring: American Society of Parenteral and Enteral Nutrition; 2010. p. 302–10.

53. Debray D, Kelly D, Houwen R, Strandvik B, Colombo C. Best practice guidance for the diagnosis and management of cystic fibrosis-associated liver disease. J Cyst Fibros. 2011;10 Suppl 2:S29–36.

54. Charlton CP, Buchanan E, Holden CE, Preece MA, Green A, Booth IW, et al. Intensive enteral feeding in advanced cirrhosis: reversal of malnutrition without precipitation of hepatic encephalopathy. Arch Dis Child. 1992;67(5):603–7.

55. Pandit C, Graham C, Selvadurai H, Gaskin K, Cooper P, van Asperen P. Festival food coma in cystic fibrosis. Pediatr Pulmonol. 2013;48(7):725–7.

56. Borowitz D, Baker RD, Stallings V. Consensus report on nutrition for pediatric patients with cystic fibrosis. J Pediatr Gastroenterol Nutr. 2002;35(3):246–59.

57. Vandeleur M, Massie J, Oliver M. Gastrostomy in children with cystic fibrosis and portal hypertension. J Pediatr Gastroenterol Nutr. 2013;57(2):245–7.
58. Rashid M, Durie P, Andrew M, Kalnins D, Shin J, Corey M, et al. Prevalence of vitamin K deficiency in cystic fibrosis. Am J Clin Nutr. 1999;70(3):378–82.
59. Feranchak AP, Gralla J, King R, Ramirez RO, Corkill M, Narkewicz MR, et al. Comparison of indices of vitamin A status in children with chronic liver disease. Hepatology. 2005;42(4):782–92.
60. Krebs NF. Update on zinc deficiency and excess in clinical pediatric practice. Ann Nutr Metab. 2013;62 Suppl 1:19–29.
61. Mohammad MK, Zhou Z, Cave M, Barve A, McClain CJ. Zinc and liver disease. Nutr Clin Pract. 2012;27(1): 8–20.
62. Narkewicz MR, Krebs N, Karrer F, Orban-Eller K, Sokol RJ. Correction of hypozincemia following liver transplantation in children is associated with reduced urinary zinc loss. Hepatology. 1999;29(3):830–3.
63. Van Biervliet S, Vande Velde S, Van Biervliet JP, Robberecht E. The effect of zinc supplements in cystic fibrosis patients. Ann Nutr Metab. 2008;52(2):152–6.
64. Guimaraes EV, Schettino GC, Camargos PA, Penna FJ. Prevalence of hyponatremia at diagnosis and factors associated with the longitudinal variation in serum sodium levels in infants with cystic fibrosis. J Pediatr. 2012; 161(2):285–9.
65. Wong F. Management of ascites in cirrhosis. J Gastroenterol Hepatol. 2012;27(1):11–20.
66. Narkewicz MR, Smith D, Gregory C, Lear JL, Osberg I, Sokol RJ. Effect of ursodeoxycholic acid therapy on hepatic function in children with intrahepatic cholestatic liver disease. J Pediatr Gastroenterol Nutr. 1998;26(1):49–55.
67. Lewindon PJ, Shepherd RW, Walsh MJ, Greer RM, Williamson R, Pereira TN, et al. Importance of hepatic fibrosis in cystic fibrosis and the predictive value of liver biopsy. Hepatology. 2011;53(1):193–201.
68. Hanna RM, Weiner DJ. Overweight and obesity in patients with cystic fibrosis: a center-based analysis. Pediatr Pulmonol. 2014;50(1):35–41.
69. Akata D, Akhan O. Liver manifestations of cystic fibrosis. Eur J Radiol. 2007;61(1):11–7.
70. Patriquin H, Lenaerts C, Smith L, Perreault G, Grignon A, Filiatrault D, et al. Liver disease in children with cystic fibrosis: US-biochemical comparison in 195 patients. Radiology. 1999;211(1):229–32.
71. Badaloo A, Reid M, Soares D, Forrester T, Jahoor F. Relation between liver fat content and the rate of VLDL apolipoprotein B-100 synthesis in children with protein-energy malnutrition. Am J Clin Nutr. 2005;81(5):1126–32.
72. Koppe SW. Obesity and the liver: nonalcoholic fatty liver disease. Transl Res. 2014;164(4):312–22.
73. Mencin AA, Lavine JE. Nonalcoholic fatty liver disease in children. Curr Opin Clin Nutr Metab Care. 2011;14(2): 151–7.
74. Panagopoulou P, Fotoulaki M, Nikolaou A, Nousia-Arvanitakis S. Prevalence of malnutrition and obesity among cystic fibrosis patients. Pediatr Int. 2014;56(1):89–94.
75. Feldstein AE, Patton-Ku D, Boutelle KN. Obesity, nutrition, and liver disease in children. Clin Liver Dis. 2014;18(1):219–31.
76. Werner A, Havinga R, Bos T, Bloks VW, Kuipers F, Verkade HJ. Essential fatty acid deficiency in mice is associated with hepatic steatosis and secretion of large VLDL particles. Am J Physiol Gastrointest Liver Physiol. 2005;288(6):G1150–8.
77. Lloyd-Still JD, Smith AE, Wessel HU. Fat intake is low in cystic fibrosis despite unrestricted dietary practices. J Parenter Enteral Nutr. 1989;13(3):296–8.
78. Kalivianakis M, Minich DM, Bijleveld CM, van Aalderen WM, Stellaard F, Laseur M, et al. Fat malabsorption in cystic fibrosis patients receiving enzyme replacement therapy is due to impaired intestinal uptake of long-chain fatty acids. Am J Clin Nutr. 1999;69(1):127–34.
79. Maqbool A, Schall JI, Garcia-Espana JF, Zemel BS, Strandvik B, Stallings VA. Serum linoleic acid status as a clinical indicator of essential fatty acid status in children with cystic fibrosis. J Pediatr Gastroenterol Nutr. 2008;47(5):635–44.
80. Marcus MS, Sondel SA, Farrell PM, Laxova A, Carey PM, Langhough R, et al. Nutritional status of infants with cystic fibrosis associated with early diagnosis and intervention. Am J Clin Nutr. 1991;54(3):578–85.
81. Macronutrients, healthful diets, and physical activity. In: Otten JL, Hellwig JP, Meyers LD, editors. DRI Dietary Reference Intakes, The guide to nutrient requirements. Washington DC: The National Academies Press; 2006. p. 71–102.
82. Baker A, Stevenson R, Dhawan A, Goncalves I, Socha P, Sokal E. Guidelines for nutritional care for infants with cholestatic liver disease before liver transplantation. Pediatr Transplant. 2007;11(8):825–34.
83. Mischler EH, Parrell SW, Farrell PM, Raynor WJ, Lemen RJ. Correction of linoleic acid deficiency in cystic fibrosis. Pediatr Res. 1986;20(1):36–41.
84. Landon C, Kerner JA, Castillo R, Adams L, Whalen R, Lewiston NJ. Oral correction of essential fatty acid deficiency in cystic fibrosis. J Parenter Enteral Nutr. 1981;5(6):501–4.

85. Steinkamp G, Demmelmair H, Ruhl-Bagheri I, von der Hardt H, Koletzko B. Energy supplements rich in linoleic acid improve body weight and essential fatty acid status of cystic fibrosis patients. J Pediatr Gastroenterol Nutr. 2000;31(4):418–23.

86. van Egmond AW, Kosorok MR, Koscik R, Laxova A, Farrell PM. Effect of linoleic acid intake on growth of infants with cystic fibrosis. Am J Clin Nutr. 1996;63(5):746–52.

87. Treem WR, Stanley CA. Massive hepatomegaly, steatosis, and secondary plasma carnitine deficiency in an infant with cystic fibrosis. Pediatrics. 1989;83(6):993–7.

88. Crill CM, Helms RA. The use of carnitine in pediatric nutrition. Nutr Clin Pract. 2007;22(2):204–13.

89. Krebs NF, Westcott JE, Arnold TD, Kluger BM, Accurso FJ, Miller LV, et al. Abnormalities in zinc homeostasis in young infants with cystic fibrosis. Pediatr Res. 2000;48(2):256–61.

90. Colomb V, Jobert-Giraud A, Lacaille F, Goulet O, Fournet JC, Ricour C. Role of lipid emulsions in cholestasis associated with long-term parenteral nutrition in children. J Parenter Enteral Nutr. 2000;24(6):345–50.

91. Foman SJ. Fat. In: Fomon SJ, editor. Nutrition of normal infants. St Louis: Mosby; 1993. p. 147–75.

92. Kneeman JM, Misdraji J, Corey KE. Secondary causes of nonalcoholic fatty liver disease. Therap Adv Gastroenterol. 2012;5(3):199–207.

Chapter 12
Gastrointestinal Complications of Cystic Fibrosis and Their Impact on Nutrition

Daniel Gelfond

Key Points

- Nutrition status in cystic fibrosis (CF) patients is closely associated with pulmonary outcomes and depends heavily on the activity of Cystic Fibrosis Transmembrane Conduction Regulator (CFTR) in the gastrointestinal tract.
- CF-related gastrointestinal complications often precede pulmonary complications and can be observed in utero or early infancy often requiring radiological or surgical interventions.
- Extent and degree of GI-related complications in CF patients varies with CFTR mutations and often most prominent with class 1 and 2 mutations.
- Nutritional deficiencies in CF patients can stream from pancreatic enzyme and bile acid insufficiency, bicarbonate deficiency to counteract gastric acidity, viscosity of the epithelial mucus, or small bowel bacterial overgrowth.
- CFTR regulates flow of bicarbonate in the gastrointestinal track that is important for pH regulation, mucin unfolding, hydration, and luminal viscosity that can impact motility and bacterial stasis
- Assessment of the gastrointestinal pH profiles and bicarbonate-dependent pH change using wireless motility capsule in patients with CF has promoted this technique as a gut specific CFTR biomarker.

  - Targeted therapy to correct CFTR gating defect in patients with G551D mutation has validated the role of this technology to establish gut specific CFTR biomarker

- Altered luminal physiology with dehydrated mucus, altered pH, immune deficiency, dysmotility, and nutrient malabsorption in CF patients predisposes to dysbiosis and small bowel bacterial overgrowth causing significant impact on overall health and quality of life in affected patients.
- Diseases of the esophagus, stomach, small intestine, and colon are not uncommon in patients with CF and often are addressed with similar therapeutic modalities as in non-CF patients.

Keywords CFTR • Gastroesophageal reflux • Gastric emptying • Small intestinal bacterial overgrowth • Distal intestinal obstruction syndrome • Constipation • Gastrointestinal cancers • Gastrointestinal motility

D. Gelfond, M.D. (✉)
WNY Pediatric Gastroenterology, 166 Washington Avenue, Batavia, NY 14020, USA

University of Rochester Medical Center, Rochester, NY USA
e-mail: dgelfond@wnypedgi.com

E.H. Yen, A.R. Leonard (eds.), *Nutrition in Cystic Fibrosis: A Guide for Clinicians*, Nutrition and Health, DOI 10.1007/978-3-319-16387-1_12, © Springer International Publishing Switzerland 2015

Introduction

Nutritional status is strongly associated with pulmonary outcomes and general health in CF patients. Maintaining an optimal weight is a significant goal of CF care [1]. The recognition and management of pancreatic involvement in patients with cystic fibrosis (CF) has played a central role in improving the nutritional status of these patients. However, recognition and management of other gastrointestinal complications of CF is also important to help improve weight gain and quality of life. Breakthrough developments in identifying the role of the cystic fibrosis transmembrane conductance regulator (CFTR) in the gastrointestinal tract have led to a better understanding of CF associated gastrointestinal diseases [2]. Recent pharmacological correctors of specific CFTR defects have provided a platform to further understand and study the role of CFTR in the gastrointestinal tract [3]. Gastrointestinal manifestations can be present in utero as well as in early neonatal life and often precede pulmonary manifestations. Recognition of early gastrointestinal symptoms often leads to further testing for diagnosing CF in infants. Inspissated secretions within the lumen of the gastrointestinal tract can lead to the intestinal obstruction of meconium ileus. In complex cases, perforation of the bowel may lead to meconium peritonitis, intestinal resection, and can further compromise nutrition and growth in children with CF. More common gastrointestinal diseases such as gastroesophageal reflux disease (GERD) have been frequently seen in both children and adults with CF and often leads to clinical discomfort and poor appetite. It is important to note that not all of the nutritional deficiencies in CF patients are secondary to insufficient caloric intake. Pancreatic diseases, in particular pancreatic insufficiency (PI) that is present at birth, will prevent adequate enzymatic breakdown of nutrients required for mucosal absorption and assimilation. Use of pancreatic enzyme replacement therapy (PERT) has been a life sustaining intervention in patients with PI. Pancreatic sufficient (PS) patients might not manifest nutritional malabsorption as seen in PI patients, but can have GI discomfort. Pancreatic diseases are covered in more detail in other chapters in this book.

Even with adequate enzymatic activity, whether endogenous or supplemental, nutritional absorption can be compromised in CF patients as a result of viscous secretions that might prevent nutrient interaction with absorptive surface of the mucosal brush border. Viscous secretions that concentrate nutrients away from the epithelial layer, can interfere with the release and efficacy of defensins, part of the innate immune system that are secreted from the crypts of the mucosal layer [4]. A compromised immune system, evidence of delayed small bowel transit [5] and small intestinal bacterial overgrowth (SIBO) may be a significant factors in poor nutritional outcomes in patients with CF. Increased viscosity of the intestinal mucus and delayed small bowel transit may also contribute to the development of constipation or distal intestinal obstruction syndrome (DIOS), which in its subacute chronic form can cause poor appetite and inadequate weight gain.

Biliary secretions are critical for fat emulsification and absorption. Liver disease seen in patients with cystic fibrosis can lead to fat malabsorption through insufficient bile secretion. More thorough discussion of liver diseases in CF is covered Chapter 11 in this book.

Other gastrointestinal diseases, such as Celiac disease, inflammatory bowel disease, and gastrointestinal cancers tend to have a higher incidence among CF patients with disease-associated impact on nutrition and growth in pediatric and adult populations.

Role of CFTR in Gastrointestinal Tact

CFTR was identified and directly linked to CF in 1989 [6]. This complex protein is a cyclic-AMP regulated chloride channel that also regulates the flow of bicarbonate (HCO_3^-) along with other ions across the apical surface of epithelial cells. Absence of CFTR or decreased functional capacity leads to electrolyte imbalance external to the surface of the epithelial membranes, leading to desiccation

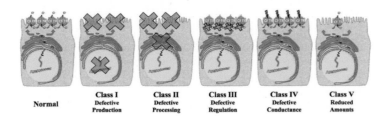

Fig. 12.1 Classification of CFTR mutations

and reduced clearance of secretions. CFTR protein is expressed on epithelial surfaces lining the gastrointestinal, integumentary, and pulmonary systems. CFTR distribution has higher abundance in the upper GI track, with highest density in the duodenum, gradually decreasing caudally [7]. CFTR is also present within pancreatic [8] and hepatobiliary systems [9]. Brunner's glands are densely present in the proximal small bowel and secrete bicarbonate-rich fluid into the crypts of the epithelial lining where it interacts with the mucin produced by epithelial goblet cells. Defective interaction between mucin and bicarbonate in CF patients can lead to thick mucus clogging the crypts and interfering with intestinal function [10]. The role of CFTR in the regulation of bicarbonate has been mostly described in CF disease, but has also been described in pancreatic diseases not associated with CF [11].

New developments in targeted therapy for specific CFTR defects have presented great therapeutic potential for a subgroup of CF patients with class III (gating) mutations (Fig. 12.1) [3, 12]. CFTR potentiator therapy with ivacaftor, a drug that targets class III mutations, provides a better insight and understanding of the pulmonary and gastrointestinal physiology in CF [13]. In particular, treatment with ivacaftor is associated with steady and significant weight gain, highlighting the central role of CFTR dysfunction in the nutritional manifestations of CF. With more therapeutic interventions developed specifically to address and correct defective cellular pathways or proteins, clinical focus in targeting CF will be aimed at early disease identification and prevention giving us the opportunity to minimize the gastrointestinal and nutritional morbidity of the disease.

Gastroesophageal Reflux and Gastric Emptying

GERD is one of the most prevalent gastrointestinal problems in CF. The principal mechanism causing GERD is an increase in the frequency and duration of transient lower esophageal sphincter relaxation (TLSR) episodes, permitting gastric contents to reflux into the esophagus. Symptoms include chest pain, heartburn, acid brash, halitosis, and dysphagia. In the USA, GERD has been reported in 30% of adult CF patients [14, 15]. There is a well-recognized relationship between GERD and chronic obstructive pulmonary disease [16]. In a 2010 survey, GERD symptoms of heartburn, acid brash, dysphagia, and dyspepsia were reported daily and occasionally in 24% and 39% of adult CF patients, respectively [17]. It has been suggested that pathologic reflux is associated with worse pulmonary outcome in patients with CF [18–20]. Despite these observations; there is poor correlation between severity of GERD symptoms and FEV_1 or FVC in adults with CF [17].

Clinical symptoms of GERD often impact nutrition by means of decreased appetite and poor caloric intake. In infants and younger children with CF, feeding refusal due to discomfort and pain associated with reflux might not be well communicated. Standard therapy with acid suppression, either histamine-2 receptor antagonist (H2RA) or proton pump inhibitor (PPI), has been used for GERD treatment. In CF patients, first-line therapy has been predominantly with PPI [21, 22]. Data from the 2013 CF Foundation Patient Registry show that more than 50% of the US CF patients are treated with PPI. This may not reflect treatment of GERD; however, since pancreatic insufficient patients are frequently prescribed acid-suppressing drugs to improve availability and efficacy of enzyme supplementation. In practice, this may preemptively address possible GER symptoms.

Although pharmacological intervention is first-line therapy, surgical intervention with fundoplication is an alternative to acid suppression in severe cases. In one study of adults with CF and reflux confirmed by 24-hour pH monitoring, laparoscopic fundoplication resulted in a small improvement in lung function, and a marked decrease in cough scores and number of pulmonary exacerbation events [23]. A separate study looking at the benefits of gastrostomy tube feedings in CF patients who failed medical therapy and required fundoplication showed statistical improvement in weight gain when gastrostomy tube feedings were used for more than 6 months [24]. This intervention may be especially important for patients who are in need of lung transplantation, as anti-reflux surgery has been shown to have a beneficial effect for patients without CF with end-stage lung disease and may improve allograft survival after transplantation [25].

Frequent emphasis on high calorie foods in CF patients can further aggravate reflux. CF dietary and nutritional supplement recommendations advise high fat diets, which can lead to prolonged gastric stasis, delayed gastric emptying, and an increased incidence of GER. However, this concern about delayed gastric emptying has not been borne out, as studies have shown similar gastric emptying time between CF patients and healthy matched controls [5, 26]. Furthermore, studies have shown no association between gastric emptying and GERD in CF patients [27].

Pancreatic Disease

Defects in the exocrine function of the pancreas in patients with CF have been subdivided into pancreatic insufficiency (PI) and pancreatic sufficiency (PS) based on the capacity to secrete pancreatic enzymes required for digestion and nutrition. More thorough discussions of PS and PI can be found in Chapter 10 and this chapter. An objective determination of pancreatic status function and routine re-evaluation is important in patients with CF, since those who are PI will need life-long PERT. A noninvasive stool assay for fecal elastase using enzyme-linked immunosorbent assay (ELISA) has been shown to be an excellent indicator of PI, with a sensitivity of 98–100% and a specificity of 93–100% [28, 29]. Serum immunoreactive trypsinogen is used in newborn screening programs to identify infants with CF, based on elevated trypsinogen from in utero pancreatic damage. Of note, even infants with PS-CF will have elevated trypsinogen. Infants born with CF-PI will have a rapid decline in the levels of serum trypsinogen in the first few years of life. Consequently, PI can be diagnosed using a blood test if serum trypsinogen is below the lower limits of normal in patients over 8 years of age [30]. Across all age groups, about 90% of patients with CF are PI. PI is usually seen in more "severe" CFTR mutations (class I, II, or III) and is present at birth in 60% of infants with CF [31].

The nutritional impact of pancreatic insufficiency is that it causes significant malabsorption of protein and fat, including fat-soluble vitamins A, D, E, and K. Deficiencies in these vitamins can range from xerophthalmia in vitamin A deficiency, osteopenia in vitamin D deficiencies, or coagulation defect with vitamin K deficiency along with other symptoms described in Chapters 4 and 5. In patients with underlying liver disease, fat malabsorption is further exacerbated by deficiency in bile salts. Malnutrition resulting from PI can have long-term sequelae with permanent stunting of stature [32, 33], cognitive dysfunction [34, 35], and a more rapid decline in pulmonary function [1, 36–40]. Over 85% of CF patients in the USA take exogenous PERT on a routine basis [21] with every meal and snack.

The nutritional efficacy of PERT relies on the physiological environment of the proximal gastrointestinal tract once present in the small bowel. To prevent denaturation and inactivation of the porcine enzyme, manufacturers encapsulated enzymes into small beads that are resistant to acid degradation. The goal is to prevent breakdown of the enzymes when in the acidic environment in the stomach and only enable their activity once in the small bowel. Microspheres are designed to dissolve at the pH of 5.5–6.0 [41, 42], which is usually achieved within the very proximal small bowel. Once gastric contents empty into the duodenum, the acidic pH is neutralized by bicarbonate-rich secretions within 10 cm of the gastro-duodenal junction. The epithelium of the small bowel, pancreatic, and biliary ducts secretes bicarbonate via a CFTR-assisted Cl^-/HCO_3^- exchange process and electrogenic secretion of HCO_3^- via a CFTR conductance pathway [43]. In patients with CF, reduced duodenal bicarbonate secretion may fail to neutralize gastric acid and thereby prevent or delay dissolution of the enteric coating until the microspheres reach more distal portions of the small bowel, thus allowing undigested food to bypass some of the absorptive surface of the intestine. This can have a profound effect on nutrition and lead to malabsorptive diarrhea. Delayed small bowel neutralization of the gastric acid with defective bicarbonate secretion has been noted in CF-PI in comparison to healthy controls in vivo [5]. Use of acid suppression in CF-PI patients on PERT might reduce gastric acidity requiring less robust bicarbonate response in the small bowel and potentially improved digestion and absorption by releasing encapsulated enzymes more proximal in the small bowel [44]. In CF patients, gastric acid suppression by PPI has been associated with a decrease in malabsorption symptoms [45–47].

Contrary to CF-PI disease, CF-PS patient have "milder" rather than "severe" CFTR genotypes and have adequate pancreatic enzyme secretion. CF-PS patients tend to have improved nutritional parameters with lower sweat chloride levels and better lung function compared to CF-PI patients. Acinar tissue in patients with PS is preserved, but there is a decreased ductal flow [48] that can lead to relatively acidic and dehydrated intestinal contents. This may account for some of the gastrointestinal symptoms seen in CF-PS patients. Decreased ductal bicarbonate and fluid secretion can also lead to intraductal enzyme activation presenting as pancreatitis in 10% of pancreatic sufficient patients. Recurrent bouts of pancreatitis in CF-PS patients can lead to chronic scarring of the ductal system and breakdown of the acinar cells causing patients to become PI. Early identification of pancreatic insufficiency in previously pancreatic sufficient patients is critical in preventing nutritional problems. In a study of 630 PS patients, 3% were found to develop PI after 5.6 years [30]. There is a rationale in advocating routine screening of the PS patients with fecal elastase and serum trypsinogen to identify early onset of pancreatic failure. Although there is no current evidence to support that the development of PI can be halted or reversed, further studies might identify triggers of developing PI.

Small Intestinal Bacterial Overgrowth

The symbiotic relationship between gastrointestinal microflora and the intestinal mucosa plays a significant role in nutrition and immune regulation. The distribution, composition, and density of the microbiome vary over a wide range across different regions of the gastrointestinal tract. The density of the microorganisms is measured as number of organisms/gram and ranges from 0 to 10^2 in the stomach, 10^2–10^3 in the proximal small bowel up to 10^7–10^8 in the terminal ileum, and 10^{12} in the colon [49]. The ability to maintain a relatively low density of the microbiota in the proximal and mid-small bowel is coordinated by multiple physiological, immunological, and chemical functions within the small bowel. Strong antegrade peristalsis, often termed the migrating motor complex, routinely sweeps all of the contents of the small bowel into the colon, thus clearing all of the residual microorganisms along with luminal contents. To assist clearance of the bacteria, intestinal mucus layer traps bacteria and is cleared during the sweeping complex. This complex is inhibited during meals to enable digestion and absorption of nutrients in the small bowel. In health, the low pH of the gastric acid will destroy a large portion of ingested microorganisms in the stomach before they enter the small bowel. Enzymatic digestion along with bile acids will further destroy bacteria in the proximal small bowel. Bactericidal properties of the immunological secretion with mucosal immunoglobulin A, along with defensins secreted from Paneth cells localized in the crypts of the small bowel, provide additional bacterial killing [4].

In CF patients, disruption of the abovementioned mechanisms with thick mucus secretions, intestinal dysmotility, chronic use of acid-suppressing agents, and antibiotics can predispose patients to intestinal stasis facilitating development of SIBO, which is seen in 30–55% of patients [50, 51]. More recent studies using wireless motility capsules along with other radioisotope studies concluded delayed small bowel transit in patients with CF to be almost twice as long as in healthy matched controls, which can further support SIBO [5, 26]. Bacterial overgrowth within the lumen of the small intestine can produce gas, toxic byproducts, and metabolites often leading to malnutrition, malabsorption, and adjacent enterocyte damage. SIBO will compete with the host for critical nutrients, alter metabolism, and inflict mucosal damage that can lead to further derangements in nutrient digestion or absorption. Bacterial overgrowth can deconjugate bile acids impairing bile acid-dependent fat absorption leading to steatorrhea and malabsorption of fats and fat-soluble vitamins. Deconjugated bile acids may exert toxic effects on enterocytes, further exacerbating damage that can lead to protein and carbohydrate malabsorption. Impaired disaccharidase activity from mucosal inflammation or from thick viscous secretions trapping access to brush border enzymes will interfere with monosaccharide availability required for intestinal absorption; the unabsorbed disaccharides are then available for bacterial degradation and fermentation. The impact on nutrition by SIBO is only in part through direct effects on enterocytes, competition for nutrients, and production of toxins. Abdominal distention from excessive fermentation and production of toxic metabolites can lead to significant clinical symptoms of abdominal pain, nausea, vomiting, diarrhea, and decreased appetite further compromising nutritional status of a host.

Diagnostic modalities such as imaging, culture of duodenal aspirates during endoscopy, and breath hydrogen testing are used to diagnose SIBO. All of these modalities have limitations in accurately diagnosing SIBO. Breath testing has been the least invasive and most practical modality to diagnose SIBO in older children and adults. Improved sensitivity to breath hydrogen testing was achieved through adding methane to a routine breath testing [52]. D-Lactic acidosis has been associated with SIBO through extrapolation that only bacteria can produce D-lactic acid in large enough volume to be detected in serum. Measurement of only the D enantiomer is only done at academic institutions and this modality has never been well-accepted as a clinical tool. Novel diagnostic developments in imaging techniques and intraluminal diagnostic devices might add to our armamentarium of tools to diagnose SIBO [53, 54].

Medical management of SIBO with broad-spectrum enteric antibiotics is the treatment of choice and may be used as empiric therapy based on symptoms and clinical suspicion. The goal of the therapy is to suppress and potentially eradicate pathogenic bacterial overgrowth that will not repopulate the small intestine once therapy is discontinued. This approach is frequently augmented with adequate bowel hydration with osmotic agents such as polyethylene glycol. Unlike antibiotics, probiotics have limited bactericidal properties, but likely will compete with the pathogenic species for colonization and nutrient availability. Discontinuation of the pharmacological agents that might be associated with development of SIBO, such as chronic antibiotics or acid suppression therapy in CF patients, can often lead to worsening clinical outcomes and has to be carefully assessed by a treating provider.

Diseases of the Small Intestine

The nutritional capacity of the small bowel is constrained not just by the surface area available for digestion and absorption of nutrients but also by specific regions of the small bowel. The small bowel is classically subdivided into duodenum, jejunum, and ileum and each region has specialized functions in terms of nutrient absorption. The duodenum plays a major role in iron absorption and the ileum is predominantly responsible for vitamin B_{12} and bile acid absorption. There is a significant overlap in nutritional and functional capabilities between different regions of the small bowel. Distal regions of the small bowel have a greater versatility to compensate for the lack of proximal small bowel capacity.

The proximal small bowel, however, has a limited capacity to perform the functions of the distal regions. This discrepancy in the regional capabilities of the small bowel and its impact on nutrition becomes relevant in surgical resections of the small bowel and diseases involving segments or specific regions of the small intestine. Postoperative strictures or distended bowel loops can facilitate SIBO. Surgical resections in CF infants with inspissated meconium ileus (MI), intestinal atresias, or in utero perforations can lead to a loss of bowel region and consequent malabsorption and nutritional compromise. A retrospective study of infants over a 20-year duration identified MI in 20% of CF confirmed cases, most requiring surgical interventions (92%) [55]. A higher incidence of MI has been observed in infants with more severe CRTR mutations with proposed pathophysiology of small bowel obstruction caused by loss of CFTR-mediated Cl^- and/or HCO_3^- transport in the intestinal epithelium along with pancreatic dysfunction [56]. However, not all patients with a given genotype will develop MI. In contrast, animal models of CF must be managed specifically to avoid bowel obstruction. Animal experiments of CFTR knock out models with transgenic intestinal expression of CFTR protein showed that expressing 20% of the wild type CFTR in the gastrointestinal tract and improving Cl^- current to at least 60% of wild type was sufficient to rescue animals from a phenotype with 100% MI [57].

Other comorbid conditions involving the small bowel such as celiac disease and inflammatory bowel disease are found to have a higher prevalence in the CF population and can further compromise small bowel function and nutrition [58, 59].

Distal Intestinal Obstructions Syndrome

DIOS, previously termed *meconium ileus equivalent*, is a complete or partial obstruction of the distal ileum with fecal material extending into cecum that can present in CF patients at any age [60]. Accumulation of this viscid fecal material adheres strongly to mucosal villi and crypts. DIOS can present as an acute event or with chronic, intermittent symptoms of abdominal pain and distention likely attributed to a partial breakdown and re-accumulation of new material over a strongly adherent mucoid mass. Symptoms include cramps, abdominal pain localized to the right lower quadrant leading to anorexia and subsequent weight loss. DIOS is seen more frequently in PI patients as well as those with a prior history of MI or prior episodes of DIOS [61]. Although DIOS is rare in PS patients, it has been reported [60]. Increased viscosity of the luminal mucus, intestinal dysmotility, and mucosal inflammation, along with defective chloride, bicarbonate, and water secretion into the gut lumen collectively contribute to DIOS. Fat malabsorption and insufficient PERT supplementation has been suggested as a pathophysiology causing DIOS, but has not been validated in a recent clinical study [62]. Even though this study did observe a significant increase in fat intake and pancreatic enzyme intake, when the ratio of enzyme supplementation was corrected for fat intake, there was no difference in the same cohort a year prior to DIOS. The impact of nutrition on pathophysiology of DIOS remains to be answered. The role of DIOS on nutrition, however, is undeniably important. Unabsorbed nutrients and distention in the distal portion of the small intestine contributes to the ileal brake, a physiological mechanism inhibiting gastric emptying, intestinal peristalsis, and reduction of intestinal secretions. All of these mechanisms along with clinical symptoms will interfere with appetite and normal enteral nutrition.

Management and urgency of clinical intervention depends on the degree of obstruction and suspicion of peritoneal irritation and symptoms. Treatment is aimed at safely disimpacting the proximal fecal mass with hyperosmolar contrast enemas (Gastrografin) [63, 64] or anterograde hyperosmotic agents (polyethylene glycol or lactulose) for milder forms of obstruction. Although surgical intervention is rarely required, timely consultation in the event of failure of medical management and acute decompensation is warranted. Persistent symptoms and signs of intestinal obstruction unresponsive to the pharmacological therapy should raise concern for abscess, fibrosing colonopathy, or neoplastic lesions within the gastrointestinal track, among others.

Emphasis is also placed on prevention of recurrent episodes of DIOS by re-educating patients on the importance of adherence to PERT with meals and snacks, routine luminal hydration along with occasional anterograde clean outs.

Constipation

Constipation is a frequent problem in patients with CF and likely shares some of the underlying mechanism with DIOS such as dysmotility and decreased luminal hydration secondary to CFTR defect. Poor appetite, excessive bloating, or abdominal pain may be the only symptoms. Patients and clinicians should be aware that most chronically constipated patients with CF have bowel movements every day [65]. DIOS starts in the ileum and extends distally into the colon while constipation starts in the recto-sigmoid and extends proximally into the colon. Both DIOS and constipation are independent of each other but can coexist. Similar to DIOS, fat malabsorption and prior history of MI were noted to be independent risk factors in pediatric CF patients with constipation [66]. Prevalence of constipation in CF patients (32%) is no different from general adult population (34–37%). CF patients with PI are on average 50% more likely to have a diagnosis of constipation in comparison to PS patients [65].

In contrast to the general population where the likely contributors to functional constipation are deficiency in dietary fiber, inadequate fluid intake, and psychosomatic causes, these factors were not associated with constipation in children with CF [66]. It is likely that CFTR dysfunction leading to relatively dehydrated intestinal contents plays an important role in facilitating constipation among CF patients. Therapeutic options in the CF patient with constipation are not different from the medical management of constipation in the general population. Treatment options include oral hyperosmotic agents such as polyethylene glycol, lactulose, or sorbitol that retain water in the intestines and facilitate softer stools. Initiation of therapy often warrants an initial clean out with a large dose of osmotic agents often in combination with stimulant agents such as senna or bisacodyl to induce colonic spasms and fecal evacuation. Magnesium-containing agents (magnesium citrate, magnesium hydroxide, or magnesium sulfate) that have both an osmotic and laxative effect and can induce colonic motility may also be used. Disturbance to electrolyte balance can be seen in chronic and large dose of magnesium preparation, so these should be used sparingly. Long-term use of dietary fiber supplementation has been advocated to maintain softer stools and establish normal defecation patterns. In general, the high calorie diet consumed by CF patients tends to have a lower dietary fiber intake; this has been suggested to have an impact on development of constipation and DIOS [67]. A closer look at the relationship between fiber intake in pediatric patients with CF and gastrointestinal complaints including DIOS did not show any relationship in 40 children [68]. Imaging modalities with abdominal X-rays may be useful in assessing fecal loading distribution of stool or response to treatment, despite carrying an inherent risk of minimal radiation exposure [66]. Clinical symptoms with a thorough history and a physical examination are usually sufficient to guide therapeutic recommendations prior to committing to additional investigations.

Gastrointestinal Cancers

Patients with CF are at increased risk for esophageal, gastric, hepatobiliary, gallbladder, small intestinal, and colon cancers relative to the US population [69]. Increased prevalence of gastrointestinal cancers has been suggested to correlate with organ specific CFTR expression, suggesting that defective expression in tissues that normally have high CFTR expression will contribute to increased inflammation and lead to increased cell turnover [69, 70]. Other factors that can contribute to an

Table 12.1 Liver disorders in patients with cystic fibrosis

Micro gallbladder	Sclerosing cholangitis
Cholelithiasis	Hepatic steatosis
Biliary tract ductal stones	Nodular regenerative hyperplasia
Focal biliary cirrhosis	Portal hypertension

increased likelihood of gastrointestinal neoplasms in CF patients are defective mucus function along with increased MUC 1, 2, and 3 expression, oxidative stress, activation of NF-κB, excessive acid exposure in the upper gastrointestinal tract, elevation of CA 19–9 and CEA and deficiencies in antioxidants (omega-3 fatty acids, vitamin E) [71]. This risk increases in post-transplant patients on immunosuppression therapy. The nutritional impact on CF patients with gastrointestinal cancers is not different from gastrointestinal cancers in the general population and management GI cancers in patients with CF does not differ from management of patients without CF. In both cases, surveillance and accurate diagnosis are crucial. Special attention to management of pulmonary issues is required in patients with CF requiring anesthesia for endoscopic or surgical interventions. The distribution and degree of neoplastic tissue, surgical interventions, and side effects of the therapeutic agents will dictate whether cancer patients are able to tolerate enteral nutrition. Alternative to enteral nutrition is parenteral nutrition, which can lead to multiple complications including sepsis.

CF-Related Liver Disease

Liver has many critical roles in the gastrointestinal, immunological, and hematological physiology and homeostasis of the body. Its most direct impact on nutrition is through bile secretion to aid in digestion and absorption of nutrients within the gastrointestinal tract. In patients with CF, the viscosity of bile is increased because of the role that CFTR has in water and bicarbonate secretion in the biliary tract. The most common mechanism of liver injury in CF patients is through cholestasis, as conjugated bile acids are backed up within the bile ducts causing portal tract and hepatocyte inflammation and tissue fibrosis. This can further compromise nutrition in patients with CF. A wide spectrum of hepatobiliary diseases can be seen in patients with CF (Table 12.1). Chapter 11 focuses in depth on CF-related liver disease and its impact on nutrition.

Conclusion

CF affects the gastrointestinal as well as the respiratory tracts. If unrecognized and untreated, the gastrointestinal manifestations can lead to poor appetite, maldigestion, and malabsorption of nutrients, and other factors that contribute to inadequate weight gain or possibly weight loss. Nutritional status, gastrointestinal factors, and pulmonary manifestations of CF are intertwined and addressing all of them can lead to improved outcomes and quality of life or our patients.

References

1. Stallings VA, Stark LJ, Robinson KA, Feranchak AP, Quinton H. Evidence-based practice recommendations for nutrition-related management of children and adults with cystic fibrosis and pancreatic insufficiency: results of a systematic review. J Am Diet Assoc. 2008;108(5):832–9. Epub 2008/04/30. eng.
2. Rowe SM, Miller S, Sorscher EJ. Cystic fibrosis. N Engl J Med. 2005;352(19):1992–2001. Epub 2005/05/13. eng.

3. Ramsey BW, Davies J, McElvaney NG, Tullis E, Bell SC, Drevinek P, et al. A CFTR potentiator in patients with cystic fibrosis and the G551D mutation. N Engl J Med. 2011;365(18):1663–72. Epub 2005/05/13. eng.
4. Wehkamp J, Fellermann K, Herrlinger KR, Bevins CL, Stange EF. Mechanisms of disease: defensins in gastrointestinal diseases. Nat Clin Pract Gastroenterol Hepatol. 2005;2(9):406–15.
5. Gelfond D, Ma C, Semler J, Borowitz D. Intestinal pH and gastrointestinal transit profiles in cystic fibrosis patients measured by wireless motility capsule. Dig Dis Sci. 2012;58(8):2275–81. Epub 2012/05/18. Eng.
6. Riordan JR, Rommens JM, Kerem B, Alon N, Rozmahel R, Grzelczak Z, et al. Identification of the cystic fibrosis gene: cloning and characterization of complementary DNA. Science. 1989;245(4922):1066–73. Epub 1989/09/08. eng.
7. Jakab R, Collaco A, Ameen N. Physiological relevance of cell-specific distribution patterns of CFTR, NKCC1, NBCe1, and NHE3 along the crypt-villus axis in the intestine. Am J Physiol Gastrointest Liver Physiol. 2011;300(1):G82–98. PubMed1152/ajpgi.00245.2010.
8. Marino CR, Matovcik LM, Gorelick FS, Cohn JA. Localization of the cystic fibrosis transmembrane conductance regulator in pancreas. J Clin Invest. 1991;88(2):712–6. PMCID: 295422. Epub 1991/08/01. eng.
9. Cohn JA, Strong TV, Picciotto MR, Nairn AC, Collins FS, Fitz JG. Localization of the cystic fibrosis transmembrane conductance regulator in human bile duct epithelial cells. Gastroenterology. 1993;105(6):1857–64. Epub 1993/12/01. eng.
10. Chen EY, Yang N, Quinton PM, Chin WC. A new role for bicarbonate in mucus formation. Am J Physiol Lung Cell Mol Physiol. 2010;299(4):L542–9. PMCID: 2957415. Epub 2010/08/10. eng.
11. LaRusch J, Jung J, General IJ, Lewis MD, Park HW, Brand RE, et al. Mechanisms of CFTR functional variants that impair regulated bicarbonate permeation and increase risk for pancreatitis but not for cystic fibrosis. PLoS Genet. 2014;10(7):e1004376. PMCID: 4102440.
12. Full Prescribing Information—KALYDECO® (ivacaftor) Tablets. http://www.accessdata.fda.gov: Vertex Pharmaceuticals Incorporated. 2014.
13. Rowe SM, Heltshe SL, Gonska T, Donaldson SH, Borowitz D, Gelfond D, et al. Clinical mechanism of the cystic fibrosis transmembrane conductance regulator potentiator ivacaftor in G551D-mediated cystic fibrosis. Am J Respir Crit Care Med. 2014;190(2):175–84.
14. Cystic Fibrosis Foundation. Patient Registry, 2010 Annual Data Report to the Center Directors. Bethesda, MD; 2010.
15. Cystic Fibrosis Foundation. Patient Registry, 2012 Annual Data Report to the Center Directors. Bethesda, MD; 2012.
16. Rabinovich RA, MacNee W. Chronic obstructive pulmonary disease and its comorbidities. Br J Hosp Med (Lond). 2011;72(3):137–45. Epub 2011/04/09. eng.
17. Sabati AA, Kempainen RR, Milla CE, Ireland M, Schwarzenberg SJ, Dunitz JM, et al. Characteristics of gastroesophageal reflux in adults with cystic fibrosis. J Cyst Fibros. 2010;9(5):365–70. Epub 2010/08/03. eng.
18. Navarro J, Rainisio M, Harms HK, Hodson ME, Koch C, Mastella G, et al. Factors associated with poor pulmonary function: cross-sectional analysis of data from the ERCF. European Epidemiologic Registry of Cystic Fibrosis. Eur Respir J. 2001;18(2):298–305. Epub 2001/09/01. eng.
19. Stringer DA, Sprigg A, Juodis E, Corey M, Daneman A, Levison HJ, et al. The association of cystic fibrosis, gastroesophageal reflux, and reduced pulmonary function. Can Assoc Radiol J. 1988;39(2):100–2. Epub 1988/06/01. eng.
20. Palm K, Sawicki G, Rosen R. The impact of reflux burden on pseudomonas positivity in children with cystic fibrosis. Pediatr Pulmonol. 2012;47(6):582–7. Epub 2011/12/14. eng.
21. Cystic Fibrosis Foundation. Patient Registry, 2011 Annual Data Report to the Center Directors. Bethesda, MD; 2011.
22. Borowitz DS, Grand RJ, Durie PR. Use of pancreatic enzyme supplements for patients with cystic fibrosis in the context of fibrosing colonopathy. J Pediatr. 1995;127(5):681–4. Epub 1995/11/01. eng.
23. Fathi H, Moon T, Donaldson J, Jackson W, Sedman P, Morice AH. Cough in adult cystic fibrosis: diagnosis and response to fundoplication. Cough. 2009;5:1. PMCID: 2634760. Epub 2009/01/20. eng.
24. Sheikh S, Quach J, McCoy K. Nissen fundoplication in patients with cystic fibrosis. Chest. 2011;140 (4_MeetingAbstracts) Suppl 4:385A. PMID: 00002953-201110004-00385.
25. Hoppo T, Jarido V, Pennathur A, Morrell M, Crespo M, Shigemura N, et al. Antireflux surgery preserves lung function in patients with gastroesophageal reflux disease and end-stage lung disease before and after lung transplantation. Arch Surg. 2011;146(9):1041–7. Epub 2011/09/21. eng.
26. Rovner AJ, Schall JI, Mondick JT, Zhuang H, Mascarenhas MR. Delayed small bowel transit in children with cystic fibrosis and pancreatic insufficiency. J Pediatr Gastroenterol Nutr. 2013;57(1):81–4.
27. Pauwels A, Blondeau K, Mertens V, Farre R, Verbeke K, Dupont LJ, et al. Gastric emptying and different types of reflux in adult patients with cystic fibrosis. Aliment Pharmacol Ther. 2011;34(7):799–807. Epub 2011/07/29. eng.
28. Walkowiak J. Faecal elastase-1: clinical value in the assessment of exocrine pancreatic function in children. Eur J Pediatr. 2000;159(11):869–70. Epub 2000/11/18. eng.
29. Beharry S, Ellis L, Corey M, Marcon M, Durie P. How useful is fecal pancreatic elastase 1 as a marker of exocrine pancreatic disease? J Pediatr. 2002;141(1):84–90. Epub 2002/07/02. eng.
30. Couper RT, Corey M, Moore DJ, Fisher LJ, Forstner GG, Durie PR. Decline of exocrine pancreatic function in cystic fibrosis patients with pancreatic sufficiency. Pediatr Res. 1992;32(2):179–82. Epub 1992/08/01. eng.

31. Bronstein MN, Sokol RJ, Abman SH, Chatfield BA, Hammond KB, Hambidge KM, et al. Pancreatic insufficiency, growth, and nutrition in infants identified by newborn screening as having cystic fibrosis. J Pediatr. 1992;120(4 Pt 1):533–40.

32. Farrell PM, Kosorok MR, Laxova A, Shen G, Koscik RE, Bruns WT, et al. Nutritional benefits of neonatal screening for cystic fibrosis. Wisconsin Cystic Fibrosis Neonatal Screening Study Group. N Engl J Med. 1997;337(14):963–9. Epub 1998/02/12. eng.

33. Farrell PM, Kosorok MR, Rock MJ, Laxova A, Zeng L, Lai HC, et al. Early diagnosis of cystic fibrosis through neonatal screening prevents severe malnutrition and improves long-term growth. Wisconsin Cystic Fibrosis Neonatal Screening Study Group. Pediatrics. 2001;107(1):1–13. Epub 2001/01/03. eng.

34. Koscik RL, Farrell PM, Kosorok MR, Zaremba KM, Laxova A, Lai HC, et al. Cognitive function of children with cystic fibrosis: deleterious effect of early malnutrition. Pediatrics. 2004;113(6):1549–58. Epub 2004/06/03. eng.

35. Koscik RL, Lai HJ, Laxova A, Zaremba KM, Kosorok MR, Douglas JA, et al. Preventing early, prolonged vitamin E deficiency: an opportunity for better cognitive outcomes via early diagnosis through neonatal screening. J Pediatr. 2005;147(3 Suppl):S51–6. Epub 2005/10/06. Eng.

36. Konstan MW, Butler SM, Wohl ME, Stoddard M, Matousek R, Wagener JS, et al. Growth and nutritional indexes in early life predict pulmonary function in cystic fibrosis. J Pediatr. 2003;142(6):624–30. Epub 2003/07/03. eng.

37. Peterson ML, Jacobs Jr DR, Milla CE. Longitudinal changes in growth parameters are correlated with changes in pulmonary function in children with cystic fibrosis. Pediatrics. 2003;112(3 Pt 1):588–92. Epub 2003/09/02. eng.

38. Steinkamp G, Wiedemann B. Relationship between nutritional status and lung function in cystic fibrosis: cross sectional and longitudinal analyses from the German CF quality assurance (CFQA) project. Thorax. 2002;57(7):596–601. PMCID: 1746376. Epub 2002/07/04. Eng.

39. Lai HJ, Shoff SM, Farrell PM. Recovery of birth weight z score within 2 years of diagnosis is positively associated with pulmonary status at 6 years of age in children with cystic fibrosis. Pediatrics. 2009;123(2):714–22. PMCID: 2775492. Epub 2009/01/28. eng.

40. Zemel BS, Jawad AF, FitzSimmons S, Stallings VA. Longitudinal relationship among growth, nutritional status, and pulmonary function in children with cystic fibrosis: analysis of the Cystic Fibrosis Foundation National CF Patient Registry. J Pediatr. 2000;137(3):374–80. Epub 2000/09/02. Eng.

41. Ferrone M, Raimondo M, Scolapio JS. Pancreatic enzyme pharmacotherapy. Pharmacotherapy. 2007;27(6):910–20. Epub 2007/06/05. eng.

42. Kraisinger M, Hochhaus G, Stecenko A, Bowser E, Hendeles L. Clinical pharmacology of pancreatic enzymes in patients with cystic fibrosis and in vitro performance of microencapsulated formulations. J Clin Pharmacol. 1994;34(2):158–66. Epub 1994/02/01. eng.

43. Clarke LL, Harline MC. Dual role of CFTR in cAMP-stimulated HCO3- secretion across murine duodenum. Am J Physiol. 1998;274(4 Pt 1):G718–26. Epub 1998/05/12. eng.

44. DiMagno EP. Gastric acid suppression and treatment of severe exocrine pancreatic insufficiency. Best Pract Res Clin Gastroenterol. 2001;15(3):477–86. Epub 2001/06/14. eng.

45. Proesmans M, De Boeck K. Omeprazole, a proton pump inhibitor, improves residual steatorrhoea in cystic fibrosis patients treated with high dose pancreatic enzymes. Eur J Pediatr. 2003;162(11):760–3. Epub 2003/09/19. eng.

46. Tran TM, Van den Neucker A, Hendriks JJ, Forget P, Forget PP. Effects of a proton-pump inhibitor in cystic fibrosis. Acta Paediatr. 1998;87(5):553–8. Epub 1998/06/26. eng.

47. Ng SM, Franchini AJ. Drug therapies for reducing gastric acidity in people with cystic fibrosis. Cochrane Database Syst Rev. 2014;7:CD003424.

48. Kopelman H, Forstner G, Durie P, Corey M. Origins of chloride and bicarbonate secretory defects in the cystic fibrosis pancreas, as suggested by pancreatic function studies on control and CF subjects with preserved pancreatic function. Clin Invest Med. 1989;12(3):207–11. Epub 1989/06/01. eng.

49. Sartor RB. Microbial influences in inflammatory bowel diseases. Gastroenterology. 2008;134(2):577–94.

50. Lewindon PJ, Robb TA, Moore DJ, Davidson GP, Martin AJ. Bowel dysfunction in cystic fibrosis: importance of breath testing. J Paediatr Child Health. 1998;34(1):79–82. Epub 1998/05/06. eng.

51. Fridge JL, Conrad C, Gerson L, Castillo RO, Cox K. Risk factors for small bowel bacterial overgrowth in cystic fibrosis. J Pediatr Gastroenterol Nutr. 2007;44(2):212–8. Epub 2007/01/27. eng.

52. Lisowska A, Wojtowicz J, Walkowiak J. Small intestine bacterial overgrowth is frequent in cystic fibrosis: combined hydrogen and methane measurements are required for its detection. Acta Biochim Pol. 2009;56(4):631–4. Epub 2009/12/10. eng.

53. Grace E, Shaw C, Whelan K, Andreyev HJ. Review article: small intestinal bacterial overgrowth—prevalence, clinical features, current and developing diagnostic tests, and treatment. Aliment Pharmacol Ther. 2013;38(7):674–88.

54. Roland BC, Ciarleglio MM, Clarke JO, Semler JR, Tomakin E, Mullin GE, et al. Small intestinal transit time is delayed in small intestinal bacterial overgrowth. J Clin Gastroenterol. 2014.

55. Farrelly PJ, Charlesworth C, Lee S, Southern KW, Baillie CT. Gastrointestinal surgery in cystic fibrosis: a 20-year review. J Pediatr Surg. 2014;49(2):280–3.

56. Carlyle BE, Borowitz DS, Glick PL. A review of pathophysiology and management of fetuses and neonates with meconium ileus for the pediatric surgeon. J Pediatr Surg. 2012;47(4):772–81. Epub 2012/04/14. eng.

57. Stoltz DA, Rokhlina T, Ernst SE, Pezzulo AA, Ostedgaard LS, Karp PH, et al. Intestinal CFTR expression alleviates meconium ileus in cystic fibrosis pigs. J Clin Invest. 2013;123(6):2685–93. PMCID: 3668832.

58. Lloyd-Still JD. Crohn's disease and cystic fibrosis. Dig Dis Sci. 1994;39(4):880–5.

59. Mihailidi E, Katakis E, Evangeliou A. Celiac disease: a pediatric perspective. Int Pediatr. 2003;18(3):141–8.

60. Houwen RH, van der Doef HP, Sermet I, Munck A, Hauser B, Walkowiak J, et al. Defining DIOS and constipation in cystic fibrosis with a multicentre study on the incidence, characteristics, and treatment of DIOS. J Pediatr Gastroenterol Nutr. 2010;50(1):38–42.

61. Colombo C, Ellemunter H, Houwen R, Munck A, Taylor C, Wilschanski M. Guidelines for the diagnosis and management of distal intestinal obstruction syndrome in cystic fibrosis patients. J Cyst Fibros. 2011;10 Suppl 2: S24–8.

62. Declercq D, Van Biervliet S, Robberecht E. Nutrition and pancreatic enzyme intake in patients with cystic fibrosis with distal intestinal obstruction syndrome. Nutr Clin Pract. 2014;30(1):134–7.

63. O'Halloran SM, Gilbert J, McKendrick OM, Carty HM, Heaf DP. Gastrografin in acute meconium ileus equivalent. Arch Dis Child. 1986;61(11):1128–30. PMCID: 1778105. Epub 1986/11/01. eng.

64. Mahmoud Zahra CF, Thomas R, Iqbal V, Borowitz D. Gastrografin enemas for treatment of distal intestinal obstruction syndrome in children and adults with cystic fibrosis. J Pharm Nutr Sci. 2014;4(2):76–80.

65. Baker SS, Borowitz D, Duffy L, Fitzpatrick L, Gyamfi J, Baker RD. Pancreatic enzyme therapy and clinical outcomes in patients with cystic fibrosis. J Pediatr. 2005;146(2):189–93.

66. van der Doef HPJ, Kokke FTM, Beek FJA, Woestenenk JW, Froeling SP, Houwen RHJ. Constipation in pediatric cystic fibrosis patients: an underestimated medical condition. J Cyst Fibros. 2010;9(1):59–63.

67. Gavin J, Ellis J, Dewar AL, Rolles CJ, Connett GJ. Dietary fibre and the occurrence of gut symptoms in cystic fibrosis. Arch Dis Child. 1997;76(1):35–7. PMCID: 1717032.

68. Proesmans M, De Boeck K. Evaluation of dietary fiber intake in Belgian children with cystic fibrosis: is there a link with gastrointestinal complaints? J Pediatr Gastroenterol Nutr. 2002;35(5):610–4.

69. Neglia JP, FitzSimmons SC, Maisonneuve P, Schoni MH, Schoni-Affolter F, Corey M, et al. The risk of cancer among patients with cystic fibrosis. Cystic Fibrosis and Cancer Study Group. N Engl J Med. 1995;332(8):494–9. Epub 1995/02/23. eng.

70. Maisonneuve P, Marshall BC, Knapp EA, Lowenfels AB. Cancer risk in cystic fibrosis: a 20-year nationwide study from the United States. J Natl Cancer Inst. 2013;105(2):122–9.

71. Alexander CL, Urbanski SJ, Hilsden R, Rabin H, MacNaughton WK, Beck PL. The risk of gastrointestinal malignancies in cystic fibrosis: case report of a patient with a near obstructing villous adenoma found on colon cancer screening and Barrett's esophagus. J Cyst Fibros. 2008;7(1):1–6. Epub 2007/09/04. eng.

Chapter 13
Nutritional Management of Cystic Fibrosis Related Diabetes Mellitus

Katie Larson Ode and Carol Brunzell

Key Points

- Cystic Fibrosis Related Diabetes Mellitus (CFRD) is a serious and common complication of cystic fibrosis. CFRD is a unique form of diabetes, which has a different cause and different natural history then the more well-known type 1 and type 2 diabetes mellitus. Therefore, CFRD requires a unique approach to nutritional therapy very different from the approach to other types of diabetes mellitus.
- CFRD is a silent disease and one of the very first manifestations may be nutritional failure. Importantly, CFRD leads to lung function decline before signs and symptoms of diabetes develop and therefore screening for this disorder is required.
- As with all forms of diabetes, nutrition therapy is essential to the care of the CF patient with CFRD. However, CF has very specific nutritional and nutrition education needs and CFRD is unique compared to other types of diabetes, which means that typical diabetic nutrition education is not sufficient and may be inappropriate for the patient with CF and diabetes.
- The underlying nutritional needs of the CF patient (high calorie, high fat, high sodium) do not change with the diagnosis of diabetes. CF patients often have variable appetite due to illness and often require oral or enteral supplementation to achieve adequate caloric intake. Therefore traditional diabetic meal plans are not practical and may be inappropriate.
- Other concerns specific to this population that affect nutrition care are alterations in sensitivity with illness, the interaction between supplemental feeding and diabetic control, pregnancy, use of steroid therapy and its complications for nutrition and diabetic control and the increased potential for disordered eating in this population coupled with the overarching need for high caloric intake.
- The only recommended treatment for CFRD is insulin, which means that carbohydrate counting and management are essential parts of the nutritional management of this disease, and assume new importance in patients who must consume a high-calorie and carbohydrate-rich diet due to the underlying nature of their disease.
- Treatment of CFRD normally results in reversal of nutritional failure and improvement in overall health in the patient with CF.

K.L. Ode, M.D., M.S. (✉)
University of Iowa Children's Hospital, 200 Hawkins Dr., 2861 JPP, Iowa City, IA 52242-1083, USA
e-mail: Katie-larsonode@uiowa.edu

C. Brunzell, R.D., L.D., C.D.E.
Diabetes Care Centers, University of Minnesota Health, Fairview,
516 Delaware Street SE, MMC 88, Minneapolis, MN 55455, USA

E.H. Yen, A.R. Leonard (eds.), *Nutrition in Cystic Fibrosis: A Guide for Clinicians*, Nutrition and Health,
DOI 10.1007/978-3-319-16387-1_13, © Springer International Publishing Switzerland 2015

Keywords Cystic fibrosis related diabetes • Type 1 diabetes • Type 2 diabetes • Insulin • Impaired glucose tolerance • Hypoglycemia • Gestational diabetes • Insulin resistance • Basal insulin • Bolus insulin • Long-acting insulin • Rapid-acting insulin • Intermediate-acting insulin • Glucocorticoids • Hemoglobin A1c • Oral glucose tolerance test • Microvascular disease • Macrovascular disease • Ketoacidosis • American Diabetes Association

Abbreviations

ADA   American Diabetes Association
AGT   Abnormal glucose tolerance
BG   Blood glucose
BMI   Body mass index
CF   Cystic fibrosis
CFF   Cystic Fibrosis Foundation
CFRD   Cystic fibrosis related diabetes
CGM   Continuous glucose monitoring
GDM   Gestational diabetes
HbA1c   Hemoglobin A1c
IGT   Impaired glucose tolerance
INDET   Indeterminate glycemia
OGTT   Oral glucose tolerance test
PERT   Pancreatic enzyme replacement therapy
T1D   Type 1 diabetes
T2D   Type 2 diabetes

Introduction

Improved treatment of cystic fibrosis (CF) has dramatically increased survival rates for those affected by CF. As people with CF are living longer, CFRD has become one of the most common complications of CF. Studies have shown that CFRD occurs in about 20% of adolescents and 40–50% of adults, but can occur at any age and is associated with worse survival. Impaired glucose tolerance (IGT) occurs in up to 75% of adults with CF [1–3]. Ideally, given the high likelihood of the development of diabetes in everyone with CF, the risk of development of diabetes should affect all nutrition education in CF.

Nutrition therapy for CFRD differs drastically from type 1 diabetes (T1D) and type 2 diabetes (T2D) in many key areas. Attaining and maintaining good nutritional status is the cornerstone of treatment in CF and has been shown to improve survival. For adults with CF, body mass index (BMI) goals are 23 kg/m^2 for males and 22 kg/m^2 for females [4]. The usual nutrition therapy guidelines for CF (high calorie, high fat, high sodium) do not change once the diagnosis of CFRD has been made. Nutrition goals for CFRD include normal growth and nutrition for children, teens, and adults with CF, and maintenance of near normal blood glucose. The recommended treatment for CFRD is insulin. Differences in nutrition therapy for CFRD, pregnancy with CFRD, gestational diabetes (GDM) in CF, IGT in CF, and treatment of hypoglycemia is essential for health care providers to understand in order to ensure best patient care [5, 6]. Because appetite can be highly variable from day to day, people with CF frequently require oral high-calorie supplements and/or enteral tube feedings to meet caloric needs [7, 8]. For these reasons, traditional diabetic meal plans are not practical. Using carbohydrate counting and insulin-to-carbohydrate ratios in conjunction with the CF eating pattern to guide insulin therapy can help to optimize glycemic control [6].

Nutritional Implications of Diabetes in CF

In CF patients who subsequently developed CFRD, compared to CF patients who were known to maintain normal glucose tolerance, the patients who subsequently developed CFRD had lower weight and BMI 4 years prior to diagnosis of CFRD, and significantly higher decline lung function 1–3 years prior to diagnosis of diabetes [9]. In follow-up, once the CFRD population was on insulin for 2 years, BMI values were similar to the non-diabetic group and lung functions improved [10]. Hyperglycemia has a negative effect on nutritional status and causes derangements in protein metabolism [11].

Diabetes Complications

People with CFRD are not at risk for macrovascular (cardiovascular) disease despite eating diets high in total and saturated fat. There has never been a CF patient reported to have died from atherosclerotic cardiovascular disease. As patients are living longer with CFRD, these recommendations may eventually change [12, 13]. Recent studies have observed an increase in obesity in the CF population, but underweight and malnutrition remain the primary nutrition focus for the majority of patients with CF [14]. However, they are at risk for the development of microvascular disease: retinopathy, neuropathy, and nephropathy, which are related to the duration and metabolic control of diabetes [15–17]. Ketoacidosis is rare, even with consistently elevated blood glucose levels as there is residual endogenous insulin secretion [18].

Etiology

The etiology of CFRD is not fully understood and the lack of understanding of the full pathophysiology of CFRD hampers development of dietary guidelines in CFRD [19]. However, it is known that CFRD is not related to either T1D or T2D, and it cannot be prevented with current therapy. CFRD is not autoimmune (as type 1 is), neither is insulin resistance a major part of the pathophysiology of CFRD at baseline (as in type 2). Rather, CFRD is primarily caused by insulin insufficiency due to progressive scarring and fibrosis of the beta cells, reduced beta cell mass, chronic and acute inflammation secondary to recurrent sinopulmonary infections, and possibly as a direct result of the causative gene mutation [18, 20–22]. Even though CFRD is not Type 2, T2D risk genes typically increase risk of CFRD [23].

Insulin is an anabolic hormone, therefore insulin deficiency leads to unintentional loss of lean body mass, adipose tissue, and malnutrition. Body weight and lean body mass are directly correlated with pulmonary function in CF. Decline in nutritional status has been shown to occur 4 years prior to diagnosis of CFRD and has been correlated with the degree of insulin deficiency at baseline, with a corresponding decline in pulmonary function and increased morbidity and mortality [24]. The majority of patients with CF die from inflammatory lung disease and CFRD accelerates this process [24, 25].

Although insulin resistance is not a primary cause of CFRD, periods of marked insulin resistance also occur in CF resulting from stress, pregnancy, illness, and glucocorticoid (steroid) therapy for pulmonary exacerbations [1].

Treatment of CFRD with insulin has been shown to be superior to oral agents in reversing protein catabolism and chronic weight loss, improving BMI, and reversing decline in pulmonary function [26].

Diagnosis

Because clinical decline begins long before clinical symptoms of diabetes appear [24], it is recommended to regularly screen CF patients for CFRD. Studies show that early diagnosis and treatment of CFRD through aggressive screening improves overall health, nutritional status, lung function, and survival [3].

Routine Screening

The most recent guidelines recommend yearly screening with Oral Glucose Tolerance testing (OGTT) (done with the patient at baseline health) starting at 10 years of age. The recommended protocol is to obtain fasting blood glucose followed by the administration of 1.75 g/kg of oral dextrose solution and then obtaining serum glucose level 120 min after administration of the solution [6]. However, some centers use alternative or modified protocols. As previously discussed, clinical decline occurs prior to the onset of full-blown diabetes. Pre-diabetic range blood sugar levels have been associated with declines in lung function [27, 28] and more rapid progression to full-blown diabetes [29]. It has been shown that abnormal glucose tolerance (AGT) can be found in children younger than 10 and the presence of AGT predicts more rapid progression to CFRD [29]. Others have found, in small studies, that treatment of pre-diabetes can improve clinical decline [30, 31]. Therefore, some centers start screening at younger ages (i.e. 6 years of age). Other centers include additional time points (such as a 1 h or 3 h glucose value), due to relationships with lung function decline [27, 32]. Some centers may use alternative techniques, such as continuous glucose monitoring (CGM) [33, 34]. Some centers will sometimes use 1 h testing and then refer for further screening [32, 35], but this is not recommended by guidelines.

Tests That Are Not Recommended for Screening

Hemoglobin A_1c (HbA_1c) is not sensitive in CF population as patients with CF may have spuriously low A_1C values and so may not reach cut-offs for screening even when they have elevated blood glucose values [36, 37]. Fasting blood sugar is also not reliable for screening as fasting hyperglycemia is a late finding in CFRD. Therefore, neither is recommended by guidelines [6].

Diagnostic Cut-Offs for Routine OGTT Screening

CFRD is diagnosed when fasting blood sugar is 126 mg/dl or higher or the 120 min blood sugar is 200 mg/dl or higher. IGT is diagnosed when 120 min glucose is less than 200 mg/dl but is more than 140 mg/dl, and the fasting blood sugar is <126 mg/dl. If intermediate time points are used, any intermediate time point with a value of 200 mg/dl or higher, with a 120 min time point <140 mg/dl, and a fasting glucose <126 mg/dl is termed Indeterminate Glycemia (INDET) (Table 13.1).

Table 13.1 Criteria for glucose tolerance category based on OGTT results

Glucose tolerance category	Fasting glucose	Midpoint glucose	120 min glucose
CFRD	< or >126 mg/dl[a]	N/A	≥200 mg/dl
IGT	<126 mg/dl	N/A	≥140 mg/dl and <200 mg/dl
INDET	<126 mg/dl	>200 mg/dl	<140 mg/dl
Normal	<100 mg/dl	<200 mg/dl	<140 mg/dl

[a]Fasting blood sugar ≥126 meets criteria for diagnosis of diabetes as a single criteria and 120 min glucose ≥200 mg/dl meets criteria for diagnosis of diabetes as a single criteria

Screening at the Time of Pulmonary Exacerbation

In patients with CF, frequent pulmonary exacerbations requiring hospitalization for intravenous (IV) antibiotics are unfortunately a relatively common occurrence. Exacerbations are a time of significant illness and inflammation. Inflammation and illness can cause marked resistance to the actions of insulin. Due to this, it is not at all uncommon for patients with CF who otherwise have normal blood sugars at baseline health to develop abnormal blood sugars during hospitalization. Therefore, the guidelines recommend standardized screening at time of hospitalization for pulmonary exacerbation in addition to routine yearly screening for CFRD. Screening at the time of pulmonary exacerbation is recommended to be done by first a.m., pre-prandial, and 2 h post-prandial bedside glucose monitoring with all meals for the first 48 h of any admission for pulmonary exacerbation. Therefore, bedside glucose monitoring would be performed 6 times daily (before breakfast, 2 h after breakfast, before lunch, 2 h after lunch, before supper, and bedtime) for the first 48 h of admission. If the blood sugar values are normal, monitoring is discontinued at 48 h. If any of the blood glucose values reach 200 mg/dl or higher, further evaluation and continued monitoring are recommended [6].

Treatment

Nutrition Therapy for CFRD

CF patients diagnosed with CFRD should continue to follow their usual high calorie, high fat, and high sodium well-balanced diet. There are **no diet restrictions** for people with CF as the majority of patients are at risk for nutritional decline due to elevated resting energy expenditure, malabsorption due to pancreatic enzyme insufficiency, and insulin insufficiency. Sugar containing beverages are requested to be taken with meals and snacks and avoided in between meals. Usual diet advice for people with T1D and T2D does not apply in CFRD. Attainment and preservation of good nutrition status is paramount for survival in CF. Monitoring carbohydrates, whether by counting grams or exchanges/choices, is the key strategy for optimal metabolic control used in conjunction with insulin therapy. Insulin therapy should be flexible to easily fit in with the patients' usual lifestyle and eating patterns [6]. Oral high calorie supplements and/or enteral tube feedings are often necessary to meet caloric requirements. There is no need to use diabetes specific oral or enteral formulas as insulin can be titrated to cover the most appropriate formula for the patient per CF team. An extremely important part of nutrition therapy is education on carbohydrate counting as it is essential that the patient and the family knows how to determine the carbohydrate content of meals and snacks so that insulin therapy can be matched to carbohydrate intake.

Insulin Therapy

CFRD is typically treated using standard basal-bolus insulin regimens, using a combination of basal and rapid-acting insulin by multiple daily subcutaneous injections, or rapid-acting insulin via an insulin pump. Insulin pump therapy has been shown to be effective in CFRD [38]. Rapid-acting insulin doses can be based on carbohydrates consumed using an insulin-to-carbohydrate ratio. Use of additional rapid-acting insulin for correction of high blood sugars added to the mealtime insulin dose is also necessary as in intensive insulin therapy for T1D and T2D. Since patients with CFRD still have some endogenous insulin secretion, treatment with insulin is similar to patients with T1D in the honeymoon period [6]. Insulin requirements for both adult and pediatric patients have been shown to be modest throughout the lifespan of patients with CF, suggesting continued residual insulin secretion [39]. Further studies have shown that total insulin requirements for the amount of carbohydrate intake in CFRD are lower when compared to patients with TID [40]. Patients with CFRD without fasting hyperglycemia (on a standard OGTT), using premeal rapid-acting insulin only without basal insulin, reversed chronic weight loss and improved nutritional status [26].

Example Regimens

15-year-old female with fasting hyperglycemia and normal BMI, weight 62 kg.

managed with insulin pump utilizing insulin aspart with settings of :

- basal rate 0.5 units/hour.
- Insulin to carbohydrate ratios: 1 unit for every 10 g of carbohydrate with breakfast, 1 unit for every 25 g with **all** snacks, and 1 unit for every 20 g with lunch and supper.
- Sensitivity set at 1 unit to drop her blood sugar by 60 mg/dl.

25-year-old male without fasting hyperglycemia and normal BMI, weight 75 kg

- insulin lispro 1 unit for every 30 g with **all** meals and snacks,
- correction dose of 0.5 units for every 50 mg/dl his blood sugar is over 150 mg/dl,
- no long-acting insulin

40-year-old female with fasting hyperglycemia, long history of CFRD, weight 50 kg

- insulin glargine 20 units daily
- insulin lispro 1 unit for every 15 g of carbohydrate with **all** meals and **all** snacks
- insulin lispro correction dose of 1 unit for every 50 mg/dl her blood sugar is over 150

All insulin should be administered **prior** to meals and snacks. All patients on insulin should check blood sugars before every meal, 2 h after each meal and at bedtime. Overnight checks should be done when long-acting insulin is added or adjusted. Post-prandial blood glucose monitoring (done 2 h after meals) is very important as those can be the only abnormal values in some patients.

These regimens above illustrate different sorts of insulin regimens that may be used. All of them require accurate carbohydrate counting on the part of the patient and the family. All regimens will need to be adjusted based on patient activity and disease status as illness and growth spurts will increase insulin requirements and exercise will decrease them. The expectation is that these regimens will be flexible and that ongoing adjustment will be required.

Insulin Therapy for Enteral Feeds

Patients with CFRD typically have nutritional decline prior to the diagnosis of diabetes [9, 41]. In the Leeds Adult CF Unit, however, this was not the case, but in their population, the proportion of patients receiving enteral tube feeding increased steadily and by 1 year prior to diagnosis of CFRD, and significantly more subjects who would develop diabetes in the future were on tube feeds compared to those who did not develop diabetes (44% of those who would develop CFRD, compared to 19% of controls). In their cohort, the diagnosis of CFRD was 4 times as likely in patients who were prescribed overnight enteral feeding. Those who subsequently developed diabetes also had increased rate of decline in the forced expiratory volume in 1 second (FEV_1) which stabilized when they were started on insulin. In children, those with CFRD had decreased weight gain compared to those without, beginning 2 years prior to diagnosis, which then normalized when they were started on insulin [8]. This study has raised concern that enteral feeds may increase the risk for CFRD. However, this study could also be interpreted to show that the usual decline in nutritional status from the pre-diabetic state can be offset with aggressive enteral nutrition support, but this does not avoid the decline in FEV_1 associated with the pre-diabetic state.

In either case, enteral support should not be held due to concerns regarding diabetes or avoided in patients with CFRD. Rather, enteral support should be started when clinically indicated and an appropriate insulin regimen to cover the enteral feed should be designed. Also, special "diabetic" formulas or supplements should not be used, rather formulas and supplements should be chosen based on those most appropriate for patients with CF and the particular clinical situation.

Insulin regimens for overnight enteral feeds are relatively simple and very effective in reversing weight loss. In some patients, insulin with overnight enteral feeds only (and not daytime carbohydrate intake) may be adequate to reverse weight loss. In our practice, for an overnight continuous feed of 8 h, we recommend determining the total carbohydrate administered by the complete feed. This is then covered by a combination of neutral protamine hagadorn (NPH) insulin and regular insulin given in a mixed dose at the beginning of the feed. Typically this can be dosed based on the patient's known carbohydrate ratio and given as 70% NPH and 30% regular insulin. This is given **in addition** to whatever insulin (including basal) the patient is already on. Blood sugar is monitored just prior to initiation of feed, and the mid-point of feed and when the feed is discontinued. Blood sugar goals on continuous feeds are non-fasting so should be in the 140–180 mg/dl range. Daytime bolus feeds are covered as if they were a meal. The carbohydrate content is ascertained, and the patient's insulin to carbohydrate ratio is used the same way as a typical meal would be covered.

For different durations of enteral feeds, insulin formulations with different durations of action can be used. Please see Table 13.2.

Table 13.2 Insulin action

Insulin	Onset of action[a]	Duration of action[a]	Peak
Rapid acting			
Aspart	10–20 min	3–5 h	1–2 h
Lispro	10–20 min	3–5 h	1–2 h
Glulisine	10–20 min	3–5 h	1–2 h
Short acting			
Regular	30 min	4–6 (up to 8) h	2–4 h
Intermediate acting			
NPH[b]	1–3 h	8–12 h	4–6 h
Long acting			
Glargine[c]	1–2 h	18–26 h	None
Detemir[c]	1–3 h	12–20 h	None (8 h)

[a]All times vary depending on dose given, location of dose, physical activity of the individual in question and insulin resistance. Insulin kinetics above are in subjects with type 1 diabetes, not subjects with CF
[b]*NPH* neutral protamine hagadorn
[c]Glargine and Detemir insulins cannot be mixed with other insulins

Example Regimens

– Overnight enteral feeds are initiated on an 18-year-old female with CFRD without fasting hyperglycemia. She is well controlled on meal boluses of insulin lispro of 1 unit for every 15 g of carbohydrate. Her 8- hour overnight continuous feed contains a total of 150 g of carbohydrate. Therefore her insulin dose for the feed is 10 units of insulin, given as a dose of 7 units of NPH mixed with 3 units of regular.
– Three daytime bolus feeds are added to the nutrition regimen of a 25-year-old male with CFRD without fasting hyperglycemia who is already on overnight feeds. The patient's carbohydrate ratio is 1 unit insulin aspart for every 10 g of carbohydrate. Each bolus feed contains 50 g of carbohydrate. Prior to each bolus, the patient is administered 5 units of insulin aspart. This is in addition to the patient's coverage of all meals and snacks with 1 unit of insulin aspart for every 10 g of carbohydrate and 10.5 units of NPH and 4.5 units of regular insulin mixed and administered prior to the 150 g 8 h continuous overnight feed.

Insulin Therapy in Illness

Patients with CFRD have many more hospitalizations for pulmonary exacerbations than CF patients without CFRD, and at much younger ages [42].

During acute illness and/or treatment with glucocorticoids, insulin requirements increase dramatically, typically two- to fourfold. Once the illness resolves, it takes about 4–6 weeks for insulin requirements to return to baseline. Close monitoring for hypoglycemia is imperative during this period and regular communication with the health care team is necessary [6].

In our practice, for patients who are eating normally, we recommend monitoring the typical 6 times daily and increasing insulin doses until normoglycemia is achieved. This may require very large doses. If the patients are ill enough that they cannot tolerate a normal diet, we recommend to monitor blood glucose every 4 h, 24 h a day. High fluid intake is encouraged. If they cannot take solid foods, the patient should take both carbohydrate-containing and carbohydrate-free fluids.

Insulin Therapy and Steroid Use

Glucocorticoid therapy causes marked insulin resistance and has been known to cause diabetes in non-CF populations. In the CF population, it can cause diabetic-range blood sugars in patients without previous diagnosis of CFRD, or markedly increased insulin needs in patients with established CFRD. It also may increase hunger and therefore increase carbohydrate intake as well.

Short-term administration of methylprednisolone causes postprandial hyperglycemia that lasts 6–12 h. Therefore, some authors have recommended the administration of NPH insulin at the time of methylprednisolone dose [42]. Rasouli et al. advocate for a dose of 0.25 units of NPH per 1 mg of methylprednisolone. If the patient has steroid-induced diabetes without pre-existing CFRD, they recommend 0.1–0.15 units of NPH per 1 mg of methylprednisolone.

For prednisone therapy, there is usually overall increase in insulin resistance, requiring increased insulin doses. The effect usually lags by about 24 h, with increased blood sugars present for 24–48 h after prednisone is discontinued. Patients on prednisone therapy usually require marked increases in insulin dosing (2–4 times base doses). Some CF patients without pre-existing CFRD may require initiation of insulin with prednisone burst therapy. Meal coverage is usually the most important, which requires teaching of carbohydrate counting.

Insulin Therapy and TPN

If TPN is needed, insulin can be given in multiple ways. First, Regular (human) insulin can be added to the bag. This is typically dosed to cover the carbohydrate content of the TPN. This is ideal as if the TPN is held or the rate is decreased, the insulin is automatically held or decreased in proportion to the amount of carbohydrate the patient receives. However, in some institutions, this is not allowed. Therefore, a subcutaneous insulin of appropriate duration can be given, dosed to cover the amount of carbohydrates in the TPN. However, if this is done, great care must be taken to replace the carbohydrates if TPN must be held or discontinued.

Example Regimen

TPN containing 95 g of carbohydrate is run as a continuous infusion over 24 h. The patient's carbohydrate ratio is 1:20. 4.5 units of regular insulin could be added to the bag, or conversely, 4.5 units of insulin glargine could be given subcutaneously when the TPN is hung. However, if the latter option is taken, if the TPN has to be discontinued, the patient must be provided with an alternate carbohydrate source until the glargine has worn off at 24 h after administration.

For types of insulin with different durations of action, please refer to Table 13.2.

Nutrition Recommendations for Pregnancy with CFRD and GDM in Women with CF

Pregnancy in CF is challenging and diabetes increases the complexity of care. Good outcomes depend on adequate pre-pregnancy nutritional status, and adequate nutrition during pregnancy. As in T1D and T2D, preconception counseling and normalization of blood glucose are necessary in women with pre-existing CFRD. In non-CF diabetic pregnancy, very small glycemic excursions can have negative impact on both the mother and the infant and therefore guidelines for management of diabetes in pregnancy are much more aggressive and request blood sugars much closer to the normal non-diabetic range than management of non-pregnant diabetics [43]. In CF, pre-existing CFRD is associated with worsened outcomes for the mother and the baby. However, there is very little published literature to support specific recommendations for the management of CFRD during pregnancy [44]. Women with CF are at higher risk for GDM because of underlying insulin deficiency, and should be screened more aggressively when planning a pregnancy. Screening is recommended as follows: women not having an OGTT within 6 months of pregnancy are to be screened as soon as possible and then re-screened during weeks 12–16 and 24–28, and if they develop GDM to be re-screened 6–12 weeks after delivery, and insulin treatment recommended [6]. All pregnant women with CF and diabetes require increased energy intake and require close monitoring of weight gain and nutritional status [44]. Standard prenatal weight gain charts can be used to determine weight gain goals. Additional calorie needs will vary based on pre-pregnancy weight, degree of pancreatic malabsorption, pulmonary status, and presence of infections. Oral supplements may be necessary to promote adequate weight gain. Suboptimal weight gain during pregnancy is a concern; therefore, current practice does not encourage the restriction of calories or carbohydrate during pregnancy. However, empty calories should be replaced with nutrient-dense foods. Aggressive initiation of insulin should be implemented rather than diet restriction. In pregnant women with CFRD or CF with GDM requiring insulin therapy, insulin should be matched to carbohydrate intake to optimize blood glucose control without restricting carbohydrate intake [6]. Insulin pump therapy is often optimal if it can be obtained, given the level of complexity of management of diabetes in pregnancy in a woman with CF. Management should be coordinated with high-risk obstetrics.

Hypoglycemia

Management of Hypoglycemia

The risk of hypoglycemia in CFRD is the same as in people with T1D and T2D requiring insulin. Since people with CFRD require pancreatic enzyme replacement therapy (PERT) with mixed nutrient foods, low blood glucose should be treated with fat-free and protein free carbohydrate sources that do not require pancreatic enzyme replacement. Absorption of fat-free carbohydrates is not compromised as patients with CF are able to secrete amylase in their saliva.

Treatment Example

Fifteen grams of rapid-acting carbohydrate should be administered and then blood sugar rechecked in 15 min. This cycle should be repeated until blood sugar is over 100 mg/dl. Examples of appropriate rapid-acting carbohydrate include: 4 oz apple juice, glucose tablets, glucose gel. If necessary, hard candies and regular soft drinks can be used, but the amount should be limited to 15 g of carbohydrate.

Reactive Hypoglycemia

Patients with CF sometimes have reactive hypoglycemia, low blood sugars happening after a meal, typically 2–3 h post-prandial. This has been clinically documented and can also be seen on 3 h OGTT [45]. This is usually considered to be secondary to the abnormal insulin secretion that is found in patients with CF, prior to progression to diabetes, although the literature has not shown a direct connection between documented hypoglycemia and progression of glucose abnormalities [46, 47]. Unfortunately, there are no guidelines or published literature to recommend treatment or screening for this condition. In our practice, we typically recommend avoidance of large carbohydrate loads with high glycemic index, especially regular soft drinks or juice, especially if taken in the absence of protein or fat.

IGT/Pre-diabetes

Nutrition Recommendations for Impaired Glucose Tolerance

Unlike the general population, IGT in CF is not due to excessive weight gain and insulin resistance, but rather underlying beta cell failure and insulin deficiency and therefore is not preventable. Due to this, nutrition guidelines for IGT in the general population are not applicable for people with CF. Weight loss is rarely recommended for people with CF. Exercise in people with CF is beneficial for overall health, and people with CF in their baseline state of health are insulin-sensitive, but exercise will not help to slow the progression towards CFRD due to progressive insulin deficiency. Most people with CF, including those with severe pulmonary disease, are capable of engaging in strength and aerobic exercise and are advised to do moderate aerobic exercise for at least 150 min per week. Spreading carbohydrates throughout the day and replacing empty calorie-carbohydrates with nutrient-dense carbohydrates are recommended. Maintenance of a healthy weight and nutritional status must be monitored closely [6].

Insulin Therapy for Impaired Glucose Tolerance/Pre-diabetes

Some authors use low-dose insulin therapy in CF patients with IGT [30] or other forms of abnormal glycemic tolerance [31, 48]. However, this is not generally recommended at this time, although it may be in the future.

Disordered Eating

Many different chronic illnesses can be associated with disordered eating, due to focus on body image caused by the illness. Chronic illnesses that require dietary management are at increased risk of causing the development of abnormal relationships with food and weight and disordered eating habits [49]. Diabetes is documented to lead to eating disorder in adolescents [50]. There are few studies of eating disorders in cystic fibrosis, but disordered eating has been documented, and some studies argue there is a higher rate than in the general population [49]. There is no literature specific to disordered eating in the context of CFRD, but it seems not irrational to speculate that the combination of both diabetes and CF may increase this risk, and it behooves the care team to be aware of and monitoring for this possibility as undetected eating disorders can derail appropriate nutrition.

Summary of Nutrition Recommendations for CFRD

See Table 13.3.

Table 13.3 Nutrition recommendations for cystic fibrosis related diabetes

Nutrient	Cystic fibrosis related diabetes
Calories	1.2–1.5 times Dietary Reference Intake (DRI) for age; individualized based on weight gain and growth. High calorie oral supplements and enteral tube feedings often necessary. Not necessary to use diabetes specific formulas
Carbohydrate	Individualized. Carbohydrates should be monitored to achieve glycemic control. Use of artificial sweeteners should be used sparingly due to lower calorie content
Fat	No restriction on type of fat. High fat necessary for weight maintenance; aim for 35–40% total calories
Protein	Approximately 1.5–2.0 times the DRI for age, no reduction for nephropathy
Sodium	Liberal, high salt diet, especially in warm conditions and/or when exercising
Vitamins, minerals	Routine supplementation with CF-specific multivitamins or a multivitamin and additional fat-soluble vitamins A, D, E, and K
Alcohol	Consult with physician due to the higher prevalence of liver disease in CF and possible use of hepatotoxic drugs
Impaired glucose tolerance	Weight loss not recommended, spread carbohydrates throughout day. Restrict sugar sweetened and other empty calorie beverages. Exercise per usual CF recommendations. Monitor nutritional status
CFRD in pregnancy and gestational diabetes mellitus	No calorie or carbohydrate restriction except sugar sweetened and other empty calorie beverages. A high calorie diet must be maintained for adequate weight gain. Aggressive use of insulin rather than diet restriction

Adapted from Moran et al. [6]

Medical and Nutrition Therapy Goals (Adapted from Moran et al. [6])

Medical Goals

- Patients with CFRD should ideally be seen quarterly by a specialized multidisciplinary team with expertise in diabetes and CF
- Patients with CFRD should receive ongoing diabetes self-management education from diabetes education programs that meet national standards for Diabetes Self-Management Education
- Patients with CFRD should be treated with insulin
- Oral diabetes agents are not as effective as insulin in improving nutritional and metabolic outcomes in CFRD and are not recommended outside the context of clinical research trials
- Patients with CFRD who are on insulin should monitor blood glucose at least 3 times a day
- Blood glucose goals for patients with CFRD are consistent with glucose goals per the American Diabetes Association (ADA) recommendations for all people with diabetes. Higher or lower goals may be indicated for some patients and that individualization is important
- A_1C measurement is recommended quarterly for patients with CFRD
- A_1C treatment goal is <7%. Higher or lower goals may be indicated for some patients and that individualization is important
- Diabetes education about the symptoms, prevention, and treatment of hypoglycemia, including the use of glucagon, is recommended for patients with CFRD and their care partners
- Blood pressure should be measured at every routine diabetes visit per ADA guidelines. Systolic blood pressure ≥130 mmHg or diastolic blood pressure ≥80 mmHg or >90th percentile for age and sex for pediatric patients should have repeat measurement on a separate day to confirm a diagnosis of hypertension
- Annual monitoring for microvascular complications of diabetes is recommended using ADA guidelines, beginning 5 years after the diagnosis of CFRD or, if the exact time of diagnosis is not known, at the time that fasting hyperglycemia is first diagnosed
- Patients with CFRD who have hypertension or microvascular complications should receive treatment as recommended by ADA for all people with diabetes, except that there is no restriction of sodium and, in general, no protein restriction
- An annual lipid profile is recommended for patients with CFRD and pancreatic exocrine sufficiency or if any of the following risk factors are present: obesity, family history of coronary artery disease, or immunosuppressive therapy following transplantation
- Patients are advised to do moderate aerobic exercise for at least 150 min per week.

Conclusion

Medical nutrition therapy is a critical aspect of the management of all forms of diabetes. It is especially critical in CFRD as nutritional status is key to the health and survival of every patient with CF. Also, CFRD is extremely common in the CF population and there is a very real chance that any given patient with CF may have diabetes at some point in his or her lifetime. Moreover, the development of CFRD leads to decreased nutritional status, decreased lung function, and increased mortality. Therefore, the nutritional management of CFRD is relevant to nearly every CF patient.

Once diabetes is diagnosed, it must be treated, and insulin therapy has been shown to reverse nutritional decline and lung function decline. Therefore, insulin is the only appropriate medication for CFRD. Other anti-diabetic medications are not indicated. Nutritional education, however, is key. Nutritional therapy of CFRD has several important differences from T1D and from T2D, primarily due to the significant nutrition needs for treatment of CF, but also due to the unique pathophysiology of CFRD. Importantly, there is no indication for restriction of carbohydrate or caloric intake and, rather, CF-specific guidelines for macronutrient composition should be followed. Appropriate enteral feeds and supplements should not be held due to CFRD, and "diabetic" formulas are not indicated. Rather, appropriate supplements and formulas indicated for CF care should be appropriately utilized. CF patients are insulin sensitive at baseline, but may develop significant insulin resistance with illness or steroid use, such that these events may cause need for insulin therapy in a patient who has not previously needed insulin. Insulin regimens should be flexible and can be designed to successfully treat patients in a variety of situations including supplemental/enteral feeds, TPN use, steroid therapy, and pregnancy.

Pre-diabetic states are very common in CF, but they cannot be prevented through carbohydrate restriction, rather, nutritional failure is often an indication that the pre-diabetic state is present and increased nutrition may be required in the peri-diabetic time period. There is no role for caloric or carbohydrate restriction in these states as; unlike in pre-diabetes related to T2D, it does not prevent progression to CFRD. Low-dose insulin therapy may be useful in these situations, but more data is needed at this point.

Despite the complexities of management of CF patients with CFRD, appropriate nutritional and insulin therapy can reverse the nutritional and clinical decline associated with CFRD and improve long-term outcomes for affected patients.

References

1. Moran A, Doherty L, Wang X, Thomas W. Abnormal glucose metabolism in cystic fibrosis. J Pediatr. 1998;133:10–7.
2. Frohnert BI, Ode KL, Moran A, Nathan BM, Laguna T, Holme B, Thomas W. Impaired fasting glucose in cystic fibrosis. Diabetes Care. 2010;33:2660–4.
3. Moran A, Dunitz J, Nathan B, Saeed A, Holme B, Thomas W. Cystic fibrosis-related diabetes: current trends in prevalence, incidence, and mortality. Diabetes Care. 2009;32:1626–31.
4. Stallings VA, Stark LJ, Robinson KA, Feranchak AP, Quinton H. Evidence-based practice recommendations for nutrition-related management of children and adults with cystic fibrosis and pancreatic insufficiency: results of a systematic review. J Am Diet Assoc. 2008;108:832–9.
5. Cystic Fibrosis Foundation (CFF). Patient Registry. 2012 Annual Data Report. Bethesda, MD; 2012.
6. Moran A, Brunzell C, Cohen RC, Katz M, Marshall BC, Onady G, Robinson KA, Sabadosa KA, Stecenko A, Slovis B. Clinical care guidelines for cystic fibrosis-related diabetes: a position statement of the American Diabetes Association and a clinical practice guideline of the Cystic Fibrosis Foundation, endorsed by the Pediatric Endocrine Society. Diabetes Care. 2010;33:2697–708.
7. Borowitz D, Baker RD, Stallings V, et al. Consensus report on nutrition for pediatric patients with cystic fibrosis. J Pediatr Gastroenterol Nutr. 2002;35:246–59.
8. White H, Pollard K, Etherington C, Clifton I, Morton AM, Owen D, Conway SP, Peckham DG. Nutritional decline in cystic fibrosis related diabetes: the effect of intensive nutritional intervention. J Cyst Fibros. 2009;8:179–85.
9. Lanng S, Thorsteinsson B, Nerup J, Koch C. Influence of the development of diabetes mellitus on clinical status in patients with cystic fibrosis. Eur J Pediatr. 1992;151:684–7.
10. Lanng S, Thorsteinsson B, Nerup J, Koch C. Diabetes mellitus in cystic fibrosis: effect of insulin therapy on lung function and infections. Acta Paediatr. 1994;83:849–53.
11. Gougeon R, Pencharz PB, Marliss EB. Effect of NIDDM on the kinetics of whole-body protein metabolism. Diabetes. 1994;43:318–28.
12. Figueroa V, Milla C, Parks EJ, Schwarzenberg SJ, Moran A. Abnormal lipid concentrations in cystic fibrosis. Am J Clin Nutr. 2002;75:1005–11.
13. Rhodes B, Nash EF, Tullis E, Pencharz PB, Brotherwood M, Dupuis A, Stephenson A. Prevalence of dyslipidemia in adults with cystic fibrosis. J Cyst Fibros. 2010;9:24–8.
14. Stephenson AL, Mannik LA, Walsh S, Brotherwood M, Robert R, Darling PB, Nisenbaum R, Moerman J, Stanojevic S. Longitudinal trends in nutritional status and the relation between lung function and BMI in cystic fibrosis: a population-based cohort study. Am J Clin Nutr. 2013;97:872–7.

15. Schwarzenberg SJ, Thomas W, Olsen TW, Grover T, Walk D, Milla C, Moran A. Microvascular complications in cystic fibrosis-related diabetes. Diabetes Care. 2007;30:1056–61.
16. Andersen HU, Lanng S, Pressler T, Laugesen CS, Mathiesen ER. Cystic fibrosis-related diabetes: the presence of microvascular diabetes complications. Diabetes Care. 2006;29:2660–3.
17. Van den Berg JMW, Morton AM, Kok SW, Pijl H, Conway SP, Heijerman HGM. Microvascular complications in patients with cystic fibrosis-related diabetes (CFRD). J Cyst Fibros. 2008;7:515–9.
18. Moran A, Diem P, Klein DJ, Levitt MD, Robertson RP. Pancreatic endocrine function in cystic fibrosis. J Pediatr. 1991;118:715–23.
19. Wilson DC, Kalnins D, Stewart C, Hamilton N, Hanna AK, Durie PR, Tullis E, Pencharz PB. Challenges in the dietary treatment of cystic fibrosis related diabetes mellitus. Clin Nutr. 2000;19:87–93.
20. Orenstein D. Cystic fibrosis. In: Rudolph A, Hostetter M, Lister G, Siegel N, editors. Rudolph's pediatrics. New York: McGraw Hill; 2002. p. 1969–80.
21. Gaskin K. Exocrine pancreatic function. In: Walker W, Goulet O, Kleinman R, Sherman P, Schneider B, Sanderson I, editors. Pediatric gastrointestinal disease. Hamilton: B.C. Decker; 2004. p. 1607–23.
22. Tofé S, Moreno JC, Máiz L, Alonso M, Escobar H, Barrio R. Insulin-secretion abnormalities and clinical deterioration related to impaired glucose tolerance in cystic fibrosis. Eur J Endocrinol. 2005;152:241–7.
23. Blackman SM, Hsu S, Vanscoy LL, Collaco JM, Ritter SE, Naughton K, Cutting GR. Genetic modifiers play a substantial role in diabetes complicating cystic fibrosis. J Clin Endocrinol Metab. 2009;94:1302–9.
24. Milla CE, Warwick WJ, Moran A. Trends in pulmonary function in patients with cystic fibrosis correlate with the degree of glucose intolerance at baseline. Am J Respir Crit Care Med. 2000;162:891–5.
25. Rosenecker J, Höfler R, Steinkamp G, Eichler I, Smaczny C, Ballmann M, Posselt HG, Bargon J, von der Hardt H. Diabetes mellitus in patients with cystic fibrosis: the impact of diabetes mellitus on pulmonary function and clinical outcome. Eur J Med Res. 2001;6:345–50.
26. Moran A, Pekow P, Grover P, Zorn M, Slovis B, Pilewski J, Tullis E, Liou TG, Allen H. Insulin therapy to improve BMI in cystic fibrosis-related diabetes without fasting hyperglycemia: results of the cystic fibrosis related diabetes therapy trial. Diabetes Care. 2009;32:1783–8.
27. Brodsky J, Dougherty S, Makani R, Rubenstein RC, Kelly A. Elevation of 1-hour plasma glucose during oral glucose tolerance testing is associated with worse pulmonary function in cystic fibrosis. Diabetes Care. 2011;34:292–5.
28. Hameed S, Morton JR, Jaffé A, Field PI, Belessis Y, Yoong T, Katz T, Verge CF. Early glucose abnormalities in cystic fibrosis are preceded by poor weight gain. Diabetes Care. 2010;33:221–6.
29. Ode KL, Frohnert B, Laguna T, Phillips J, Holme B, Regelmann W, Thomas W, Moran A. Oral glucose tolerance testing in children with cystic fibrosis. Pediatr Diabetes. 2010;11:487–92.
30. Bizzarri C, Lucidi V, Ciampalini P, Bella S, Russo B, Cappa M. Clinical effects of early treatment with insulin glargine in patients with cystic fibrosis and impaired glucose tolerance. J Endocrinol Invest. 2006;29:RC1–4.
31. Dobson L, Hattersley AT, Tiley S, Elworthy S, Oades PJ, Sheldon CD. Clinical improvement in cystic fibrosis with early insulin treatment. Arch Dis Child. 2002;87:430–1.
32. Waugh N, Royle P, Craigie I, Ho V, Pandit L, Ewings P, Adler A, Helms P, Sheldon C. Screening for cystic fibrosis-related diabetes: a systematic review. Health Technol Assess. 2012;16. iii–iv, 1–179.
33. Jefferies C, Solomon M, Perlman K, Sweezey N, Daneman D. Continuous glucose monitoring in adolescents with cystic fibrosis. J Pediatr. 2005;147:396–8.
34. Khammar A, Stremler N, Dubus J-C, Gross G, Sarles J, Reynaud R. Value of continuous glucose monitoring in screening for diabetes in cystic fibrosis. Arch Pediatr. 2009;16:1540–6.
35. Franco WB, Brown RF, Bremer AA. Use of "glucola alternatives" for cystic fibrosis-related diabetes screening. J Cyst Fibros. 2011;10:384–5.
36. Holl RW, Buck C, Babka C, Wolf A, Thon A. HbA1c is not recommended as a screening test for diabetes in cystic fibrosis. Diabetes Care. 2000;23:126.
37. Godbout A, Hammana I, Potvin S, Mainville D, Rakel A, Berthiaume Y, Chiasson J-L, Coderre L, Rabasa-Lhoret R. No relationship between mean plasma glucose and glycated haemoglobin in patients with cystic fibrosis-related diabetes. Diabetes Metab. 2008;34:568–73.
38. Hardin DS, Rice J, Rice M, Rosenblatt R. Use of the insulin pump in treat cystic fibrosis related diabetes. J Cyst Fibros. 2009;8:174–8.
39. Sunni M, Bellin MD, Moran A. Exogenous insulin requirements do not differ between youth and adults with cystic fibrosis related diabetes. Pediatr Diabetes. 2013;14:295–8.
40. Scheuing N, Thon A, Konrad K, et al. Carbohydrate intake and insulin requirement in children, adolescents and young adults with cystic fibrosis-related diabetes: a multicenter comparison to type 1 diabetes. Clin Nutr. 2015;34:732–8.
41. Marshall BC, Butler SM, Stoddard M, Moran AM, Liou TG, Morgan WJ. Epidemiology of cystic fibrosis-related diabetes. J Pediatr. 2005;146:681–7.

42. Rasouli N, Seggelke S, Gibbs J, et al. Cystic fibrosis-related diabetes in adults: inpatient management of 121 patients during 410 admissions. J Diabetes Sci Technol. 2012;6:1038–44.
43. Metzger BE, Lowe LP, Dyer AR, et al. Hyperglycemia and adverse pregnancy outcomes. N Engl J Med. 2008;358:1991–2002.
44. Michel SH, Mueller DH. Nutrition for pregnant women who have cystic fibrosis. J Acad Nutr Diet. 2012;112:1943–8.
45. Hirsch IB, Janci MM, Goss CH, Aitken ML. Hypoglycemia in adults with cystic fibrosis during oral glucose tolerance testing. Diabetes Care. 2013;36:e121–2.
46. Radike K, Molz K, Holl RW, Poeter B, Hebestreit H, Ballmann M. Prognostic relevance of hypoglycemia following an oral glucose challenge for cystic fibrosis-related diabetes. Diabetes Care. 2011;34, e43.
47. Battezzati A, Battezzati PM, Costantini D, Seia M, Zazzeron L, Russo MC, Daccò V, Bertoli S, Crosignani A, Colombo C. Spontaneous hypoglycemia in patients with cystic fibrosis. Eur J Endocrinol. 2007;156:369–76.
48. Hameed S, Morton JR, Field PI, et al. Once daily insulin detemir in cystic fibrosis with insulin deficiency. Arch Dis Child. 2012;97:464–7.
49. Quick VM, Byrd-Bredbenner C, Neumark-Sztainer D. Chronic illness and disordered eating: a discussion of the literature. Adv Nutr. 2013;4:277–86.
50. Powers MA, Richter S, Ackard D, Gerken S, Meier M, Criego A. Characteristics of persons with an eating disorder and type 1 diabetes and psychological comparisons with persons with an eating disorder and no diabetes. Int J Eat Disord. 2012;45:252–6.

Chapter 14
Nutrition Pre and Post Lung Transplant

Teresa Schindler

Key Points

- Malnutrition is common in CF patients prior to transplant
- Patients with a BMI <18.5, depletion of fat free mass, or hypoalbuminemia, may have worse outcomes post-transplant
- While nutritional status generally improves after transplant, CF patients face many complications which have nutritional implications

Keywords Cystic fibrosis • Lung transplantation • Nutrition

Introduction

While the life expectancy for individuals with cystic fibrosis (CF) continues to improve, respiratory failure continues to be the main cause of mortality for those afflicted with the disease. Lung transplantation offers those with end-stage lung disease a survival advantage and improved quality of life compared to those who do not receive a transplant. Optimizing nutritional status prior to transplantation can improve post-transplant outcomes, however this can be quite challenging to accomplish.

Despite noted improvements in nutritional status for CF patients after lung transplantation, they face multiple unique nutritional considerations.

Overview of Lung Transplantation in CF

According to the CF Foundation Registry, over 200 lung transplants were performed in individuals with CF in 2011, and about 2800 people with CF have received a lung transplant since 1990 [1]. Cystic fibrosis is the third major indication for lung transplantation, after emphysema and pulmonary fibrosis [2].

T. Schindler, M.S., R.D.N. (✉)
Pediatric Pulmonology, Rainbow Babies and Children's Hospital Case Medical Center,
11100 Euclid Ave, Cleveland, OH 44106, USA
e-mail: Terri.schindler@uhhospitals.org

E.H. Yen, A.R. Leonard (eds.), *Nutrition in Cystic Fibrosis: A Guide for Clinicians*, Nutrition and Health, 207
DOI 10.1007/978-3-319-16387-1_14, © Springer International Publishing Switzerland 2015

Table 14.1 lists the indications for lung transplantation for cystic fibrosis. Absolute contraindications to lung transplantation are listed in Table 14.2. The vast majority of those transplanted receive a bilateral double lung transplant; a small minority (<5%) require liver and lung transplantation [3].

Survival rates for lung transplant recipients regardless of indication are lower compared to most other solid organ transplants. Compared to other solid organ transplants, lung transplant recipients experience higher rates of re-hospitalizations as well: 43.7% in the first year and 36% in the second year [3]. Compared to individuals receiving lung transplants for other indications, median accrual survival is slightly better in individuals with CF: 7.5 years for all recipients, and 10.4 years for those who survive the first year [2].

In 2005, the Lung Allocation Score (LAS) was implemented to improve the outcomes of those who are listed for transplant as well as those who receive a transplant. The LAS calculation (see Table 14.3) is a score that reflects risk of wait-list mortality while avoiding transplants in those who have a very poor likelihood of survival [3].

Expected wait time in the US varies according to age, blood type, height, geography, and LAS (for those age 12 years and older) [2, 3]. Approximately 65% of candidates are transplanted within a year of listing. However, the wait can vary greatly depending on the area of the country in which the person is listed [3].

Although wait-list mortality has decreased significantly since implementation of the LAS, it is important to optimize and stabilize nutritional status prior to transplant. The median body mass index (BMI) prior to transplant is 19.2 kg/m^2, with 39% of those who had a BMI below 18.5 kg/m^2 [4].

Table 14.1 Indications for lung transplant referral [4, 5]

1.	FEV$_1$ < 30% predicted and/or rapid decline in FEV$_1$
2.	Recurrent, massive hemoptysis
3.	Relapsing or complicated pneumothorax
4.	Respiratory infections necessitating an ICU admission
5.	Malnutrition, diabetes, female gender, oxygen requirement, and poor quality of life/functional incapacity and/or an increasing need for intravenous antibiotic therapy may also be important indications for early referral

Table 14.2 Absolute contraindications to lung transplantation (some factors may vary depending on location) [4, 6]

- Malignant disease in the past 2 years
- Lack of medical insurance
- Untreatable severe dysfunction of another important organ system (heart, liver, kidney) not amenable to surgical correction/combined transplant
- Chronic, incurable extrapulmonary infection
- Severe deformations of chest and spine
- Severe or symptomatic osteoporosis
- Lack of adherence to therapies
- Untreated mental disorders combined with lack of cooperation
- Addictive disorder currently or during the past 6 months (including tobacco, alcohol, substance abuse)
- Lack of social support system

Table 14.3 Factors used in Lung Allocation Score (LAS)

• Age
• BMI
• Presence/absence of diabetes
• Functional status
• FVC
• O2 requirement
• 6 min walk distance
• Mechanical ventilation
• PCO2
• Diagnosis

Impact of Nutritional Status on Transplant Outcomes

Malnutrition is a common condition for individuals with CF with end-stage lung disease. The cause of malnutrition is multi-factorial. Factors leading to malnutrition in end-stage lung disease include elevated resting energy expenditure (REE), poor appetite, and frequent pulmonary exacerbations. For example, mean REE was 132% predicted in pediatric patients awaiting lung transplantation (majority with CF) [7]. In addition, frequent episodes of increased respiratory symptoms can cause poor appetite and intake, and delayed gastric emptying is a common complication of end-stage disease in CF [8].

Extremes of body weight have been shown to negatively affect lung transplant outcomes. Specifically, adult CF patients with a BMI <18.5 kg/m^2 have a significantly higher risk of post-transplant mortality than adult CF patients with a normal or higher BMI [9, 10]. Other markers of nutritional status have been used to determine post-transplant outcomes, including Fat Free Mass (FFM) and serum albumin. Depletion of FFM was strongly associated with increased mortality while awaiting lung transplant and longer post-transplant intensive care unit stays [11]. A retrospective study in 2014 by Hollander et al. confirmed previous studies in which a low BMI ($\leq$18.5 kg/m^2) and low FFM index appear to impair survival in lung transplant candidates with CF [4]. Hypoalbuminemia (serum albumin <3 mg/dl) was associated with an increased risk of early mortality in post-transplant patients [12].

Despite evidence that supports optimal nutritional status prior to transplant, malnutrition may not be an absolute contraindication to transplantation, depending on the transplant center. Reversing malnutrition can be a difficult endeavor, and aggressive nutrition support is not without risks. In fact, Belkin et al. found that use of a nutritional intervention was associated with increased risk of death in patients with CF awaiting lung transplantation [13]. See Table 14.4 for enteral nutrition support considerations in pre-transplant patients.

There have been mixed reports regarding the effectiveness of dietary interventions in the pre-transplant period. Despite dietetic interventions including oral supplements, tube feedings or both, Hollander and colleagues did not see an improvement in BMI and FFM in the pre-transplant time period [4].

Nutrition Support in the Pre-Transplant Period

Ambulatory patients should continue a high calorie, high fat diet and be encouraged to consume regular meals and snacks to meet high energy demands. Small, frequent meals may be better tolerated, especially during a pulmonary exacerbation and if delayed gastric emptying is present. Reviewing methods to boost calories in foods and beverages can be helpful, as well as providing lists of high

Table 14.4 Post-gastrostomy tube placement and nutrition support considerations and recommendations in pre and post-transplant patients

1. Adequate pain control, particularly to ensure proper airway clearance
2. Monitor stool elimination pattern; consider laxative prophylaxis, particularly if narcotics are used for pain control
3. Provide alternative methods for airway clearance (vest therapy and chest physiotherapy are often not tolerated in the immediate post-placement period)
4. Monitor for hyperglycemia (glucose checks half way through feedings and at end of feedings once up to full rate)
5. Intact formula trial [25, 26]
6. Reflux precautions unless patient has fundoplication
7. Soft diet if patient is post fundoplication
8. Monitor for re-feeding syndrome in severely malnourished patients
9. Avoid over-feeding patients with CO^2 retention/mechanically ventilated patients [27]
10. Penn State Equation (PSU 2003) can be used to calculate energy needs for intubated patients (Academy of Nutrition and Dietetics Evidence Analysis Library (*Critical Illness Guidelines*) April 2012; include additional calories (approximately 15% of total calories) to compensate for malabsorption for patients with pancreatic insufficiency [28]
11. Non-enteric coated Viokace® can be crushed and added to formula, or enzyme beads may be suspended in nectar-thick fluids and administered with tube feedings for patients with pancreatic insufficiency [29, 30]

calorie snacks for between-meal consumption. An appetite stimulant may be helpful for patients with anorexia [14], and encouraging the use of supplemental oxygen when needed may help lower energy expenditure in patients with severe lung disease.

For patients with cystic fibrosis related diabetes (CFRD), optimizing blood sugar control can help improve nutritional status. Patients who do not have known CFRD should be screened preoperatively by oral glucose tolerance test if they have not had CFRD screening in the last 6 months [15]. It is important to provide patients with anticipatory guidance about the increased likelihood of developing temporary hyperglycemia necessitating insulin therapy during the immediate post-transplant period, and the recommendation to continue routine monitoring for CFRD on an annual basis or earlier if symptoms such as unexplained weight loss develop after transplantation.

The use of oral nutritional supplements in CF is common, however there is limited evidence to support their use. A 2014 Cochrane systematic review on this topic indicated that oral supplements do not confer additional benefit in the nutritional management of moderately malnourished children with CF, and that further controlled trials are needed to establish a role in the management of patients with advanced lung disease [16]. Possible factors relating to variable success with oral supplements may include flavor fatigue and decreased food intake when supplements are taken with meals. Alternating types and flavors of supplements and consuming them after meals and/or at the end of the day may improve the efficacy of oral nutritional supplements.

Gastrostomy tube (GT) placement for enteral feedings is another option for improving nutritional support. Data regarding the effectiveness of gastrostomy tube feedings are conflicting. A study from 2004 indicated that mortality was significantly increased when FEV_1 predicted was less that 50% at the time of gastrostomy insertion [17]. However a more recent study found that FEV_1 at the time of GT placement did not correlate with FEV_1 slope change after GT placement [18]. There is also conflicting data regarding effectiveness of gastrostomy tube feedings in patients with severe lung disease with regard to improving both FEV_1 and BMI [18–21]. Since most studies were relatively small and did not include prospective randomization, they were not included in a 2012 Cochrane review of enteral tube feedings in cystic fibrosis [22].

Gastroesophageal reflux disease (GERD) is reported in 30% of CF patients according to the CFF registry, and is associated with worse pulmonary outcomes [23, 24]. Considering the potential, significant impact of GERD on pulmonary outcomes, screening prior to GT placement and tube feeding often includes upper GI, pH probe, and gastric emptying study. Careful post-gastrostomy tube placement monitoring should also be considered (Table 14.4 and Fig. 14.1).

Pre-transplant CF Nutrition Assessment (18 and older)

Social:

FEV1   **Exercise/activity level:**

Nutrition Concerns / Questions:

Financial/psychosocial considerations:

Pt goal for wt (pre-tx): ↑ ↓ ↔**Comment:**

Transplant center: **LAS if listed:**

Additional Diagnoses: *CFRD +/- IGT +/- CFLD +/- Osteoporosis/penia +/- Kidney stones +/- DIOS +/- Pancreatitis +/- Fracture +/- Sinus dz* +/-Food allergy +/-Colonoscopy+/-Other/describe:* *interfering w/smell/taste

	Current Date:	Prior Date:
Ht (cm)		
Wt (kg)		
BMI		

Oral Intake Pattern	Appetite => ☐ Baseline ☐ Increased ☐ Decreased

Tube Feeds (kcal)	
Oral Supplements	
Calcium Intake	

Medications / Vitamins

☐ **Pancreatic Enzymes**

    Enzyme Dose: units lipase/kg/ largest meal;

    Total: units lipase /kg/day

    EnzymeProgram:

    ☐ **CF Specific Vitamins**

    Dose: Soft / chew / liquid

☐ **Other vitamins/minerals :**

☐ **Acid Blocker:**

Other Pert Medications / Appetite Stimulants/ Insulin / ADHD /CAM/Herbal:

Subjective report of adherence to enzymes/vitamins/supplements/tube feeds

GI / Absorption				
Sx: *Abdominal Pain*	*GERD Constipation*	*Nausea*	*Vomiting*	*None*
# stools/d/description =>				
Reflux screen				
Gastric emptying				
CFRD / Endocrine				
IF CFRD: Endo MD and year diagnosed:				
Last Seen:				
Blood sugar Range:				
? Lows/ Reactive hypoglycemia:				

Labs / Date	Results	Interventions
GFR or CrCl		
LFTs		
Vitamin A		
Vitamin E		
Vitamin D		
PT / INR or PIVKA		
DEXA		
OGTT		
Fasting Glu / Hgb A$_1$C		
Other		

Fig. 14.1 Pre-transplant nutrition assessment. Used with permission from University Hospitals Case Medical Center

Evaluation:

Nutrition Risk Assessment	Low Risk BMI>20	Moderate Risk BMI 19.9-18.6	High Risk BMI ≤18.5 Alb <3 BMI>30

Estimated energy and protein needs:
Estimated energy and protein intake:

Nutritional Diagnosis:
Nutrition Prescription:
       Goals / Plan:

Nutrition Intervention:
       Education/Materials Provided:

Monitoring and Evaluation:

Signature:

Fig. 14.1 (continued)

Post-Transplant Considerations

Immediate Post-Transplant Period

In the immediate post-operative period, patients are managed in the intensive care unit until stable enough to be transferred to a transplant unit or step-down unit. They may or may not need nutrition support during this time, depending on how quickly they are extubated and complications they may encounter. If enteral tube feedings are required, it is important to include additional calories for malabsorption when estimating energy needs, and plan for enzyme replacement therapy (see # 11 Table 14.4).

Oropharyngeal dysphagia is a common complication after thoracic surgical procedures, including lung transplantation, and can increase the risk of aspiration pneumonia [31]. Assessment for this complication is recommended prior to allowing the patient to resume oral intake after transplant. This complication may delay introduction of food and/or fluids and necessitate enteral tube feedings or the use of commercial thickeners until the dysphagia resolves.

Other gastrointestinal complications that can interfere with intake include distal intestinal obstruction syndrome (DIOS), gastric bezoars, delayed gastric emptying, and side effects from post-transplant medications. DIOS has been reported to occur in 10–20% of patients after transplant; in one study, the complication was particularly common in the early post-transplant time period [32, 33]. Monitoring stool patterns, using laxatives as needed, and ensuring patients are restarted on appropriate enzyme therapy can help reduce the risk of developing DIOS. Gastric bezoars, concretions of ingested matter in the GI tract manifesting as foreign bodies, are a complication after transplant, particularly for patients with cystic fibrosis. Dellon et al. in a retrospective study found that 11% of cystic fibrosis patients developed bezoars with a mean incidence of 34 days from transplant [34]. Delayed gastric emptying may develop or worsen post-transplant. Raviv et al. documented delayed gastric emptying in 50% of all lung transplant candidates prior to transplantation; this increased to 74% at 3 months post-transplant and decreased slightly to 63% at 12 months post-transplant [35]. Diets that are higher in fat and fiber may not be well tolerated during this time period due to delayed gastric emptying, and optimizing blood sugar control should help minimize the adverse effects of hyperglycemia on gastric emptying. Anti-rejection medications, particularly mycophenolate mofetil, as well as anti-microbial antibiotics may cause considerable gastrointestinal upset and diarrhea, further leading to decreased intake. Certain anti-rejection medications such as tacrolimus and cyclosporine are lipid-based and should be taken consistently either with or without enzyme replacement therapy to maintain stable levels.

Stress from major surgery, infection, and medications such as prednisone all significantly increase the risk of either new onset diabetes or worsened blood sugar control for those with existing CFRD. It is very common for patients to need insulin for the first time or much higher doses than what was required in the past in the immediate post-operative time period [15]. Patients who are discharged from the hospital without the diagnosis of diabetes should continue to be screened annually for CFRD [15] (Fig. 14.2).

Nutritional considerations 6 or more months out from transplant are unique. GERD is a particular concern as it may be more common in patients with cystic fibrosis and is associated with increased risk of chronic rejection [36]. Bronchiolitis obliterans syndrome (BO/BOS/OB), commonly referred to as chronic rejection, is the major cause of mortality in patients after lung transplantation [2].

Which vitamin and mineral supplements, as well as doses, are recommended in post-transplant patients is unknown. Routine, annual monitoring of fat soluble vitamin levels should continue post-transplant. Increased vitamin A and E levels have been reported in CF patients after lung transplantation; hypervitaminosis A is particularly concerning as toxicity can cause increased intracranial pressure, osteoporosis, and liver damage [37]. Standard CF vitamins may need to be discontinued since these

Post-transplant CF Nutrition Assessment (18 and older)		
Social:		
Nutrition Concerns / Questions:		
Pt goal for wt (short and long term): ↑ ↓ ↔ **Comment:**		
Transplant or CF center (circle): **Date of transplant:**		
Additional Diagnoses: *CFRD +/- IGT +/- CFLD +/- Osteoporosis/penia +/- Kidney stones +/- DIOS +/- Pancreatitis +/- Fracture +/- Sinus dz* +/- Food allergy +/- Colonoscopy +/- Other/describe:****interfering w/smell/taste**		
?Fundoplication (date): **? BOS (date):**		
	Current Date:	**Prior Date:**
Ht (cm)		
Wt (kg)		
BMI		

Oral Intake Pattern	**Appetite =>** □ **Baseline** □ **Increased** □ **Decreased**		
Tube Feeds (kcal)			
Oral Supplements			
Calcium Intake			
Dietary restrictions			
Medications / Vitamins			
□ **Pancreatic Enzymes**			
Enzyme Dose: units lipase/kg/ largest meal;			
Total: units lipase /kg/day			
EnzymeProgram: □ **CF Specific Vitamins:**			
Other:			
Dose: Soft / chew / liquid			
□ **Other vitamins/minerals :**			
□ **Acid Blocker:**			
Other Pert Medications / Appetite Stimulants/ Insulin / ADHD /CAM/Herbal/anti-rejection:			

Fig. 14.2 Post-transplant nutrition assessment (after discharge). Used with permission from University Hospitals Case Medical Center

Following food safety guidelines? Y   N

GI / Absorption		
Sx: *Abdominal Pain GERD Constipation Nausea Vomiting None*		
# stools/d =>	**Description:**	**? in stool pattern ?blood**
Reflux screen		
Gastric emptying		

CFRD / Endocrine □ OGTT screening completed □ N/A	
IF CFRD: Endo MD and year diagnosed:	
Last Seen:	
Blood sugar Range:	
? Lows / Reactive hypoglycemia	

Labs / Date	Results	Interventions
GFR or CrCl		
LFTs		
Vitamin A		
Vitamin E		
Vitamin D		
PT / INR or PIVKA		
DEXA		
OGTT		
Fasting Glu / Hgb A$_1$C		
Other		

Evaluation:

Nutrition Risk Assessment	Low Risk BMI>20	Moderate Risk BMI 19.9-18.6	High Risk BMI ≤18.5 Alb <3 BMI > 30

Estimated energy and protein needs:
Estimated energy and protein intake:

Nutritional Diagnosis:
Nutrition Prescription:
    Goals / Plan:

Nutrition Intervention:
    Education/Materials Provided:

Monitoring and Evaluation:

Signature:

Fig. 14.2 (continued)

products contain significant doses of vitamins A and E compared to most general over-the-counter multivitamin products. Optimizing vitamin D levels may be important as low serum vitamin D levels are associated with increased rates of rejection and infection after lung transplantation [38]. Additionally, vitamin K_2 supplementation showed a favorable effect on lumbar spine bone mineral density in post lung transplant patients [39]. Adequate calcium, vitamin D, and vitamin K intake as well as weight-bearing exercise should be encouraged to help negate the effects of corticosteroids on bone health in the post-transplant period.

    Renal dysfunction is another common complication that can occur in adults with CF after lung transplantation and may require new dietary restrictions. A cohort study reviewing CFF patient registry data from 2000–2008 showed a 2-year risk of 35% for developing renal dysfunction; risk factors included pre-transplant renal function impairment, increased age, female gender, and CF related diabetes [40]. Restrictions in potassium and phosphorus may be necessary, and patients who develop renal insufficiency may be particularly high risk for developing hypervitaminosis A.

Gastrointestinal malignancies are a particular concern for CF patients post-transplant. Immunosuppressive agents, in addition to the inherent increased risk of GI malignancy associated with cystic fibrosis, are believed to be the major causes of the increased incidence of GI malignancies in this post lung transplant population [41]. Colorectal cancer appears to be the most common malignancy, with one study showing a sevenfold increased risk of advanced adenomas [42]. More aggressive screening for colorectal cancer is likely warranted for this population. In particular, it is important to consider investigating malignancy as the cause of unexplained symptoms such as changes in bowel habits, progressive weight loss, and/or anemia.

Food safety is important to review with all solid-organ transplant recipients. Immunosuppression leads to increased risk of food-borne infections such as Salmonella and listeriosis [43, 44]. The Academy of Nutrition and Dietetics offers general food safety tips, and the Food and Drug Administration (FDA) offers a food safety handout designed specifically for patients who have received solid organ and bone marrow transplants http://www.fda.gov/downloads/Food/ResourcesForYou/Consumers/SelectedHealthTopics/UCM312793.pdf.

Finally, for most patients with CF, significant improvements in weight gain and BMI are noted between 3 and 24 months after transplant, with most increase noted in underweight patients [4, 45]. There is no evidence to specify an optimal BMI for cystic fibrosis patients who are post lung transplant; the 2008 published guidelines with BMI goals of 23 for males and 22 for females are based on correlation to FEV_1 in pre-transplant patients [46]. However, knowing that complications are quite common after transplant, it would seem prudent to recommend achieving and maintaining a normal BMI for age. Some patients may become overweight if they continue to follow the typical high fat, high calorie CF diet; monitoring BMI trend is important.

Conclusion

Lung transplantation offers survival and quality of life advantage to patients with cystic fibrosis; however they face many nutrition-related challenges before and after the transplant process. It is important for nutrition professionals to be aware of the unique gastrointestinal and nutritional issues that individuals with cystic fibrosis face, and continue to offer nutrition guidance throughout the transplant process.

References

1. Cystic Fibrosis Foundation Patient Registry 2012 annual data report. Bethesda. Cystic Fibrosis Foundation; 2013.
2. Hirche TO, Knoop C, Hebestreit H, et al. ECORN-CF Study Group. Practical guidelines: lung transplantation in patients with cystic fibrosis. Pulm Med. 2014;62:1342.
3. Scientific Registry of Transplant Recipients 2012 National data report. The SRTR is administered by the Chronic Disease Research Group of the Minneapolis Medical Research Foundation, with oversight and funding from the Health Resources and Services Administration; 2013.
4. Hollander FM, van Pierre DD, de Roos NM, van de Graaf EA, Iestra JA. Effects of nutritional status and dietetic interventions on survival in cystic fibrosis patients before and after lung transplantation. J Cyst Fibros. 2014;13:212–8.
5. Liou TG, Adler RD, Huang D. Use of lung transplantation survival models to refine patient selection in cystic fibrosis. Am J Respir Crit Care Med. 2005;171:1053–9.
6. Yankaskas JR, Mallory GB, Consensus Committee. Lung transplantation in cystic fibrosis: consensus conference statement. Chest. 1998;113:217–26.

7. Kalnins D, Pencharz PB, Grasemann H, Solomon M. Energy expenditure and nutritional status in pediatric patients before and after lung transplantation. J Pediatr. 2013;163:1500–2.
8. Bodet-Milin C, Querellou S, Oudoux A, et al. Delayed gastric emptying scintigraphy in cystic fibrosis patients before and after lung transplantation. J Heart Lung Transplant. 2006;25:1077–83.
9. Lederer DJ, Wilt JS, D'Ovidio F, et al. Obesity and underweight are associated with an increased risk of death after lung transplantation. Am J Respir Crit Care Med. 2009;180:887–95.
10. Singer JP, Peterson ER, Snyder ME, et al. Body composition and mortality after adult lung transplantation in the United States. Am J Respir Crit Care Med. 2014;190:1012–21.
11. Schwebel C, Pin I, Barnoud D, et al. Prevalence and consequences of nutritional depletion in lung transplant candidates. Eur Respir J. 2000;16:1050–5.
12. Baldwin MR, Arcasoy SM, Shah A, et al. Hypoalbuminemia and early mortality after lung transplantation: a cohort study. Am J Transplant. 2012;12:1256–67.
13. Belkin RA, Henig NR, Singer LG, et al. Risk factors for death of patients with cystic fibrosis awaiting lung transplantation. Am J Respir Crit Care Med. 2006;173:659–66.
14. Nasr SZ, Drury D. Appetite stimulants use in cystic fibrosis. Pediatr Pulmonol. 2008;43:209–19.
15. Moran A, Brunzell C, Cohen R, et al. Clinical care guidelines for cystic fibrosis-related diabetes. Diabetes Care. 2010;12:2697–716.
16. Smyth RL, Rayner O. Oral calorie supplements for cystic fibrosis. Cochrane Database Syst Rev. 2014;11:CD000406.
17. Oliver MR, Heine RG, Ng CH, Volders E, Olinsky A. Factors affecting clinical outcome in gastrostomy-fed children with cystic fibrosis. Pediatr Pulmonol. 2004;37:324–9.
18. Best C, Brearly A, Gaillard P, et al. A pre-post retrospective study of patients with cystic fibrosis and gastrostomy tubes. J Pediatr Gastroenterol Nutr. 2011;53:453–8.
19. Efrati O, Mei-Zahav M, Rivlin J, et al. Long term nutritional rehabilitation by gastrostomy in Israeli patients with cystic fibrosis: clinical outcome in advanced pulmonary disease. J Pediatr Gastroenterol Nutr. 2006;42:222–8.
20. Walker SA, Gozal D. Pulmonary function correlates in the prediction of long-term weight gain in cystic fibrosis patients with gastrostomy tube feedings. J Pediatr Gastroenterol Nutr. 1998;27:53–6.
21. White H, Morton AM, Conway SP, Peckham DG. Enteral tube feeding in adults with cystic fibrosis; patient choice and impact on long term outcomes. J Cyst Fibros. 2013;12:616–22.
22. Conway S, Morton A, Wolfe S. Enteral tube feeding for cystic fibrosis. Cochrane Database Syst Rev. 2012;12:CD001198.
23. Navarro J, Rainisio M, Harms HK, et al. Factors associated with poor pulmonary function: cross-sectional analysis of data from the ERCF. European Epidemiologic Registry of Cystic Fibrosis. Eur Respir J. 2001;18:298–305.
24. Stringer DA, Sprigg A, Juodis E, et al. The association of cystic fibrosis, gastroesophageal reflux, and reduced pulmonary function. Can Assoc Radiol J. 1988;39:100–2.
25. Erskine JM, Lingard CD, Sontag MK, Accurso FJ. Enteral nutrition for patients with cystic fibrosis: comparison of a semi-elemental and nonelemental formula. J Pediatr. 1998;132:265–9.
26. Pelekanos JT, Holt TL, Ward LC, Cleghorn GJ, Shepherd RW. Protein turnover in malnourished patients with cystic fibrosis: effects of elemental and nonelemental nutritional supplements. J Pediatr Gastroenterol Nutr. 1990;10:339–43.
27. Talpers SS, Romberger DJ, Bunce SB, Pingleton SK. Nutritionally associated increased carbon dioxide production. Excess total calories vs high proportion of carbohydrate calories. Chest. 1992;102:551–5.
28. Concepts in CF Care Consensus Conferences: pediatric nutrition for patients with cystic fibrosis. Cystic Fibrosis Foundation; 2008.
29. Written communication from Actavis Pharmaceuticals regarding *in vitro* Viokace® validation studies.
30. Ferrie S, Graham C, Hoyle M. Pancreatic enzyme supplementation for patients receiving enteral feeds. Nutr Clin Pract. 2011;26:349–51.
31. Atkins BZ, Peterson RP, Daneshmand MA, et al. Impact of oropharyngeal dysphagia on long-term outcomes of lung transplantation. Ann Thorac Surg. 2010;90:1622–9.
32. Morton JR, Ansari N, Glanville AR, Meagher AP, Lord RV. Distal intestinal obstruction syndrome (DIOS) in patients with cystic fibrosis after lung transplantation. J Gastrointest Surg. 2009;13:1448–53.
33. Gillijam M, Chaparro C, Tullis E, et al. GI complications after lung transplantation in patients with cystic fibrosis. Chest. 2003;123:37–41.
34. Dellon ES, Morgan DR, Mohanty SP, Davis SP, Aris RM. High incidence of gastric bezoars in cystic fibrosis patients after lung transplantation. Transplantation. 2006;81:1141–6.
35. Raviv Y, D'Ovidio F, Pierre A, et al. Prevalence of gastroparesis before and after lung transplantation and its association with lung allograft outcomes. Clin Transplant. 2012;26:133–42.
36. Mendez BM, Davis CS, Weber C, Joehl RJ, Fisichella PM. Gastroesophageal reflux disease in lung transplant patients with cystic fibrosis. Am J Surg. 2012;204:e21–6.
37. Stephenson A, Brotherwood M, Robert R, et al. Increased vitamin A and E levels in adult cystic fibrosis patients after lung transplantation. Transplantation. 2005;79:613–5.

38. Lowery EM, Bemiss B, Cascino T, et al. Low vitamin D levels are associated with increased rejection and infections after lung transplantation. J Heart Lung Transplant. 2012;31:700–7.
39. Forli L, Bollerslev J, Simonsen S, et al. Dietary vitamin K2 supplement improves bone status after lung and heart transplantation. Transplantation. 2010;89:458–64.
40. Quon BS, Mayer-Hamblett N, Aitken ML, Goss CH. Risk of post lung transplant renal dysfunction in adults with cystic fibrosis. Chest. 2012;142:185–91.
41. Meyer KC, Francois ML, Thomas HK, et al. Colon cancer in lung transplant recipients with CF: increased risk and results of screening. J Cyst Fibros. 2011;10:366–9.
42. Gory I, Brown G, Wilson J, et al. Increased risk of colorectal neoplasia in adult patients with cystic fibrosis: a matched case–control study. Scand J Gastroenterol. 2014;49:1230–6.
43. Centers for Disease Control and Prevention. Outbreak of Salmonella serotype Javinia infections, Orlando, FL, June 2002. MMWR Morb Mortal Wkly Rep 2002;51:683–4.
44. Goulet V, Hebert M, Hedberg C, et al. Incidence of listeriosis and related mortality among groups at risk of acquiring listeriosis. Clin Infect Dis. 2012;54:652–60.
45. Dirk H, Ralf E, Roland H, Stefan DA. Reversability of cachexia after bilateral lung transplantation. Int J Cardiol. 2008;133:46–50.
46. Stallings VA, Stark LJ, Robinson KA, Feranchak AP, Quinton H. Evidence-based practice recommendations for nutrition-related management of children and adults with cystic fibrosis and pancreatic insufficiency: results of a systematic review. J Am Diet Assoc. 2008;108:832–9.

Chapter 15
Pregnancy, Nutrition, and Cystic Fibrosis

Michelle Brotherwood

Key Points

- As life expectancy increases in cystic fibrosis so does the incidence of women with CF becoming pregnant. To date there are no consensus guidelines about managing these patients. It is important to have a multidisciplinary approach including a registered dietitian to optimize the patient's health.
- Weight gain can be a challenge in pregnancy for women with CF who have high calorie needs and malabsorption. This can be exacerbated by GI symptoms common in pregnancy that can affect intake.
- All medications need to be reviewed for their safety in pregnancy. Vitamin levels need to be monitored each trimester as Vitamin A can be of particular concern in pregnancy.
- Women with CF who become pregnancy are at a higher risk of gestation diabetes and screening this early (starting at 8–10 weeks) is recommended. Those women who have diabetes prior to conception should be closely monitored to optimize their blood sugar control
- Breastfeeding may be an option but should be discussed with the healthcare team

Keywords Pregnancy • Weight gain • Gestational diabetes • Vitamins • Enzymes • Breastfeeding

Introduction

With increased life expectancy and improved health outcomes the number of pregnancies occurring in women with cystic fibrosis (CF) is on the rise and is now considered a viable option for many women. The first successful pregnancy in cystic fibrosis was reported in 1960 [1] and the numbers reported have been increasing each year. Published data shows that the outcomes for both women with CF and their babies have improved considerably over time [2–5]. Several studies suggest that pregnancy itself does not affect women's survival or disease related outcomes [2, 5–7]. However, there are very few research studies looking at prenatal care for women with CF and as a result, there are no current consensus guidelines for nutritional management of population [7]. In practice, as outlined in this chapter, care

M. Brotherwood, R.D., C.D.E. (✉)
Pulmonary, Children's Hospital Los Angeles, 4650 Sunset Blvd, Mailstop #8, Los Angeles, CA 90026, USA
e-mail: mbrotherwood@gmail.com

E.H. Yen, A.R. Leonard (eds.), *Nutrition in Cystic Fibrosis: A Guide for Clinicians*, Nutrition and Health, DOI 10.1007/978-3-319-16387-1_15, © Springer International Publishing Switzerland 2015

is provided based on current CF nutrition recommendations and nutrition recommendations for the general population during pregnancy. This chapter will review nutrition guidelines for pre, during, and post pregnancy as well as breastfeeding for the woman with CF.

Pre-pregnancy Nutrition & Evaluation

There may be a misconception among some women with CF, their families and even among some healthcare providers that women with CF are not able to get pregnant or successfully sustain a pregnancy. There is some conflicting data in the literature. Some studies show decreased fertility compared to the general population [8] and other studies show that there is no difference [9]. However, pregnancy has been seen in women with CF who have very low lung function and even post-transplant [2]. Ideally, the pregnancy is planned, which helps to optimize the woman medically, nutritionally, and mentally for this challenging time [7, 10].

The counseling and support that the medical team, including a CF dietitian, provides to the woman considering pregnancy is extremely important [7, 10]. It is imperative that the clinician has the most up-to-date and accurate information that is shared in a hopeful, non-judgmental but realistic way [11]. A woman's decisions about her own pregnancy should be supported, regardless of personal feelings, so that a great team and patient relationship can continue [7]. Nutrition topics to address should include nutrition intake, expected weight gain, safety of medications in pregnancy, social support, financial considerations, breastfeeding, and caring for a child while ensuring the woman's health is also being managed [7]. There may be value in connecting a woman considering pregnancy to other women with CF (via email, social media, or phone) who have had successful pregnancies to offer support and answer questions.

As with any pregnancy, rate of weight gain and total weight gained during a pregnancy are clinically very important measures to follow for both the health of the mother and baby [12, 13]. A British study did show that weight below the 10th percentile placed women at risk for infertility, preterm birth, and increased complications during delivery [13]. There is some evidence to suggest that severe malnutrition, as measured by a body mass index (BMI) <18 kg/m^2, is considered a relative contraindication to pregnancy given the resulting fetal outcomes [14]. In cystic fibrosis, the pre-pregnancy nutrition goal, as with all women with CF, should focus on improving BMI to the current CFF recommendation of ≥22 mg/kg^2.[15]. This can be achieved by optimizing oral intake of calories and with the use of oral supplements and/or gastrostomy tube (GT) feeds [7, 16]. Other suggestions for nutrition interventions to optimize nutrition are discussed in greater detail in this book. Infant outcomes are improved with better nutritional status of the mother [2, 7, 17]. Maternal health post-partum is directly related to nutritional status during pregnancy [2, 17]. A survey of mothers with CF in the UK has shown that those who received nutritional advice before conceiving had a significantly greater weight gain during pregnancy and gave birth to significantly heavier babies [10]. It is also important at this time to establish baseline vitamin levels as vitamin A can be of concern in pregnancy [18]. This will be discussed in more detail later in this chapter. Folic acid supplementation is also very important at this time as discussed later in this chapter. Finally, establishing baseline glycemic status in a woman considering pregnancy is very important as there may be undiagnosed hyperglycemia [19].

Pregnancy Tracking and Clinic Visits

It is important that each individual CF care center (both adult and pediatric) develop a protocol and guidelines for pregnancy, or at the very least have a discussion together about this issue, with the hope of standardizing treatment and optimizing patient care. It is recommended that the dietitian assess and counsel women at regular clinic visits throughout pregnancy. Nutrition assessments should occur at least once a trimester, more often with complicated cases [7, 10]. During these visits, anthropometric information such as height, weight history, and weight gain during pregnancy should be monitored [7]. Furthermore, it is essential to record a dietary history, patient's use of nutritional supplements and vitamin/mineral preparations as well as associated symptoms such as nausea/vomiting. A pregnancy flowchart is a useful tool to track nutrition throughout the pregnancy. See example in Fig. 15.1.

Other Medication and Tests

In the planning stages of pregnancy, it is very important to review medications with a physician and pharmacist, to ensure they are safe in pregnancy [7]. Not all medications used in CF have been tested for safety during pregnancy. Each drug is classified into one of four categories in pregnancy [18, 20]:

A. Drugs that have been used widely during pregnancy and are assumed safe for the fetus
B. Drugs not known to cause harm to the human fetus but with insufficient experience to consider them safe.
C. Drugs that could theoretically cause harm to the fetus by their pharmacological actions
D. Drugs known or believed to cause harm to the fetus. Pregnancy category C medications include pancrelipase (use caution but not considered to cause a risk to the pregnancy), albuterol (but unknown whether harm can be caused), vitamin K (use caution).

Enzymes in Pregnancy

Women who are pancreatic insufficient must continue to use pancreatic replacement therapy (PERT) as directed during their pregnancy. The dose may not need to be adjusted with pregnancy but should be assessed at each visit or with symptoms of malabsorption. When examining PERT and pregnancy, there has been a concern addressed over the use of phthalates as an ingredient in the digestive enzymes themselves. Phthalates are used as a plasticizer in enteric-coatings of solid oral drug products to maintain flexibility, but can be used for different functions in other drugs [21, 22]. Phthalates are used in pancreatic enzymes as an enteric coating to protect the enzyme from the acid environment of the stomach. Animal research is available describing the impact of phthalates. Some phthalates demonstrate no toxicity, while others demonstrate problems related to developmental and reproductive toxins in laboratory animals [21]. In December 2012 the Food and Drug Administration (FDA) distributed "Guidance for Industry: Limiting the use of certain phthalates as excipients in Center for Drug Evaluation and Research (CDER) regulated products." The recommendation stated that although there is limited human data the FDA has determined that there is evidence that the exposure to dibutyl phthalate (DBP) and di (2-ethylhexyl) phthalate (DEHP) from pharmaceuticals presents a potential risk of developmental and reproductive toxicity. The FDA recommended that the pharmaceutical industry avoid the use of DBP and DEHP as excipients in CDER-regulated drug and biologic products. Prior to the guidance many pancreatic enzymes used DBP or DEHP as the enteric coating; they are no longer in pancreatic enzymes [22].

The FDA concluded that hypromellose phthalate (HPMCP) could be included in their "unofficial" listing of items Generally Recognized as Safe (GRAS). The FDA is aware of the use of HPMCP in pancreatic enzymes [22].

Phthalates have been found in the urine of patients taking pancreatic enzymes as first discovered by Keller et al. in 2009 [23]. As a result of the Keller et al.'s paper, there was a great concern in the

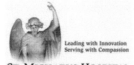

ST. MICHAEL'S HOSPITAL
A teaching hospital affiliated with the University of Toronto

Adult Cystic Fibrosis Program
Nutrition Evaluation: Pregnancy

Patient Name:_____

Age:_____ Due date:_____

Patient ID
_____

	Pre-Pregnancy	1st Trimester (1-13 weeks)	2nd Trimester (13-27 weeks)	3rd Trimester (27-40 weeks)
Date				
Weeks Gestation				
Height				
Weight				
BMI				
Weight gain				
MAC				
TS				
MAMC				
ALB				
HGB				
Ferritin				
Serum vitamin A				
Serum vitamin E				
Serum vitamin D				
OGTT: FBS				
2 hr				
Oral glucose challenge				
Calcium intake				
Calcium supplements				
Vitamin supplements				
Requirements: KCAL				
GI Symptoms				
Oral supplements				
Nutrition Support				

GI ISSUES

Pancreatic Status: PI / PS
Enzyme therapy: Type:_____ ____/meal ____/snack
Hx of GI complications: _____

_____

Other: (ie. Financial, social support)_____

_____

Fig. 15.1 Adult Cystic Fibrosis Program Nutrition Evaluation. Used with permission from Adult CF clinic at St. Michael's Hospital in Toronto, Canada

CF community and the FDA was approached to provide guidance on the use of phthalates in enzymes. As a result DBP and DEHP were removed from enzymes and replaced with HPMCP. The risk of malnutrition for someone who has CF resulting from avoiding enzymes is real; therefore, the CFF recommends that patients who require enzymes as part of their CF care should continue taking the medication [24].

A body of data indicates toxicity of DBP and DEHP, especially for the developing fetus; therefore, healthcare providers question the use of pancreatic enzymes containing phthalates by pregnant women. Based on the available data there is no indication that the phthalate in currently available enzyme products produces adverse effects. To date there are no papers describing fetal anomalies in infants born to women taking pancreatic enzymes. Women who have CF and take enzymes should continue taking their enzymes, including during pregnancy [25].

In considering the issue of phthalates in digestive enzymes, there are enteric coated enzymes on the market which do not contain any phthalates [24]. It seems reasonable that if a woman with CF is able to switch enzymes, without any issues related to malabsorption, a non-phthalate containing enzyme is a good option given the ongoing need for research in this area.

Weight Gain

Regular monitoring of weight gain is extremely important during pregnancy [7]. Currently, there are no CF specific guidelines of expected weight gain in pregnancy and therefore the standard pregnancy weight gain recommendations apply in this patient population based on pre-pregnancy baseline BMI. See Table 15.1 [26].

The challenge for many women with CF is that they are starting out with a low pre-pregnancy BMI, therefore any work to optimize weight gain prior to conception is beneficial in this often very motivated group. In the general population, pregnancy increases calorie needs in the second trimester by 350 kcal/day and increases to 450 kcal/day in the third trimester (there is no increased need in the first trimester from pregnancy itself) [27]. Nutrition counseling should include creative ways to meet high calorie needs with a patient centered approach without guilt or judgment. The use of high calorie oral nutrition supplements can be extremely helpful at this time to meet the high calorie needs and should be used liberally as tolerated [7, 28]. If the woman has a skin level gastrostomy tube prior to pregnancy, it is suggested that it is changed to a variable length tube to allow for the abdomen to swell. During pregnancy increased volume of feeds or the addition of daytime bolus feeds may be beneficial to meet increased calorie needs [7, 28].

More aggressive nutrition intervention may be needed if weight gain is poor and/or if there are concerns over the growth of the baby [28]. Nasogastric (NG) feeds are an option to supplement oral intake although for some women this may affect their ability to clear their sputum and exacerbate reflux. This method, in general, to be a well-tolerated and less invasive way to increase calories and

Table 15.1 Recommended weight gain during pregnancy

Pre-pregnancy BMI	Recommended range of total weight gain (pounds)
<18.5 (underweight)	28–40
18.5–24.9 (normal weight)	25–35
25–29.9 (overweight)	15–25
≥30 (obese)	11–20

Adapted from Institute of Medicine (US) Weight Gain During Pregnancy: reexamining the guidelines. Washington, DC. National Academies Press; 2009 most women are very motivated for a healthy pregnancy and are agreeable to NG feeds. Another option can be parenteral nutrition (PN), if the woman is admitted to hospital (and already has PN access). PN does not displace calories from food or supplements and does not have GI side effects, however it is not without risks. If the woman is eating mixed meals, PN can be given as IV lipids to provide a concentrated source of calories. This approach has been used at by some CF centers with success (unpublished data).

GI Issues

The usual gastrointestinal problems of pregnancy, such as reflux and constipation, may be particularity troublesome for women with CF and should be managed aggressively to ensure that there is not an impact weight gain [7, 16]. It is important to ask women often if they are experiencing these side effects and offer advice on any nutrition interventions that may help.

Constipation and distal ileal obstruction syndrome (DIOS) are already common in people with CF and can be made worse by pregnancy and iron supplementation (which is often prescribed in pregnancy) [28]. Measures should be taken to manage these symptoms as per CF standard of care with PEG 3350 (ex.Miralax) and golytely bowel clear outs as needed [16, 28]. Probiotics from natural food sources are safe in pregnancy and can help with these symptoms. If probiotics are being considered as a medication, this should be discussed with the medical team, including the obstetrician, before initiation. Reflux, a common GI symptom in CF, can be exacerbated in pregnancy and affect intake [25, 29].

Medications used to treat reflux are generally considered safe in pregnancy [20] and should be considered. Hyperemesis is a serious medication condition that requires close attention and management by the medical team [27].

Vitamin and Mineral Supplementation

The combination of CF and pregnancy presents unique challenges and considerations for vitamin and mineral supplementation. Controversy exists around the recommendation for women to stay on their CF specific multivitamin during pregnancy. It is very important in pregnancy to have fat soluble vitamin levels tested, ideally prior to conception to ensure optimal serum levels. Serum fat soluble vitamin levels should be tested each trimester [7, 16].

Folic Acid

Folic acid is important in the prevention of neural tube birth defects, which affect the brain and spinal cord of the fetus. Neural tube defects develop in the first 28 days after conception, before many women know they are pregnant. It is recommended that any woman who could get pregnant take 400 micrograms (mcg) of folic acid daily, starting before conception and continuing for the first 12 weeks of pregnancy. These guidelines are the same in the CF population [7, 12, 30]. Commercially available CF specific multivitamins, developed specifically for this population, contain folic acid ranging between 200 and 400 mcg (2 soft gels). The amount of folic acid in CF specific multivitamins alone may not meet needs, additional supplementation may be necessary. Folic acid is available as a single supplement and does not need to come as part of a prenatal multivitamin. Many foods are rich in folic acid including green leafy vegetables, nuts, beans, citrus fruits, and many fortified foods. However folic acid intake from food may not be adequate, given the risk to the fetus, it is advisable to take a supplement with the 400 mcg of folic acid to help prevent neural tube defects [12, 30].

Vitamin E

The role and importance of vitamin E in pregnancy is not well described in the literature. Serum levels should be monitored and additional supplementation prescribed to reach therapeutic levels [7, 28].

Vitamin K

Vitamin K deficiency can lead to increased risk of bleeding which may negatively impact a pregnancy. If possible, a serum level measuring prothrombin induced by vitamin K absence-II (PIVKA II) should be measured to assess vitamin K status [28]. If this is not possible, measure of blood coagulation using prothrombin time (PT) or international normalized ration (INR) can be used. Vitamin K should be supplemented as per CF care guidelines during pregnancy [7, 28].

Vitamin D

Vitamin D is extremely important both in CF and pregnancy and CF. Serum vitamin D levels should be monitored closely to reach a level of >30 ng/mL (>75nmol/L) prior to and during pregnancy [7, 12, 31]. A vitamin D deficiency during pregnancy can cause growth retardation and skeletal deformities and may also have an impact on birth weight [12]. A deficiency of vitamin D has also been linked to a greater risk of pregnancy complications, including preeclampsia, and a higher likelihood of a delivery via cesarean section [12, 39]. For most women with CF, additional Vitamin D_3 supplementation is needed in addition to what is found in their CF specific multivitamins [28, 31]. While there are no consensus guidelines on the upper limit of safety of Vitamin D supplementation in pregnancy, 10,000 IU/day of cholecalciferol (Vitamin D_3), the upper limit used in non-pregnant CF patients, is believed to be appropriate. Serum vitamin D levels should be closely monitored each trimester [28, 31, 39].

Vitamin A

Vitamin A supplementation presents the greatest concern and area for debate when it comes to pregnancy in CF. Most patients with CF who are pancreatic insufficient require additional supplementation of vitamin A, from CF specific multivitamins, in order to achieve therapeutic levels [16, 28]. In pregnancy, Vitamin A is essential for embryogenesis; however, high dietary supplementation of retinol in the non-CF population has been associated with birth defect [7, 12, 32, 33]. These studies evaluated the association between the amount of ingested vitamin A and birth defects. Serum vitamin A levels were not monitored in these studies but the assumption is that high vitamin A intake would result in high serum levels [32, 33]. The World Health Organization guidelines indicate an increased risk with >10,000 IU retinol per day [18]. As a result, this level of vitamin A intake has become the consensus guideline recommendation for upper limit of safety in pregnancy [32, 33]. It is also important to remember that low vitamin A levels can also be harmful to a baby's growth and development [12]. The recommended adult dose of currently available CF specific multivitamins (2 soft gels) contain between 28,000 and 36,344 IU of Vitamin A (retinal and beta carotene) [34], although most have 88–92% of Vitamin A as beta carotene [20]. Unlike preformed vitamin A, beta carotene is not known to be teratogenic or lead to reproductive toxicity. Even large supplemental doses (20–30 mg/day) of beta carotene or diets with high levels of carotenoid-rich food for long periods are not associated with toxicity and therefore is felt to be safer in pregnancy [32]. A study by Stephenson et al. showed that pregnant women on CF specific multivitamins maintained serum levels of vitamin A within normal limits and no birth defects were noted.

If CF specific multivitamins are discontinued because of concerns of high vitamin A intake, it is extremely important to monitor serum levels pre-pregnancy and during each trimester to avoid fat soluble vitamin deficiency. It is suggested that this decision should be made together with the obstetrics and CF care center and blood work results shared and communicated to the patient.

Calcium

Calcium is also an important micronutrient for a pregnant woman [12, 27]. It can help prevent loss of bone density, which can already be low with CF, as the baby uses calcium for its own bone growth. A brief diet history on calcium intake during pregnancy is recommended to ensure that intake is adequate [16]. At this time, the recommendation remains >1500 mg/day of calcium intake/day and should be supplemented if dietary intake is inadequate [12, 27, 28].

Iron

Iron requirements go up significantly during pregnancy, primarily because of the increased blood volume [12]. A full iron panel including ferritin should be drawn prior to and during pregnancy and microcytic anemia corrected with supplementation. Be aware of the gastrointestinal side effects of iron supplementation which can affect intake and contribute to constipation [12].

CFRD and Gestational Diabetes

Both pre-existing CFRD and gestational diabetes are important considerations in pregnancy. Women with CF who become pregnant are at increased risk of gestational diabetes which can affect the health of the baby [2, 7, 19]. Women with CFRD who become pregnant need to optimize their blood glucose control. Blood glucose levels can be affected by hormones, gastrointestinal issues, and stress [19]. Hyperglycemia can affect the developing fetus throughout the pregnancy. In early pregnancy, a mother's diabetes can result in birth defects and an increased rate of miscarriage. Many of the birth defects that occur affect major organs such as the brain and heart. During the second and third trimester, ongoing hyperglycemia can lead to over-nutrition and excess growth of the baby and may affect the infant's risk of developing type 2 diabetes later in life [19, 33, 35]. Also, hypoglycemia can exacerbate the difficulties many women with CF have in achieving a positive protein balance and sufficient weight gain during pregnancy. In addition, when high blood sugar from the mother causes high insulin levels (hyperinsulinemia) in the baby, the baby's blood sugar can drop very low after birth, because it is no longer receiving large amounts of glucose from the mother [35].

Gestational Diabetes

In pregnancy, insulin secretion is enhanced with normal to decreased insulin sensitivity in the non-CF population. Any insulin resistance that develops in late pregnancy is compensated for by the increased secretion. Women with CF have been studied in pregnancy and shown to be unable to match this increased insulin and hence are at higher risk of gestational diabetes and enhanced protein catabolism with impaired weight gain [36]. Gestational diabetes occurs in 14–33% of pregnancies in CF for those who have previously had normal glucose tolerance (incidence in non-CF: 3–7%—depending on ethnicity). The main difference between CF and non-CF women is when gestation diabetes is first discovered. With CF, it can be identified as early as 8 weeks gestation and requires insulin (normally seen by ~24–28 weeks in non-CF population [19].

The Cystic Fibrosis Foundation guidelines recommend an oral glucose tolerance test (OGTT) if considering pregnancy to determine baseline glucose status. Once pregnant, it is recommended to repeat OGTT (if not previously done in the past 6 months). During the pregnancy, it is recommended to repeat OGTT at the end of both the first (12–16 weeks) and second trimester (24–28 weeks) (suggest 1 h & 2 h post prandial values) given how early gestation diabetes is shown to occur in women with CF [7].

CFRD Prior to Pregnancy

For women who have known CFRD, detailed education about target blood sugars and risk during pregnancy is important at this time [7, 19, 33, 35]. Target HbA$_1$C prior to conception of <7% is recommended, although ideally the target in pregnancy is <6.1% [19]. Given that most women are highly motivated with compliance at this time, you can suggest a 3-month trial of optimizing HbA$_1$C prior to considering pregnancy may be helpful to see if this goal can be achieved. It is important to have a referral to an endocrinologist with knowledge in gestational diabetes, even if the patient is followed at a pediatric hospital [19].

Whether from gestational diabetes or CFRD, optimizing blood sugars during pregnancy is extremely important and needs to be balanced with the high calorie requirements for weight gain [7, 19, 36]. Maintaining high calorie intake and using rapid/short acting insulin is treatment of choice. This can be achieved with injections or with the use of an insulin pump. Carbohydrate counting is the most effective way to control hyperglycemia and maintain a high calorie intake. Foods high in simple sugars and oral nutrition supplements can still be consumed but should be taken with a meal so that the total carbohydrate can be added into the insulin to carbohydrate ratio [19]. High calorie but lower carbohydrate snacks can be recommended between meals to avoid hyperglycemia but maintain calories such as cheese, nuts, seeds, or meat. It is very important that CF appropriate nutrition counseling be given, and that the women are counseled not to limit portions and as is common in gestational diabetes without CF [19].

Blood glucose guidelines are different in pregnancy with blood glucose targets of 60–120 mg/dl (3.3–6.7 mmol/l) [19, 37]. It is normal to see a rise in insulin requirements as pregnancy proceeds up to 36 weeks gestation but those needs can decrease rapidly at the end of pregnancy and blood glucose levels should be monitored. It is recommended that women check their blood sugars before and 2 h after every meal [19, 37]. Insulin requirements may be disturbed by hyperemesis, delayed gastric motility, and/or use of steroid therapy. In extreme cases of uncontrolled hyperglycemia [19, 37], in-patient care may be needed.

Other Nutrition Considerations

As with any pregnancy, the same nutrition advice applies in CF regarding abstaining from alcohol, limiting caffeine and fish consumption, food borne illness, and food safety [12]. This advice should be given in the pre-conception time period if possible and re-enforced with education handouts. Ideally, none of these changes to a woman's dietary intake will significantly affect her total calorie/fat intake [7]. If a woman is a vegetarian or vegan, particular attention may need to be made to protein intake as well as certain vitamins/minerals [12].

Breastfeeding

Breastfeeding remains the optimal choice for infant nutrition but for a variety of reasons this can be a challenge in CF [12]. Limited literature is available on the composition of breast milk in women with CF, however, Shiffman et al. concluded that milk secreted by women with CF appears to be physiologically normal and safe for the infant [38]. It should be noted that during a pulmonary exacerbation, the concentrations of milk macronutrients were shown to be reduced [12].

For many women with CF, keeping up with their own high calorie needs is very difficult. The extra calorie requirements (300–800 kcal/day) needed to sustain breastfeeding may require additional nutrition interventions [12]. A number of CF related medications can be passed through breast milk. Medications used during breastfeeding should be reviewed for safety [7]. It is also important to consider social supports & nutritional status before/during pregnancy as breastfeeding can be challenging for a woman who already herself has a complicated burden of treatment [7]. Above all, patient choice/preference must be considered the most important part of a decision to breastfeed. The mom's decision should be fully supported by the entire team.

Conclusion

The nutrition management of pregnancy in CF presents a number of challenges. Despite a lack of evidence and guidelines to optimize nutrition management there are many successful outcomes reported. Careful nutrition assessment and interventions can allow for successful pregnancies.

References

1. Siegel D, Siegel S. Pregnancy and delivery in a patient with cystic fibrosis of the pancreas. Obstet Gynecol. 1960;16:439–40.
2. Gillijam M, Antoniou M, Shin J, et al. Pregnancy in cystic fibrosis: fetal and maternal outcome. Chest. 2000;118: 85–91.
3. Edenborough FP, Stableforth DE, Webb AK, et al. Outcome of pregnancy in women with cystic fibrosis. Thorax. 1995;50:170–4.
4. Burden C, Ion R, Chung Y, et al. Current pregnancy outcomes in women with cystic fibrosis. Eur J Obstet Gynecol Reprod Biol. 2012;164(2):142–5.
5. Ødegaard I, Stray-Pedersen B, Hallberg K. Maternal and fetal morbidity in pregnancies of Norwegian and Swedish women with cystic fibrosis. Acta Obstet Gynecol Scand. 2002;81(8):698–705.
6. Schechter, MS, Quittner, AL, Konstan, MW, et al. Long-term Effects of Pregnancy and Motherhood on Disease Outcomes of Women with Cystic Fibrosis. Ann Am Thorac Soc. 2013;10(3):213–9.

7. Edenborough FP, Borgo G, Knoop C, et al. Guidelines for the management of pregnancy in cystic fibrosis. J Cyst Fibros. 2008;7(1):S2–32.
8. Schram CA, Stephenson AL, Hannam TG, et al. Cystic Fibrosis (cf) and ovarian reserve: a cross-sectional study examining serum anti-mullerian hormone (AMH) in young women. J Cyst Fibros. 2014; pii: S1569-1993(14)00219-7 [Epub ahead of print].
9. Ahmad A, Ahmed A, Patrizio P, et al. Cystic fibrosis and fertility. Curr Opin Obstet Gynecol. 2013;25(3):167–72.
10. Morton A, Wolfe S, Conway SP. Dietetic intervention in pregnancy in women with CF—the importance of pre-conceptional counselling. Israel J Med Sci. 1996;32:S271.
11. McArdle JR. Pregnancy in cystic fibrosis. Clin Chest Med. 2011;32(1):111–20.
12. Berzy D, Mehta A, Carlson S, et al. Pregnancy. Manual of clinical dietetics. Chicago: American Dietetic Association; 2000.
13. Boyd JM, Mehta A, Murphy DJ. Fertility and pregnancy outcomes in men and women with cystic fibrosis in the United Kingdom. Hum Reprod. 2004;19:2238–43.
14. Lau EM, Moriarty C, Ogle R, et al. Pregnancy and cystic fibrosis. Pediatr Respir Rev. 2010;11:90–4.
15. Stallings VA, Stark LF, Robinson KA, Feranchak AP, Quinton H. Evidence-based practice recommendations for nutrition-related management of children and adults with cystic fibrosis and pancreatic insufficiency: results of a systematic review. J Am Diet Assoc. 2008;108:832–9.
16. Cystic Fibrosis Trust Nutrition Working Group. Nutritional management of cystic fibrosis. London: Cystic Fibrosis Trust; 2002.
17. Kent NE, Farquharson DF. Cystic fibrosis in pregnancy. CMAJ. 1993;149:809–13.
18. World Health Organization. Vitamin A dosage during pregnancy and lactation. Recommendations and report of a consultation; 1998. Document NUT/98.4.
19. Moran A, Brunzell C, Cohen RC, et al. Clinical care guidelines for cystic fibrosis-related diabetes: a position statement of the American Diabetes Association and a clinical practice guideline of the Cystic Fibrosis Foundation, endorsed by the Pediatric Endocrine Society. Diabetes Care. 2010;33(12):2697–708.
20. Lexicomp Online®, Pediatric & Neonatal Lexi-Drugs®, Hudson, OH: Lexi-Comp, Inc.; 29 January 2015. http://webstore.lexi.com/s.nl/ctype.KB/it.I/id.342/KB.3234/.f.
21. Enright BP, McIntyre BS, Thackaberry EA, et al. Assessment of hydroxypropyl methylcellulose, propylene glycol, polysorbate 80, and hydroxypropyl-β-cyclodextrin for use in developmental and reproductive toxicology studies. Birth Defects Res B Dev Reprod Toxicol. 2010;89(6):504–16.
22. Food and Drug Administration. Guidelines for industry; limiting the use of certain phthalates as excipients in CDER-regulated products. December 2010.
23. Keller BO, Davidson AG, Innis SM. Phthalate metabolites in urine of CF patients are associated with use of enteric-coated pancreatic enzymes. Environ Toxicol Pharmacol. 2009;27(3):424–7. doi:10.1016/j.etap.2008.12.005. Epub 2009 Jan 14.
24. Cystic Fibrosis Foundation. Phthalates and pancreatic enzymes (position statement). March 2012 (website publication).
25. Suzanne H. Michel, MPH, RD, LDN. Excerpt on phthalates and pregnancy for women with cystic fibrosis. (unpublished work, used with permission) 2014.
26. Weight gain during pregnancy. Committee Opinion No. 548. American College of Obstetricians and Gynecologists. Obstet Gynecol. 2013;121:210–2.
27. Hark L, Catalano PM. Nutritional management during pregnancy. Obstetrics: normal and problem pregnancies. 6th ed. Philadelphia, PA: Saunders Elsevier; 2012 (Chapter 7).
28. Pencharz PB, Durie PR. Nutritional management of cystic fibrosis. Annu Rev Nutr. 1993;13:111–36.
29. Borowitz D, Gelfond D. Intestinal complications of cystic fibrosis. Curr Opin Pulm Med. 2013;19(6):676–80. doi:10.1097/MCP.0b013e3283659ef2.
30. Lassi ZS, Salam RA, Haider BA, et al. Folic acid supplementation during pregnancy for maternal health and pregnancy outcomes. Cochrane Database Syst Rev. 2013;3:CD006896.
31. Tangpricha V, Kelly A, Stephenson A, et al. An update on the screening, diagnosis, management, and treatment of vitamin D deficiency in individuals with cystic fibrosis: evidence-based recommendations from the Cystic Fibrosis Foundation. J Clin Endocrinol Metab. 2012;97(4):1082–93.
32. Johnson EJ, Russell RM. Beta-carotene. In: Coates PM, Betz JM, Blackman MR, et al., editors. Encyclopedia of dietary supplements. 2nd ed. London and New York: Informa Healthcare; 2010. p. 115–20.
33. Werler MM, Lammer EJ, Mitchell AA. Teratogenicity of high Vitamin A intake. N Engl J Med. 1996;334:1195–7. author reply 1197.
34. http://www.yasoo.com/products/aquadeks/
35. Suhonen L, Hiilesmaa V, Teramo K. Glycaemic control during early pregnancy and foetal malformations in women with type I diabetes mellitus. Diabetologia. 2000;43:79–82.

36. Hardin DS, Rice J, Cohen RC, et al. The metabolic effects of pregnancy in cystic fibrosis. Obstet Gynaecol. 2005;106:367–75.
37. Clinical Practice Guidelines Expert Committee, Canadian Diabetes Association. Clinical Practice Guidelines, 2003.
38. Shiffman ML, Seale TW, Flux M, et al. Breast-milk composition in women with cystic fibrosis: report of two cases and a review of the literature. Am J Clin Nutr. 1989;49(4):612.
39. Mahomed K, Gulmezoglu AM. Vitamin D supplementation in pregnancy. Cochrane Database Syst Rev 1999, Issue 1. Art No.: CD000228.

Chapter 16
Nutrition for Pancreatic Sufficient Individuals with Cystic Fibrosis

John F. Pohl and Catherine M. McDonald

Key Points

- Cystic fibrosis (CF) is typically associated with exocrine pancreatic insufficiency (PI)
- Although patients with CF and PS typically have milder CF transmembrane conductance regulator (CFTR) gene mutations, they are still at risk of malnutrition without careful monitoring.
- Tests for pancreatic exocrine status, including the fecal elastase-1 (FE-1) immunosorbent assay, should be used to determine exocrine status as well as to monitor for progression to a PI status.
- CF patients with PS are at risk of pancreatitis and testing for this scenario should be considered if clinically warranted.

Keywords Pancreas • Sufficiency • Elastase • Celiac • Pancreatitis

Introduction

Cystic fibrosis (CF) is typically associated with exocrine pancreatic insufficiency (PI) and nutritional care of the CF patient with exocrine pancreatic sufficiency (PS) is less well described. Although patients with CF and PS typically have milder CF transmembrane conductance regulator (CFTR) gene mutations, they are still at risk of malnutrition without careful monitoring. Tests for pancreatic exocrine status should be used to determine exocrine status as well as to monitor for progression to a PI status. Such tests include the fecal elastase-1 (FE-1) immunosorbent assay which is associated with excellent sensitivity and specificity. Clinicians also should be aware that CF patients with PS are at risk of pancreatitis and testing for this scenario should be considered if clinically warranted.

According to the 2012 Cystic Fibrosis Foundation's Patient Registry Annual Data Report, 87.3% of people with CF use pancreatic enzyme supplements for pancreatic exocrine insufficiency, suggesting approximately 12.7% of CF patients are pancreatic sufficient (PS) [1]. Other estimates of PS with cystic fibrosis range between 11 to 15% [2, 3]. Generally, PS is associated with milder CFTR

J.F. Pohl, M.D. (✉) • C.M. McDonald, Ph.D., R.D.N.
Division of Pediatric Gastroenterology, Department of Pediatrics, Primary Children's Hospital,
University of Utah, Salt Lake City, UT 84112, USA
e-mail: john.pohl@hsc.utah.edu

E.H. Yen, A.R. Leonard (eds.), *Nutrition in Cystic Fibrosis: A Guide for Clinicians*, Nutrition and Health,
DOI 10.1007/978-3-319-16387-1_16, © Springer International Publishing Switzerland 2015

phenotypes and better nutritional status [4–7]. However, persons with CF PS are not exempt from gastrointestinal and/or nutritional problems. Pancreatic status is not a predictor of mortality after adjusting for CFTR genotype, lung function, and BMI [4–7]

Nutrition Goals

Regardless of pancreatic status, the primary goal for any infant, children, or adolescent with CF is to attain and maintain normal growth for age [6–8]. Infants should achieve weight-for-age and length-for-age percentiles similar to the non-CF population by 2 years [8]. A body mass index (BMI) of at least 50 percentile is recommended for children and adolescents with CF [8, 9]. Among CF children aged 5–10 years, a positive correlation is noted between BMI and PS [4].

All adults with CF should maintain an absolute BMI greater than 20 kg/m^2 (preferably 22 kg/m^2 for females and 23 kg/m^2 for males [9, 10]).

Assessment of Nutritional Status

A thorough nutritional assessment, regardless of exocrine pancreas status, is recommended for all CF patients, and a registered dietitian/nutritionist with expertise in CF nutrition care is imperative in the care of these patients [8–12]. The Cystic Fibrosis Foundation recommends that a nutritional assessment occurs at least annually in the outpatient setting [8, 9]. In children, length/height, weight, and BMI should be determined using Center for Disease Control growth charts [13]. Growth monitoring for PS children and weight/BMI monitoring for PS adults should be conducted according to Cystic Fibrosis Foundation recommendations for clinical care [11]. Other nutritional parameters, including fat-soluble vitamin and micronutrient status, should be monitored and maintained within normal limits for age [10]. Whether PS or PI, the goal of nutritional treatment for infants, children, and adolescents with CF is to maintain normal growth for age [8, 9]. Maintaining appropriate BMI in pediatric CF patients is associated with better forced expiratory volume in 1 s (FEV$_1$), so utilization of newborn CF screening and serial determinations of BMI over time is necessary [14, 15].

The Cystic Fibrosis Foundation evidence-based guidelines for management of infants with CF do not differentiate between PS and PI for treatment recommendations for feedings, vitamins, and other micronutrients [8]. As with any infant, breastfeeding is recommended for infants with CF, regardless of pancreatic status. If infants with CF are formula fed, standard infant formulas (as opposed to hydrolyzed protein formulas) should be used [8]. Calorie-dense feedings should be used if weight loss occurs or inadequate weight gain is observed [8]. The introduction of complementary foods should be delayed until at least 4–6 months of age per guidelines of the American Academy of Pediatrics [16]. As children progress toward school-age years as well as adolescence, caloric requirements will increase again as children become involved with physical activities [17].

Not all adult CF PS patients maintain adequate nutrition. Descriptions of underweight (BMI < 18.5 kg/m^2) range from 3.8 to 6.7% in CF PS adults [6, 7]. However, PS and milder CF genotypes are associated with an increased propensity for overweight (BMI 25–29) and obesity (BMI $\geq$ 30) than CF PI [6]. Although a positive association exists between pulmonary function and BMI, the potential benefit of overweight or obesity for any person with CF may be offset by the known risks, such as cardiovascular disease and metabolic syndrome [6, 11].

CF PS patients may be at the same risk of hyperlipidemia as the general population [12]. Although overweight and obesity are more common in CF PS patients, hypertriglyceridemia is associated with elevated BMI in CF regardless of pancreatic status [18]. The Cystic Fibrosis Foundation currently does not have specific recommendations for lipid monitoring for CF PS patients other than those for the general pediatric and adult populations [12, 19].

Individualized medical nutrition therapy should address each patient's specific needs. Persons with CF PS may have lower energy requirements compared with those with more severe genotypes [6]. High-calorie, high-fat diets may not be appropriate for CF PS children and adults [6]. Further studies are needed to delineate more specific nutrition requirements for those patients with PS and milder expressions of CF.

Vitamin and Mineral Status

The CF patient with pancreatic sufficiency (PS) should be able to maintain normal fat-soluble vitamin levels (vitamins A, D, E, and K) due to preservation of exocrine pancreatic function, and it is less common for fat-soluble vitamin deficiencies to occur in this specific population [20]. Regardless, fat-soluble vitamin levels should be obtained annually in all CF patients. Vitamin A is typically measured as a serum retinol level, and low levels of this vitamin can lead to night blindness [21, 22]. Vitamin D is measured in its hepatic-derived form known as 25-hydroxyvitamin D or calcifediol, and normal levels of this vitamin are needed for osteoporosis prevention and reduction of CF respiratory exacerbations [23–25]. Vitamin D is synthesized by exposure to sunlight, is affected by northern latitude climates where there is decreased ultraviolet B radiation, and is associated with lower levels during the winter season of these geographic locations [26]. Vitamin E (alpha tocopherol) is measured often through high-performance liquid chromatography and can be associated with neuropathy at low levels although neuropathy is rarely observed in CF patients [27]. Prothrombin time and partial thromboplastin time are used as indicators of vitamin K status although testing, including measuring plasma proteins induced by vitamin K absence factor II and percentage of serum undercarboxylated osteocalcin can be used to directly measure vitamin K in experimental settings [20, 28].

In a similar manner, CF patients with PS should not have any water-soluble vitamin or mineral deficiencies. Iron, zinc, and copper deficiencies have been described in CF patients, but such studies have not delineated associated exocrine pancreas status [29]. Iron deficiency occurs in CF and can be associated with worsening lung disease, including *Pseudomonas aeruginosa* infections although healthy CF children also can have iron deficiency [30]. In particular, *P. aeruginosa* can acquire iron from its host's hemoglobin [31]. Serum ferritin is an acute-phase reactant and can be elevated in CF patients with associated inflammation, such as in the setting of a pulmonary exacerbation [30]. Salt supplementation also may be needed in both PS and PI CF infants to prevent failure to thrive [32]. Calcium supplementation should be given concurrently with vitamin D use in order to facilitate calcium absorption. It is unknown if there is a maximum dosing of vitamin D that enhances calcium absorption in CF patients although high dosing for Vitamin D dosing is recommended [33]. Magnesium deficiency has been reported in CF pediatric patients, and hypomagnesemia can be associated with decreased respiratory muscle strength although specific deficiency is not commonly reported in the CF population [34]. Folic acid, copper, thiamine (vitamin B1), riboflavin (vitamin B2), pyridoxine (vitamin B6), and cobalamin (vitamin B_{12}) can be associated with neuropathy; however, it is unclear if neuropathy in the setting of CF is due to these specific deficiencies [27].

In particular, CF patients with a history of ileum resection (as in a meconium ileus presentation) can have impaired absorption of vitamin B_{12}. Vitamin B_{12} from the diet is combined with R protein in the saliva and intrinsic factor in the stomach. Pancreatic proteases break down R protein to facilitate binding of Vitamin B_{12} linked intrinsic factor to its receptor in the terminal ileum. In the setting of CF, pancreatic insufficiency (PI) can affect vitamin B_{12} absorption which is further complicated in any CF patient with ileal resection [35]. Of note, high vitamin B_{12} levels from excessive vitamin B_{12} intake have been associated with a decline in forced expiratory volume at 1 s (FEV_1) in pediatric CF patients, but the cause of this finding is unknown and it is unclear if CF patients with PS have this same outcome as those patients who have PI [36].

Table 16.1 Testing methods of exocrine pancreatic insufficiency [38]

Stool smear	Test is not recommended. False positives can occur with petroleum lubricants
72-h fecal fat collection	Fecal fat output greater than 7% is considered positive. Test is time consuming. Constipation can cause false negatives. Stool must be collected in container and not in toilet
Steatocrit	Crude technique for determining fat malabsorption in stool by centrifuging in hematocrit tubing. Test is not recommended
Stool trypsin or chymotrypsin measurement	Enzymes are degraded easily in stool, so false negatives are possible. Test is not recommended
Breath testing	This test is typically done by hydrogen breath testing. Test is difficult for young children to do. False positives occur in bacterial overgrowth or intestinal dysmotility
Duodenal pancreatic enzyme collection	This test is accurate but very invasive. Intravenous secretin or cholecystokinin can increase sample yield. Low pH can decrease pancreatic enzyme levels due to degradation
Fecal pancreatic elastase-1 testing	This test has excellent sensitivity and specificity. Only a small amount of stool is needed. FE-1 levels can be decreased in diarrhea or intestinal inflammation. Other causes of pancreatic exocrine insufficiency can demonstrate a low FE-1 level (i.e., Shwachman–Diamond Syndrome)

Assessing Pancreatic Status

Most CF children are tested for PI at the same time they are diagnosed with CF, and standard testing for CF includes sweat testing, DNA screening, or newborn screening through immunoreactive trypsinogen. PI is diagnosed in the majority of CF patients [37]. PS patients should be tested for exocrine PI if there is evidence of pancreatic dysfunction such as diarrhea due to malabsorption, steatorrhea, abdominal pain, or weight loss. Several tests of variable sensitivity and specificity exist to diagnose PI including the stool smear utilizing the Sudan stain, the 72-h stool collection to determine fractional excretion of fecal fat, steatocrit, measurement of trypsin and chymotrypsin, breath testing, and duodenal intubation to obtain pancreatic enzymes after intravenous administration of secretin or cholecystokinin (Table 16.1). Duodenal intubation to obtain pancreatic enzymes is considered the most accurate test, although it is invasive and difficult to perform. On the other hand, fecal elastase-1 (FE-1) is an easy test to perform with associated excellent sensitivity and specificity. FE-1 is excreted from the pancreas and into the stool and has the advantage of not being affected by bacterial degradation or use of pancreatic enzyme replacement therapy [38]. FE-1 is measured using a human monoclonal enzyme-linked immunosorbent assay and has no special storage requirements. FE-1 measurements are significantly lower in PI patients compared to PS patients and can help delineate exocrine pancreatic status [2]. Currently, measurement of FE-1 is considered standard of care to diagnose pancreatic exocrine status and is recommended as annual testing in all CF PS patients [39].

It should be noted that other diseases associated with exocrine PI can be associated with a low FE-1 measurement, including Shwachman–Diamond Syndrome [40]. Low FE-1 levels are also associated with intestinal resection as in "short bowel syndrome," intestinal inflammation, and many gastrointestinal diseases associated with diarrhea. False-positive FE-1 testing in these clinical scenarios occur as a result of diarrhea symptoms [41, 42]. Celiac disease also has been associated with a low FE-1. The cause of low FE-1 in celiac disease is likely multi-factorial including diarrhea associated with celiac disease, villous atrophy leading to decreased pancreatic enzyme production, and elevated peptide YY associated with celiac disease leading to decreased pancreatic enzyme production. It is unknown if pancreatic enzyme replacement therapy is helpful in such patients with celiac disease [43]. However, FE-1 typically returns to normal levels after intestinal mucosa regeneration occurs on a gluten-free diet [44].

Table 16.2 Nutritional parameters to be followed in CF patients [54]

Growth parameters (length/height, weight, BMI)
Fecal elastase (to be checked annually in the PS patient)
Vitamin A (measure serum retinol)
Vitamin D (measure 25-hydroxy vitamin D or calcifediol)
Vitamin E
Vitamin K (measure prothrombin time and partial thromboplastin time)
Vitamin B_{12} (if history of surgery to terminal ileum, measure serum methylmalonic acid)
Serum electrolytes, especially serum sodium
Calcium
Zinc
Iron (consider serum iron, iron binding capacity, transferrin saturation, ferritin). Remember that ferritin is an acute-phase reactant in the setting of acute inflammation
Glucose (oral glucose tolerance test if concern for cystic fibrosis-related diabetes)
Essential fatty acid screen

Annual Assessment

CF patients with PS need to have exocrine pancreatic status and nutritional parameters followed carefully (Table 16.2). Most CF patients with PS will progress to PI in the first 2 years of life although a decline in pancreatic exocrine function can occur more gradually [45, 46]. It is recommended that CF patients with PS undergo annual FE-1 testing as part of their annual CF laboratory testing [47]. If a CF patient converts to PI, pancreatic enzyme replacement therapy with the addition of gastric acid suppression therapy (H_2 receptor antagonist or proton pump inhibitor) should be considered per established guidelines as outlined by the Cystic Fibrosis Foundation [48]. Although uncommon in the setting of CF, other causes of PI may need to be considered, if clinically warranted (Table 16.3) [38].

Another consideration in the setting of a CF PS who has symptoms of abdominal pain, diarrhea, malabsorption, and weight loss is the possible diagnosis of celiac disease. Celiac disease can present with symptoms similar to PI, and testing for celiac disease should occur with any CF PS patient or CF PI patient who has continued symptoms despite being on pancreatic enzyme replacement therapy [49]. Clinical studies have demonstrated that the percentage of patients with celiac disease in CF patient populations ranges from 1.2 to 2.13% which is considered a higher prevalence compared to the general population [49–51]. The diagnosis of celiac disease requires screening blood work, including the tissue transglutaminase IgA antibody titer followed by esophagogastroduodenoscopy with duodenal biopsies if serum antibody titers are positive[49]. Typical duodenal biopsies in the setting of celiac disease will reveal a spectrum of villous atrophy, crypt hyperplasia, and increased intraepithelial lymphocytes based on the Marsh-Oberhuber classification system [52]. A gluten-free diet, with the help of a dietitian with experience in both cystic fibrosis and celiac disease, is critical to provide dietary education for these diseases. Guidelines for celiac disease diagnosis and management are readily available from many gastroenterology societies [53, 54].

Pancreatitis in the Setting of Exocrine Pancreatic Sufficiency

CF PS patients are at risk of acute pancreatitis (AP). In particular, CF patients with PS or CF patients with borderline sweat tests are predisposed to AP [55]. Mutations to the (CFTR) gene lead to pancreatitis in CF PS patients as well as in some non-CF patients with heterozygous CFTR mutations. The mechanism of AP development may be due to decreased bicarbonate secretion in the

Table 16.3 Causes of pancreatic insufficiency in children [38]

Cystic fibrosis (most common cause of pancreatic insufficiency)
Shwachman–Diamond syndrome (second most common cause of pancreatic insufficiency)
Chronic pancreatitis (anatomical obstruction, hereditary pancreatitis, etc.)
Johanson–Blizzard syndrome
Pearson's bone marrow syndrome
Congenital rubella syndrome
Pancreatic isolated enzyme defects
Pancreas agenesis/hypoplasia

Reproduced with permission from Practical Gastroenterology, Practical Gastroenterology Publishing, Inc.

pancreatic duct in which a subsequent decrease in pH leads to premature activation of trypsin and loss of tight junction integrity leading to a process of pancreatic autodigestion. Interestingly, patients with mild CF phenotypes (including CF PS patients) have a greater risk of AP, presumably due to their retaining of some residual pancreatic duct flow [56]. AP can be seen in CF PS patients, although CF PI patients can present with AP with similar elevations in serum amylase and lipase if residual functioning pancreatic tissue is present. Rarely, AP also is an initial presenting symptom of CF [57]. Heterozygote CFTR mutations are a common cause of chronic pancreatitis (CP) and should be considered in any patient, regardless of CF status, who presents with acute recurrent pancreatitis (ARP) or CP. Additionally, CFTR mutations can potentially interact with other genetic causes of ARP or CP, such as mutations of SPINK1, PRSS1, and CTRC, which can further exacerbate pancreatitis symptoms [58].

In summary, CF PS patients should follow the same nutritional guidelines set out for CF PI patients. Pancreatic exocrine function can decline over time and careful monitoring for this scenario is needed to avoid nutritional complications arising from untreated evolving PI. Annual testing for exocrine pancreatic function with a FE-1 stool assay is recommended. CF PS patients should also be monitored for development of acute pancreatitis.

Conclusion

Although CF patients with PS are not common, it should be understood that such patients are at risk of developing PI over time. Subsequently, these patients need careful monitoring of their nutritional status as well as making sure they are not developing exocrine PI. Testing for PI, such as measuring FE-1, should be considered for any CF PS patient who is losing weight or showing signs of malabsorption. CF PS patients are at risk of acute pancreatitis (AP) and chronic pancreatitis (CP), and any CF PS patient who presents with significant abdominal pain should have a serum amylase, serum lipase, and appropriate imaging (such as an abdominal ultrasound) obtained.

References

1. Cystic Fibrosis Foundation Patient Registry. 2012 annual data report. Bethesda, MD: Cystic Fibrosis Foundation; 2013.
2. Borowitz D, Baker SS, Duffy L, Baker RD, Fitzpatrick L, Gyamfi J, et al. Use of fecal elastase-1 to identify misclassification of pancreatic functional status in patients with cystic fibrosis. J Pediatr. 2004;145:322–6.
3. Couper RTL, Corey M, Moore DJ, Fisher LG, Forstner GG, Drurie PR. Decline of exocrine pancreatic function in patients with pancreatic sufficiency. Pediatr Res. 1992;32:179–82.

4. Bradley GM, Blackburn SM, Watson CP, Doshi VK, Cutting GR. Genetic modifiers of nutritional status in cystic fibrosis. Am J Clin Nutr. 2012;96:1299–308.

5. McKone EF, Goss CH, Aitken ML. CFTR genotype as a predictor of prognosis in cystic fibrosis. Chest. 2006;130:1441–7.

6. Stephenson AL, Mannik LA, Walsh S, Brotherwood M, Robert R, Darling PB, et al. Longitudinal trends in nutritional status and the relation between lung function and BMI in cystic fibrosis: a population-based cohort study. Am J Clin Nutr. 2013;97:872–7.

7. Dray X, Kanaan R, Bienvenu T, Desmazes-Dufeu N, Dusser D, Marteau P, et al. Malnutrition in adults with cystic fibrosis. Eur J Clin Nutr. 2005;59:152–4.

8. Borowitz D, Robinson KA, Rosenfeld M, Davis SD, Sabadosa KA, Spear SL, et al. Cystic fibrosis foundation evidence-based guidelines for management of infants with cystic fibrosis. J Pediatr. 2009;155:S73–93.

9. Borowitz D, Baker RD, Stallings V. Consensus on nutrition for pediatric patients with cystic fibrosis. J Pediatr Gastroenterol Nutr. 2002;35:246–59.

10. Smyth AR, Bell SC, Bojcin S, Bryon M, Duff A, Flume P, et al. European cystic fibrosis society standards of care: best practice guidelines. J Cyst Fibros. 2014;13:S23–42.

11. Stallings VA, Stark LJ, Robinson KA, Feranchak AP, Quinton H, Clinical Practice Guidelines on Growth and Nutrition Subcommittee, Ad Hoc Working Group. Evidence-based practice recommendations for nutrition-related management of children and adults with cystic fibrosis and pancreatic insufficiency: results of a systematic review. J Am Diet Assoc. 2008;108:832–9.

12. Yankaskas JR, Marshall BC, Sufian B, Simon R, Rodman D. Cystic fibrosis adult care consensus conference report. Chest. 2004;125:1S–39.

13. Centers for Disease Control Growth Charts. Available at http://www.cdc.gov/growthcharts/. Last Accessed 24 Nov 2014.

14. Martin B, Schechter M, Jaffe A, Cooper P, Bell S, Ranganathan S. Comparison of the US and Australian cystic fibrosis registries: the impact of newborn screening. Pediatrics. 2012;129(2):e348–55.

15. Peterson M, Jacobs D, Milla C. Longitudinal changes in growth parameters are correlated with changes in pulmonary function in children with cystic fibrosis. Pediatrics. 2003;112(3 Pt 1):588–92.

16. Grimshaw KEC, Maskell J, Oliver EM, Morris ECG, Foote KD, Mills C, et al. Introduction of complementary foods and the relationship to food allergy. Pediatrics. 2013;132:e1529–38.

17. Karlberg J, Kjellmer I, Kristiansson B. Linear growth in children with cystic fibrosis. I. birth to 8 years of age. Acta Paediatr Scand. 1991;80(5):508–14.

18. Ishimo M-C, Belson L, Ziai S, Levy E, Berthiaume Y, Coderre L, Rabasa-Lhoret R. Hypertriglyceridemia is associated with insulin levels in adult cystic fibrosis patients. J Cyst Fibros. 2013;12:271–6.

19. US preventive services task force. Final recommendation statement lipid disorders in adults (cholesterol, dyslipidemia): screening. Available at http://www.uspreventiveservicestaskforce.org/Page/Document/RecommendationStatementFinal/lipid-disorders-in-adults-cholesterol-dyslipidemia-screening.Last Accessed 19 Nov 2014.

20. Rana M, Wong-See D, Katz T, Gaskin K, Whitehead B, Jaffe A, et al. Fat-soluble vitamin deficiency in children and adolescents with cystic fibrosis. J Clin Pathol. 2014;67:605–8.

21. Brei C, Simon A, Krawinkel M, Naehrlich L. Individualized vitamin A supplementation for patients with cystic fibrosis. Clin Nutr. 2013;32(5):805–10.

22. Roddy M, Greally P, Clancy G, Leen G, Feehan S, Elnazir B. Night blindness in a teenager with cystic fibrosis. Nutr Clin Pract. 2011;26(6):718–21.

23. Sheikh S, Gemma S, Patel A. Factors associated with low bone mineral density in patients with cystic fibrosis. J Bone Miner Metab. 2014;33(2):180–5.

24. Javier R, Jacquot J. Bone disease in cystic fibrosis: what's new? Joint Bone Spine. 2011;78(5):445–50.

25. Gilbert C, Arum S, Smith C. Vitamin D deficiency and chronic lung disease. Can Respir J. 2009;16(3):75–80.

26. Rosecrans R, Dohnal J. Seasonal vitamin D changes and the impact on health risk assessment. Clin Biochem. 2014;47(7–8):670–2.

27. Chakrabarty B, Kabra S, Gulati S, Toteja G, Lodha R, Kabra M, et al. Peripheral neuropathy in cystic fibrosis: a prevalence study. J Cyst Fibros. 2013;12(6):754–60.

28. Bertolaso C, Groleau V, Schall J, Maqbool A, Mascarenhas M, Latham N, et al. Fat-soluble vitamins in cystic fibrosis and pancreatic insufficiency: efficacy of nutrition intervention. J Pediatr Gastroenterol Nutr. 2014;58(4):443–8.

29. Yadav K, Singh M, Angurana S, Attri S, Sharma G, Tageja M, et al. Evaluation of micronutrient profile in North Indian children with cystic fibrosis: a case–control study. Pediatr Res. 2014;75(6):762–6.

30. Uijterschout L, Nuijsink M, Hendriks D, Vos R, Brus F. Iron deficiency occurs frequently in children with cystic fibrosis. Pediatr Pulmonol. 2014;49(5):458–62.

31. Marviq R, Damkiaer S, Khademi S, Markussen T, Molin S, Jelsbak L. Within-host evolution of pseudomonas aeruginosa reveals adaption toward iron acquisition from hemoglobin. MBio. 2014;5(3):e00966–14.

32. Coates A, Crofton P, Marshall T. Evaluation of salt supplementation in CF infants. J Cyst Fibros. 2009; 8(6):382–5.

33. Ferguson J, Chang A. Vitamin D supplementation for cystic fibrosis. Cochrane Database Syst Rev. 2014;5:CD007298.

34. Gontijo-Amaral C, Guimaraes E, Camargos P. Oral magnesium supplementation in children with cystic fibrosis improves clinical and functional variables: a double-blind, randomized, placebo-controlled crossover trial. Am J Clin Nutr. 2012;96(1):50–6.

35. Kotilea K, Quennery S, Decroes V, Hermans D. Successful sublingual cobalamin treatment in a child with short bowel syndrome. J Pediatr Pharmacol Ther. 2014;19(1):60–3.

36. Maqbool A, Schall J, Mascarenhas M, Dougherty K, Stallings V. Vitamin B12 status in children with cystic fibrosis and pancreatic insufficiency. J Pediatr Gastroenterol Nutr. 2014;58(6):733–8.

37. Weintraub A, Blau H, Mussaffi H, Picard E, Bentur L, Kerem E, et al. Exocrine pancreatic function testing in patients with cystic fibrosis and pancreatic sufficiency: a correlation study. J Pediatr Gastroenterol Nutr. 2009;48(3):306–10.

38. Pohl J, Easley D. Pancreatic insufficiency in children. Pract Gastroenterol. 2003;27(10):38–48.

39. Luth S, Teyssen S, Forssmann K, Kolbel C, Krummenauer F, Singer M. Fecal elastase-1 determination: 'gold standard' of indirect pancreatic function tests? Scand J Gastroenterol. 2001;36(10):1092–6.

40. Gokce M, Tuncer M, Cetin M, Gumruk F. Molecular diagnosis of Schwachman–Diamond syndrome presenting with pancytopenia at an early age: the first report from Turkey. Indian J Hematol Blood Transfus. 2013;29(3):161–3.

41. Carroccio A, Verghi F, Santini B, Lucidi V, Iacono G, Cavataio F, et al. Diagnostic accuracy of fecal elastase 1 assay in patients with pancreatic maldigestion or intestinal malabsorption: a collaborative study of the Italian Society of Pediatric Gastroenterology and Hepatology. Dig Dis Sci. 2001;46(6):1335–42.

42. Salvatore S, Finazzi S, Barassi A, Verzelletti M, Tosi A, Melzi d'Eril G, et al. Low fecal elastase: potentially related to transient small bowel damage resulting from enteric pathogens. J Pediatr Gastroenterol Nutr. 2003;36(3):392–6.

43. Evans K, Leeds J, Morley S, Sanders D. Pancreatic insufficiency in adult celiac disease: do patients require long-term enzyme supplementation? Dig Dis Sci. 2010;55(10):2999–3004.

44. Walkowiak J, Herzig K. Fecal elastase-1 is decreased in villous atrophy regardless of the underlying disease. Eur J Clin Invest. 2001;31(5):425–30.

45. O'Sullivan BP, Baker D, Leung KG, Reed G, Baker SS, Borowitz D. Evolution of pancreatic function during the first year in infants with cystic fibrosis. J Pediatr. 2013;162:808–12.

46. Walkowiak J, Nousia-Arvanitakis S, Agguridaki C, Fotoulaki M, Strzykala K, Balassopoulou A, et al. Longitudinal follow-up of exocrine pancreatic function in pancreatic sufficient cystic fibrosis patients using fecal elastase-1 test. J Pediatr Gastroenterol Nutr. 2003;36(4):474–8.

47. Doull I. What and when to collect from infants with cystic fibrosis. Arch Dis Child. 2007;92(10):831–2.

48. http://www.cff.org/UploadedFiles/treatments/CFCareGuidelines/Nutrition/Consensus-Statement-Pancreatic-Enzyme-Replacement-March-1995.pdf. Last Accessed 19 Nov 2014.

49. Pohl J, Judkins J, Meihls S, Lowichik A, Chatfield B, McDonald C. Cystic fibrosis and celiac disease: both can occur together. Clin Pediatr. 2011;50(12):1153–5.

50. Fluge G, Olesen H, Gilljam M, Meyer P, Pressler T, Storroston O, et al. Co-morbidity of cystic fibrosis and celiac disease in Scandinavian cystic fibrosis patients. J Cyst Fibros. 2009;8(3):198–202.

51. Walkowiak J, Blask-Osipa A, Lisowska A, Oralewska B, Pogorzelski A, Cichy W, et al. Cystic fibrosis is a risk factor for celiac disease. Acta Biochim Pol. 2010;57(1):115–8.

52. Dickson B, Streutker C, Chetty R. Coeliac disease: an update for pathologists. J Clin Pathol. 2006;59(10):1008–16.

53. Institute AGA. AGA Institute medical position statement on the diagnosis and management of celiac disease. Gastroenterology. 2006;131(6):1977–80.

54. Hill I, Dirks M, Liptak G, Colletti R, Fasano A, Guadalini S, et al. Guideline for the diagnosis and treatment of celiac disease in children: recommendations of the North American Society for Pediatric Gastroenterology, Hepatology and Nutrition. J Pediatr Gastroenterol Nutr. 2005;40:1–19.

55. Terlizzi V, Tosco A, Tomaiuolo R, Sepe A, Amato N, Casale A, et al. Prediction of acute pancreatitis risk based on PIP score in children with cystic fibrosis. J Cyst Fibros. 2014;13(5):579–84.

56. Ooi C, Durie P. Cystic fibrosis transmembrane conductance regulator (CFTR) gene mutations in pancreatitis. J Cyst Fibros. 2012;11(5):355–62.

57. De Boeck K, Weren M, Proesmans M, Kerem E. Pancreatitis among patients with cystic fibrosis: correlation with pancreatic status and genotype. Pediatrics. 2005;115(4):e463–9.

58. Masson E, Chen J, Audrezet M, Cooper D, Ferec C. A conservative assessment of the major genetic causes of idiopathic chronic pancreatitis: data from a comprehensive analysis of PRSS1, SPINK1, CTRC and CFTR genes in 253 young French patients. PLoS One. 2013;8(8):e73522.

Chapter 17
Behavioral Interventions and Anticipatory Guidance

Jamie L. Ryan, Stephanie S. Filigno, and Lori J. Stark

Key Points

- For more than a decade, the nutritional guidelines set forth by the CF Foundation have recommended a behavioral assessment of mealtime behaviors in youth with CF to identify factors associated with nutritional management and to promote optimal growth through early intervention.
- Adherence to nutritional guidelines in CF is poor with fewer than 25% of children reaching the minimum recommended 120% DRI for energy. Of the factors associated with dietary adherence, disruptive child mealtime behavior coupled with ineffective parenting strategies are salient predictors of lower calorie intake and lower weight status.
- The Behavioral Pediatrics Feeding Assessment Scale is a psychometrically sound measure of mealtime behavior that can be completed by parents during a standard nutritional assessment and used to inform treatment recommendations.
- A series of studies have demonstrated the many positive effects of a behavioral plus nutrition intervention in children with CF, referred to as Be-In-CHARGE, including increased calorie consumption and weight gain and improved parent–child interactions.
- As part of Be-In-CHARGE, parents are taught several child behavioral management strategies and how to apply them at meals. Examples include how to effectively use parent attention to encourage increased energy intake and behavioral cooperation, setting specific action-oriented goals for each meal as a way to gradually increase calories over time, and tracking calories to monitor intake patterns and provide feedback toward progress with goals.
- Providing anticipatory guidance about developmentally normative behavior and mealtime challenges is important to help parents know what to expect as the child gets older and when more intensive behavioral intervention may be necessary.

J.L. Ryan, Ph.D.
Division of Behavioral Medicine and Clinical Psychology, Cincinnati Children's Hospital Medical Center,
Center for Adherence and Self-Management, 3333 Burnet Ave., MLC 7039, Cincinnati, OH 45229-3039, USA
e-mail: jamie.ryan@cchmc.org

S.S. Filigno, Ph.D. • L.J. Stark, Ph.D., A.B.P.P. (✉)
Division of Behavioral Medicine and Clinical Psychology, Cincinnati Children's Hospital Medical Center,
3333 Burnet Ave., MLC 3015, Cincinnati, OH 45229-3039, USA
e-mail: stephanie.filigno@cchmc.org; lori.stark@cchmc.org

E.H. Yen, A.R. Leonard (eds.), *Nutrition in Cystic Fibrosis*, Nutrition and Health,
DOI 10.1007/978-3-319-16387-1_17, © Springer International Publishing Switzerland 2015

Keywords Dietary adherence • Behavioral assessment • Behavioral intervention • Child development • Child behavior management

Abbreviations

BPFAS   Behavioral Pediatric Feeding Assessment Scale
CF   Cystic fibrosis
CFF   Cystic Fibrosis Foundation
DRI   Dietary reference intake
RCT   Randomized clinical trial
RDA   Recommended dietary allowance

Introduction

The present chapter provides an overview of behavioral strategies and their use in managing the nutritional needs of children with cystic fibrosis (CF) and is divided into six major sections. First, the nutritional recommendations and consensus guidelines developed by the CF Foundation are reviewed. Second, behavioral factors associated with dietary adherence are discussed. Knowledge of common barriers to reaching nutrition goals can guide the clinical assessment and be used in conversations between clinicians and families. Third, the use of behavioral assessment in identifying behavioral targets for treatment is described. Including a brief face-valid measure of mealtime challenges can help in determining the need for intervention.

Next, the outcomes of behavioral intervention studies targeting CF nutrition are reviewed. These positive findings are the basis for recommendations to integrate behavioral components with nutrition, including monitoring of energy intake, goal setting, and using child behavioral management strategies at meals. Fifth, a description of key behavioral strategies and recommendations for intervention to increase dietary adherence are proposed. Each strategy is described such that clinicians could apply these skills when working with families to improve nutrition. Finally, developmental issues to consider when addressing the nutritional needs of children with CF are provided.

Nutritional Recommendations

Advancements in CF treatment have contributed to an increased life expectancy and early nutrition intervention is one of the key clinical initiatives that has contributed to this outcome [1]. To help children with CF reach the 50th percentile for growth (weight for length <2 years and body mass index >2 years), nutritional recommendations include the consumption of 120–150% of the recommended dietary allowance (RDA) of energy for healthy peers [2, 3]. Maintaining a high-calorie, high-fat diet is essential for normal growth, which in turn is associated with improved clinical outcomes [4–6].

For more than 10 years, the CF Foundation has recommended a preventative approach to nutritional care in CF, including consideration of behavioral, nutritional, and medical components associated with nutritional management, in order to promote optimal health and quality of life for children with CF. In addition to providing children with CF recommendations for energy intake,

Consensus Committees assembled by the CF Foundation have emphasized growth and nutritional status monitoring and early intervention to optimize normal growth and prevent nutritional failure. Early consensus-based guidelines focusing on children at risk for or diagnosed with nutritional failure were informed, in part, by the findings of observational studies documenting behaviors incompatible with eating in children with CF from infancy through school-age. Specifically, behavioral assessment of mealtime feeding behaviors was recommended to identify factors associated with nutritional management and appropriate targets for intervention [3].

Following a series of behavioral intervention studies and a systematic review of the evidence, updated clinical care guidelines recommended that intensive behavioral intervention be combined with nutrition education to promote weight gain in children aged 1–12 years, particularly when growth deficits were present [7]. For children younger than 1 year of age, nutritional guidelines recommended that CF teams encourage positive eating behaviors early in development through the dissemination of handouts on anticipatory guidance for managing behavior at meals (available to clinicians on PortCF) at the 4- and 8-month visit, and at routine visits every 2–3 months after the age of 2 years [8]. Overall, a behavioral approach to CF nutrition has been encouraged by the CF Foundation and reinforced in consensus-based guidelines; this initiative will soon be extended to preschoolers as guidelines specific to this age range are scheduled to be disseminated in the near future.

Adherence to Nutritional Recommendations

Given the robust association between weight status and lung function [4–6], adherence to nutritional recommendations is critical to optimizing growth and survival for children with CF [9, 10]. In this context, adherence is defined as "the extent to which a person's behavior coincides with medical or health advice" [11]. Despite the establishment of consensus-based guidelines for nutritional care in CF [3], adherence to calorie intake recommendations are poor ranging from 12 to 20% [12–14], with fewer than 25% of children with CF receiving the minimum recommended 120% DRI for energy [12, 15, 16].

Factors associated with dietary adherence in CF have been examined to identify targets for intervention. Perhaps the most salient predictor of a family's ability to adhere to nutritional recommendations in CF is child mealtime behavior and parent–child mealtime interactions. Specifically, mealtime observations and parent-report of disruptive behavior among toddler, preschool, and school-age children with CF have found behaviors incompatible with eating (e.g., whining, crying, delaying meals by excessive talking, leaving the table, spitting out food) to be higher when compared to children without CF [17–19]. In an attempt to manage these behaviors and complete the feeding task, there is an increased use of ineffective parenting practices (e.g., pleading, coaxing, physically feeding the child, prolonging mealtime) [20]. While some of these approaches are typical even among parents of children without CF, these strategies are counterproductive to meeting dietary recommendations and can reinforce difficult child eating behaviors. In general, more disruptive mealtime behaviors are predictive of lower calorie intake [17, 21] and lower weight status [18]. Even when parents are successful in reaching nutritional goals during mealtime, opportunities for positive family interactions may be compromised [22].

A related barrier to dietary adherence is deficits in nutritional knowledge specific to CF, such as the importance of offering snacks, taking enzyme medications before eating, and boosting caloric intake [12, 23]. While nutrition education is an important first step in addressing deficits in CF-specific knowledge, it is not sufficient to increase caloric intake [24]. Therefore, behavioral intervention appears necessary to improve adherence to nutritional recommendations, global family functioning during mealtimes, and growth outcomes in children with CF.

Behavioral Assessment of Feeding Concerns

In line with the Consensus Committee's initiative focused on the prevention of nutritional failure in children with CF [3, 7], early evaluation of adherence barriers including behaviors incompatible with eating is critical to identifying children at risk for poor intake and growth and thus requiring intensive intervention. The Behavioral Pediatrics Feeding Assessment Scale (BPFAS) [17] has been recommended for use in CF clinical care to evaluate behavior at mealtimes [3]. The BPFAS is a parent-report measure developed for use with children ages 7 months to 7 years [25] and consists of 35 items that assess the frequency of child and parent behaviors and if the behavior is a problem during meals. Behaviors reported on the BPFAS have been associated with health outcomes, such as energy intake [17] and weight gain [21] in children with CF. Behavioral concerns endorsed on the BPFAS have also been linked to clinically important behaviors observed at mealtimes (i.e., meal length, leaving table, talking, negotiating, coaxing, and feeding child) [26]. This measure does not require any specific training and can easily be incorporated into standard nutritional assessment. Direct observation of mealtime interactions (i.e., video-recorded or in-person) is another method for evaluating child eating behavior and parent–child interactions. While this approach may not always be feasible in a busy clinic setting, it has the benefit of providing an opportunity for the therapist to model behavioral strategies directly with the child and coaching parents how to use the skills in the immediate moment.

Behavioral Intervention Outcomes

The CFF consensus recommendations were largely informed by a strong program of research started after initial studies found that parents described mealtimes as a "battle ground" [27] and reported typical parenting strategies to manage child behavior at mealtime were not effective [15, 19]. Subsequent studies applied behavioral theory to develop and test the effectiveness of behavioral interventions targeting nutrition in CF. Table 17.1 provides an overview of study characteristics and outcomes of behavioral interventions for children with CF.

In a series of programmatic studies, each with increasing methodological rigor, Stark and colleagues have examined the effects of a behavioral plus nutrition education intervention (i.e., Be-In-CHARGE) on dietary adherence among children with CF [27–31]. First, in a small sample of five mildly malnourished children with CF (5–12 years old) and their parents [27], a multiple baseline design was used to examine the effectiveness of the behavioral intervention on increasing caloric intake. The intervention consisted of six 90-min group sessions. Parents were first taught how to measure and record their child's calorie intake to establish their baseline intake and to set and monitor the caloric goals during intervention. Each intervention session targeted increasing daily calorie intake at one meal, starting with snack, and proceeding across breakfast, lunch and dinner, thereby gradually increasing the total daily caloric intake by a predetermined amount by the end of treatment.

In addition to providing nutritional education including examples of nutritious high-calorie foods and ways to introduce new foods, each session focused on introducing a child behavior management skill to promote increased calorie consumption. Key components included praise for eating, ignoring child complaints or disruptive behaviors, using contingency management techniques (e.g., star chart), implementing a token system for meeting weekly calorie goals, and setting rules for mealtime (e.g., limit meals to 20 minutes) [27]. The pretest–posttest design indicated a 25–43% increase in total daily caloric intake and significant improvements in weight and height; both were maintained at the 9-month follow-up [27]. The multiple baseline design demonstrated that the average caloric intake of a meal did not change until the meal was targeted, thereby demonstrating that the increase in caloric intake was due to the intervention and not other factors. A replication study added relaxation training in the

Table 17.1 Overview of behavioral intervention studies in CF nutrition

Study	Sample	Intervention(s)	Behavioral strategies	Primary outcome	Secondary outcome
Stark et al. (1990)	$N=5$ 5–12 years	BM+NE	Self-monitoring, contingency management, goal setting, shaping	Increased daily caloric intake (M, 76% of RDA to 116% for three children; M, 135–186% for two children); Posttreatment RDA maintained at 9-month follow-up for 3/5 children	Increased weight gain (M, 25–26 kg) and height; No significant changes in pulmonary functioning from pre- to post-treatment
Stark et al. (1993)	$N=3$ 3–8 years	BM+NE	Self-monitoring, differential attention, contingency management, goal setting, relaxation training	Increased daily caloric intake (M, 102% of RDA to 148%); Calorie consumption maintained at 24-month follow-up	Increased weight gain, height growth, and body fat; Remained above baseline at 24 months
Stark et al. (1996)	$N=10$ 5–10 years	BM+NE ($n=5$); WLC ($n=4$)	Self-monitoring, differential attention, contingency management, contracting, goal setting, feedback, limit setting	BM+NE: Greater increased daily caloric intake (M, 1,032 vs. 244) and weight gain (M, 1.7 vs. 0.0 kg); Maintained at 6-month follow-up	BM+NE: Improved weight z-scores (−1.18–0.74); Declined weight z-scores for WLC; No changes in pulmonary functioning resting energy expenditure, or activity level pre- to post-treatment
Stark et al. (2003)	$N=7$ 6–12 years	BM ($n=3$); NE ($n=4$)	Self-monitoring, differential attention, contingency management, goal setting, feedback	BM: Greater increased daily caloric intake (M, 1036 vs. 408); Maintained for both conditions at 24-month follow-up (M, 964 vs. 313 calories/day)	BM: Greater weight gain (M, 1.42 vs. 0.78 kg); No differences at 24-month follow-up; No group differences in parent–child interactions or coping
Stark et al. (2009)	$N=79$ 4–12 years	BM+NE ($n=33$); NE ($n=34$)	Self-monitoring, differential attention, contingency management, contracting, goal setting, feedback, limit setting	BM+NE: Greater increased daily caloric intake (M, 872 vs. 489) and weight gain (M, 1.47 vs. 0.92 kg); No differences at 24 months	BM+NE: Greater increased % of estimated energy requirement (M, 148 vs. 127%) and BMI z-score (0.38 vs. 0.18); EER maintained at 24 months
Powers et al. (2005)	$N=14$ 18–48 months	BM+NE ($n=4$); SC ($n=6$)	Self-monitoring, differential attention, contingency management, limit setting	BM+NE: Greater increased daily caloric intake (842 vs. −131 kcal); Maintained at 3- and 12-month follow-up	Improved weight (M, 1.4 kg/6 months) and height (M, 5.1 cm/6 months) velocities pretreatment to 3-months and post-treatment to 12-months (M, 2.5 kg/12 months and 8.3 cm/12 months)
Hourigan et al. (2013)	$N=4$ 21–31 months	Adapted BM+NE	Self-monitoring, differential attention, contingency management, limit setting	Increased caloric intake and weight gain for two malnourished toddlers	Preliminary support for decreased disruptive behavior

middle of the intervention to help with reported abdominal discomfort associated with eating and found similar improvements for three young children with CF (3–8 years old). The 32–60% increase in total calorie consumption was achieved and maintained at the 2-year follow-up and greater than expected weight gain was observed at follow-up periods for some children [28].

The scientific rigor of the aforementioned case series single subject design studies was enhanced using a randomized group design in a sample of nine children with CF ranging between 5 and 10 years of age [29] where the behavioral intervention was compared to a wait-list control. As hypothesized, children in the behavioral intervention plus nutrition education group evidenced greater calorie intake (increased daily calories: 1032 vs. 244) and weight gain (1.7 vs. 0 kg) pre- to post-treatment compared to the wait-list control group [29].

While these studies demonstrate the utility of a combined behavioral and educational approach in managing the nutritional needs of children with CF, there is evidence suggesting that behavioral intervention alone may play a valuable role in increasing dietary adherence. For example, behavioral intervention has been associated with an increase in positive parent–child mealtime interactions (e.g., parent attention to positive eating behavior) and a decrease in child disruptive behaviors and parental attention to child behaviors incompatible with eating [32]. To examine the unique contributions of behavioral intervention in a sample of seven school-age children with CF (6–12 years), a subsequent pilot randomized clinical trial (RCT) was conducted in which families were randomly assigned to either behavioral intervention or enhanced nutrition education. Both conditions were seen for the same number of treatment sessions, received the same nutritional information related to calorie content, calorie goals, and recommendations for goal attainment, but only the behavioral intervention group was taught child behavior management strategies and given feedback on their child's progress [30]. While both conditions were effective in increasing caloric intake, children in the behavioral intervention group demonstrated greater improvements in calorie consumption (average of 1036 vs. 408 cal/day), gained twice as much weight, and were more likely to improve their weight percentile for their age compared to the enhanced nutrition education group [30]. Average weekly caloric intake decreased for both conditions at the 2-year follow-up, but remained above baseline and was less variable for children in the behavioral intervention group.

Following the pilot RCT a multi-site RCT was conducted comparing behavioral intervention plus nutrition education ($n=33$) and nutrition education alone ($n=34$) in school-age children with CF [31]. The behavior plus nutrition intervention was more effective than nutrition education alone at increasing daily calorie intake (872 vs. 489 cal/day) and weight (1.47 vs. 0.92 kg). The two groups were comparable at 24-month follow-up with children in both treatment groups maintaining the recommended 120% estimated energy requirement, likely due to the fact that the nutrition education condition included energy intake monitoring strategies, not typically included in standard care, which allowed for maintenance of daily intake into follow-up [31]. This finding suggests that incorporating behavioral components into standard nutrition counseling (e.g., setting caloric goals that gradually increase, monitoring child caloric intake, and providing tailored dietary recommendations and feedback on progress toward reaching calorie goals via graphs), even when the parent–child interaction is not a focus of treatment, may be associated with increased adherence to nutritional recommendations.

The benefits of behavioral intervention have also been seen in children with CF as young as 18 months [33]. In an RCT including 10 toddlers, ages 18 months to 4 years, parents of children in the behavioral plus nutrition education group reported significantly higher calorie intake pre- to post-treatment (increased daily calories: 842 vs. 131) and were more likely to meet the clinical goal of 120% RDA per day compared to children receiving usual care [33]. Furthermore, more children in the intervention group reached or exceeded the benchmark for normal weight and height velocity compared to the control group. Consistent with findings in older children, treatment effects were maintained at 12-month follow-up.

Overall, several behavioral strategies (e.g., praise, ignoring, contingency management, and token systems) have been associated with increased dietary adherence, improved growth status, and increases in positive mealtime interactions among children with CF and their parents. A description of behavioral strategies highlighted in Be-In-CHARGE and how they can be used to manage child behavior and promote calorie consumption is provided below and summarized in Table 17.2. Additional information on Be-In-CHARGE can be found in the protocol available online at www.oup. com/us/pediatricpsych.

Application of Behavioral Strategies to Improve Nutrition

Differential Attention

A basic building block of behavioral child management is differential attention in which desired behaviors are attended to via praise and undesirable behaviors are ignored. By attending to and reinforcing appropriate eating behaviors, the goal is to increase the frequency of these behaviors (e.g., the child takes more bites or sits cooperatively longer). By simultaneously ignoring or not attending to inappropriate behaviors, the inappropriate behaviors decrease over time while appropriate behaviors increase [34]. Differential attention can be particularly challenging for parents of children with CF, as it is difficult for parents who feel such pressure for their child to gain weight and therefore eat, not to coax or plead with their child to eat just part of the meal when the child is complaining about the food or about not being hungry. However, parent attention is a form of reinforcement and when given following problematic behavior will lead to an increase in these behaviors (e.g., complaints about food or not being hungry) again in the future to get their parent's attention.

To increase desired eating behaviors, these behaviors must be attended to instead. Parent attention is reinforcing to children. The most effective reinforcement is verbal praise that positively evaluates and describes the specific behavior being targeted (e.g., "You're doing a great job eating your crackers"). Behaviors to praise include, but are not limited to, sitting at the table, loading the fork with food, taking bites, eating quickly, chewing, and swallowing. Praise is most effective when it is genuine, given immediately after the desired behavior, specific and varied. Some parents may be uncomfortable praising their child's behavior, particularly for behaviors "they are supposed to be doing," or not be familiar with ways to reinforce the behavior. Providing handouts on different ways to phrase praise and types of praise (e.g., thumbs up, pat on the back, hug) and practicing during clinic visits can help families become more comfortable using this important skill at home.

Once parents understand how parent attention can function as reinforcement, ignoring child behaviors incompatible with eating gets a little easier. For instance, a parent must acknowledge that scolding their child or even telling their child to eat, while perceived by parents as negative, provides powerful parent attention and rarely results in the desired outcome, the child eating their meal cooperatively. Common behaviors to ignore include whining, complaints about the food or being full, requests to eat less or requests for eat foods that were not prepared, excessive talking that delays eating, and questions about being ignored [35]. Because ignoring problematic behavior can be difficult, parents can be recommended to turn their head away from the child, talk to another family member, or leave the room when the child begins to engage in the behavior. It is likely that strained mealtime interactions have become a part of the family's daily routine, and the child is accustomed to a predictable parent response and outcome. Thus it is important to emphasize the need for consistency in using the behavioral skills and preparing parents that the child may test limits and engage in the undesirable behavior at increased rates or try additional inappropriate behaviors (e.g., yelling they do not like a food) when ignoring is first implemented, can help parents stay focused on the end goal, which is to out-wait the child until he or she engages in the desirable behavior.

Table 17.2 Behavioral strategies and application in CF nutrition

Behavioral strategy	Purpose	Key elements	Example
Differential attention	*Praising*: Increase desired behavior *Ignoring*: Decrease behavior incompatible with eating	*Praising*: Specify desired behavior with positive evaluation; Provide immediately after behavior; Be enthusiastic; Vary responses; Behaviors include sitting at the table, loading utensil with food, taking bites *Ignoring*: Remove attention to problem behavior; Address temporary extinction burst; Behaviors include whining, complaints about food or being full, requests to eat less or other foods, excessive talking or questions	*Praising*: Verbal—"Nice job eating so quickly." "I like that you came to the table for dinner right away." "I'm happy with how many bites you have taken"; Nonverbal—high five, thumbs up, hug *Ignoring*: Silence, turn or look away, get up from the table, leave the room
Contingency management	Establish clear expectations for desired behavior and the positive/negative consequences	Develop system to monitor target behavior; List of possible rewards; Vouchers or tokens for older children and adolescents; Provide tangible reward (reinforcer) immediately after desired behavior; Withhold reward for problem behavior	"You ate your whole snack really fast. You can go color." "You stayed at the table for 20 minutes. Now you can put a sticker on your chart."
Behavioral contracts	Systematic approach to increase motivation and engagement in behavior change	Written agreement describing: key people and their roles; 1–2 target behaviors; goal; monitoring method; consequences (positive/negative); date to re-evaluate terms	*Key people*: Patient, caregiver(s) *Target behavior*: 1 snack/day *Goal*: 2 snack/day for 5/7 days *Roles*: Patient will eat snack and place sticker; Mom/dad will provide 2 or more snacks/day and reward goal attainment *Monitor*: Sticker chart *Consequence*: 5 or more stickers for a movie night *Re-evaluate*: 1 week
Self-monitoring	Increase awareness of consumption and eating behavior; Identify barriers to calorie goals; Feedback on treatment progress	Diet diary includes type of food, amount prepared and consumed, method of preparation, enzymes and multivitamins; Completed daily	See Fig. 17.1
Goal setting	Monitor progress; Promote independence	*Specific*: Answers who, what, when, where, and how *Measurable*: Can be seen and tracked; Answers how much/many *Attainable*: Independent steps; Short-term versus long-term goals *Realistic*: Considers capability and willingness *Timely*: Set time frame to complete goal and motivate (typically 1–2 weeks)	'I will eat 250 more calories at snack this week.' 'I will take my enzymes before each meal on 5 out of 7 days.'
Limit setting	Decrease behaviors that cannot be ignored; Increase parental control	Clear rules and consequences; Explain in advance; Keep rules short and simple; Use of "if/when-then" statements to describe positive and negative consequences; Rehearse new rules to check the child's understanding; Consistently respond to behavior	*Rule and rationale*: "You have 20 minutes to eat lunch so you can get a lot of energy and go do other things." *Positive consequence*: "If you quickly (state calorie goal), we will let you leave the table and go play video games." *Negative consequence*: "If you do not (state calorie goal) in 20 minutes, you cannot play video games and will not get any food until our next meal."

Contingency Management

Similar to differential attention, contingency management is based on the principle that behavior occurs in a predictable way, and increases or decreases in response to the consequence that follows it. From this perspective, more desirable behavior (e.g., playing video games) is made contingent on engaging in behavior that is less appealing (e.g., meeting dinner energy goal). In other words, the child only receives a desired reward after completing the expected task. Typically contingencies are used to encourage children to eat all the food on their plate or eat enough to meet their calorie goal. Developing a contingency management plan allows parents and children to openly discuss expectations for meals and what the child can earn by meeting the stated expectations. It also teaches children to make informed choices and removes the parent–child struggle from the meal, because the parent can allow the removal of a reward contingent upon not meeting a calorie goal to eventually motivate the child to work harder to achieve the goal in order to get the desired reward. A monitoring plan (e.g., star chart) can help track the child's progress and provides a visual aid for children to see how close they are to receiving the reward.

In order for contingency management to be effective, it is important to avoid giving the reward if it is not earned (e.g., child consumes 75% of the energy goal instead of the complete goal), as inconsistency increases the probability that the child will try to reduce the expectation next time. Acknowledging that children's interests frequently change and some rewards may not be available immediately after the desired behavior, it is helpful to develop a list of possible rewards ahead of time. Rewards or privileges do not need to cost much (e.g., one to one time with a parent, choice of desert, movie night, going to the park), especially if they are to be delivered after each meal/snack in the beginning, but they need to be in proportion to the expected behavior and something the child values and will be motivated to earn. Children may be extremely resistant to changing their eating behavior; therefore, rewarding desired behavior after each meal and snack helps maintain their motivation until it becomes more comfortable and incorporated into the daily routine. Over time with consistently experiencing the "if-then" pattern, the reward for desired eating behavior moves from daily to weekly and is eventually faded out altogether.

Contracting

Behavioral contracting is a more formal and systematic approach to implementing contingency plans and has been effective in increasing treatment adherence in children with CF [36–38]. Contracts are useful because they serve as a written reminder of the agreed upon terms and can be referred back to if there are questions, thus reducing possible family conflict at mealtime. By their very nature, contracts displayed in a common area (e.g., refrigerator, kitchen table, counter) are a visual support tool and can help remind parents and children of their responsibilities. For older children and adolescents, being involved in the negotiation process promotes independence and can increase their motivation to follow the terms of the contract [39].

Self-Monitoring

Self-monitoring (i.e., tracking behavior) is an effective tool for behavior change and serves many purposes [40]. First, measuring one's behavior requires close attention to things that might otherwise be overlooked, such as the type and amount of food consumed for a snack, and provides more accurate estimates of caloric intake. Similarly, this increased attention may lead to increased calorie consumption. Second, self-monitoring data provides rich information to be used in setting calorie goals, providing tailored feedback on the types of foods to increase, identifying barriers to following nutritional recommendations, and generating possible solutions to overcome these difficulties. For example, a detailed diet diary can help families and providers work more efficiently to identify deficits in nutrition knowledge (i.e., calorie content) and environmental factors interfering with reaching the calorie goal (i.e., mealtime duration) in order to choose the most appropriate intervention. Most importantly, monitoring a child's energy intake and comparing it against energy goals gives parents a clear stopping point for their child's food intake and thus when a child consumes sufficient calories to meet the goal the parent can feel accomplished. When there are no energy goals or caloric monitoring parents are often in the position of feeling they failed regardless of how much their child ate, because they are never sure how much is enough.

In order for self-monitoring to be used effectively, accurate data collection is critical. Thus, it is important for parents and possibly older children to learn the following: reading food labels and understanding serving portions, measuring food and liquid in various forms, and recording hidden foods (e.g., sugar added to oatmeal or butter on cooked vegetables) and meals/snacks eaten away from home (i.e., school lunch). Dietary monitoring can be time-consuming at first, particularly as families learn how to get an accurate calorie amount and determine how to incorporate it into their daily routine. Smartphone and web-based applications, such as MyFitnessPal™ and calorieking.com, can save families a lot of time and effort because expansive databases are used to identify the specific food in the correct measurement and automatic calculation of calories. These applications also have the capability of reading UPC scans and thus saving more time for families because they do not have to type in the food to search for it. For families who prefer to track calories on paper diaries, it is important to help them identify an appropriate place to keep the diet diary so that it is seen regularly and serves as a cue to record each meal and snack.

Tracking calories can be an important source of information for families who are concerned that their child "does not eat," as children with CF may be consuming as much as children without CF [16]; however, the pressure for the child to eat [41] and grow leads to parent perceptions of poor intake. Monitoring allows for the opportunity to identify specific times that warrant clinical attention, such as snacks or dinner, or increasing calories following an illness. Moreover, tracking calories provides the basis for goal setting, an essential component of behavioral interventions. See Fig. 17.1 for an example of how dietary data can be used to reinforce consistent use of behavioral strategies in overcoming temporary declines in calorie intake in order to reach total daily calorie goals. The clinical utility of self-monitoring relies on feedback and illustrating to parents the association between monitoring observations and dietary changes. A graphical representation of the data can be used to reinforce efforts to track daily calorie intake, monitor treatment progress, and identify ongoing barriers preventing goal attainment. Graphic presentation with the average weekly caloric intake as well as the daily calories also allows parents to see overall success and decrease the focus on any particular day that may be low.

Goal Setting

Making dietary changes can seem daunting, but a collaborative goal setting process can help families organize nutritional recommendations and skills into practical and manageable steps. Setting calorie goals one meal at a time provides a means to monitoring the child's progress and reinforce increased calorie intake. It also allows parents to feel comfortable stopping offers of food by giving them a clear target for each meal/snack. To increase the chance of reaching the desired outcome, goals need to be specific and action-oriented. Establishing how the goal will be measured provides a concrete indicator

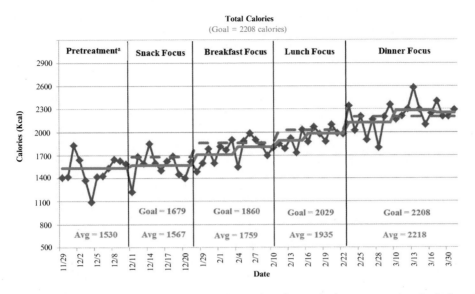

Fig. 17.1 Illustration of data obtained from a daily diet diary and use for monitoring progress toward calorie goals over time. *Red*, calorie goal; *Blue*, total daily calories; *Green*, average calorie intake. [a]Baseline measurement of caloric intake after starting self-monitoring and before setting calorie goals

of whether the goal is accomplished. While children with CF are advised to consume more than 120% of the RDA, changing learned eating patterns quickly to reach calorie recommendations is nearly impossible. Reinforcing success in reaching small attainable goals can increase the child's self-efficacy and encourage increased calorie consumption over time. Consistent with Be-In-CHARGE [30, 31], snack is chosen as a starting point because there are several opportunities for snack during the day and children may be more likely to accept snacks as each snack can be a small amount of food, therefore making early treatment success more likely. Next, one meal is targeted per week with a goal of increasing calories at the targeted meal by approximately 250 cal. The child and parent's motivation and ability to reach the calorie goal should be considered when determining whether the goal is realistic or needs to be modified. Lastly, a calorie goal can be refined after a specified time period to determine if the goal is appropriate. For example, if after 4 weeks of meeting a calorie goal a child does not gain the expected amount of weight, the calorie goal could be increased.

Parental Limit Setting

As previously stated, often a child's first response when parent attention is removed during planned ignoring is to increase the frequency and/or intensity of behavior, or attempt to get their parents' attention another way. For example, the child may get up from the table before the meal is over. To help parents maintain control over the mealtime, it is necessary to establish rules and consequences for meals. Rules for meals are simple, made in advance, and explicitly state the relationship between a specific behavior and its consequence, which may involve access or removal of privileges.

In order for children with CF to meet nutritional recommendations, it is important for them to be seated at the table during a meal and consume enough food to meet calorie goals. Instructing children to remain at the table until a parent or caregiver gives them permission to leave allows the adult to be in control during meals. As recommended in the Be-In-CHARGE protocol, children who leave the table prematurely should be escorted back to the table in a calm manner and without any discussion or other attention, such as making eye contact. Parents are encouraged to praise the child throughout the meal and make the association between staying at the table and positive consequences (i.e., "I like the way you are sitting at the table with the family.") to prevent the child from leaving.

Relatedly, setting a time to end the meal is necessary for several reasons. Previous observational studies found that meals for children with CF lasted an average of 10 min longer than meals for children without CF (27 vs. 17 min), and the second half of the meal included more behaviors incompatible with eating [42]. Contrary to general weight-loss management strategies, children with CF are encouraged to eat quickly because the brain and stomach register feeling full after roughly 20 min and longer mealtimes are less likely to be an effective long-term strategy for improving overall consumption and growth [19, 43]. Thus, a 20-min time limit encourages children to eat quickly and can be used to motivate them to reach calorie goals and earn their reward. If the child does not consume enough calories within 20 min, parents are encouraged to remove the food and not allow access to food until the next meal or snack. It is important that food not be given until the next scheduled meal to increase the likelihood that the child will eat what is offered at the next meal.

In sum, child behavioral management strategies have been found to be effective in improving behavior at meals and increasing dietary adherence in children with CF. Strategies can be tailored to the needs of the child and family, applied to related aspects of nutritional care in CF (e.g., taking enzymes as prescribed), and easily incorporated into standard nutritional counseling when comprehensive behavioral intervention is not feasible.

Developmental Considerations

Preschool

Compared to infancy when eating behaviors are relatively predictable and parents are largely responsible for the feeding schedule, the toddler and preschool period can pose unique challenges for parents of children with and without CF. Parents may notice a decline in their child's appetite or increased picky eating and be inclined to persist and push for high-calorie intake. They may be comforted to learn that preferences for certain tastes are innate and others evolve over time, thereby explaining why infants and toddlers readily accept sweet foods (e.g., fruits and juices) and reject new foods with a bitter taste (e.g., vegetables) [44]. Being aware of this normal course of food acceptance and fussy eating, parents of children with CF can gradually introduce new foods by combining them with already preferred foods or making access to preferred foods contingent on tasting novel foods. Repeated exposure in a nonthreatening setting is necessary, as preschoolers taste a new food up to 16 times before it is accepted [45]. Similar to other areas of a child's development, parental attitudes and behaviors can influence early childhood experiences that begin to shape long-term eating patterns and behaviors. A child's food preferences and eating behaviors are largely reflected by what is provided and modeled early in life [46, 47]. Accordingly, parents play a critical role in making high-calorie, high-fat foods available and easily accessible to encourage children to try a wide range of foods.

School-Age

For many parents, preparing children to start school can be exciting yet anxiety provoking as the transition means less parental control. Notably, parents of school-age children with CF report an inability to monitor their child's eating habits in school, with some children being offered portions smaller than recommended and parents feeling pressured to compensate at home [41]. Educating the school about the nutritional needs of children with CF and establishing a positive working relationship can help relieve parental concerns and promote child nutritional management. For example, a Section 504 Plan can be developed allowing a child to carry or have access to extra snacks, have additional time to eat lunch, and take enzymes and nutritional supplements as needed to increase daily calories [48].

During the school-age period, children's cognitive abilities are rapidly expanding and they are better able to form and express their thoughts and illness beliefs. This represents an ideal time to address any misconceptions or fears that might interfere with the child's willingness to follow nutritional recommendations [49]. Specifically, peer influences and the need for social acceptance are developmentally appropriate topics worth discussing in order to problem-solve around perceived barriers and meet nutrition goals [50–52].

Adolescence

Adolescence is a transitional period marked by increasing autonomy and independence, and the desire to establish an individual identity separate from the family unit. Developing a sense of self through experimentation with different roles is typical among adolescents [53], but the risks and health implications are much greater for adolescents with CF, as treatment burden increases in response to a progressing illness and the regimen interferes with school-related or social activities [41, 54]. Consequently, up to 60% of adolescents with CF report being non-adherent to varying regimen components [55, 56]. Among females with CF, perceived visible differences during puberty (e.g., short stature or low body mass) have been associated with body dissatisfaction and maladaptive eating attitudes [57, 58] and may help explain the tendency to be less adherent to a high-fat diet. Parental awareness and continued involvement are needed to ensure the competing demands in normal adolescent development and pediatric disease management do not adversely impact health outcomes in an already vulnerable population.

To prepare adolescents with CF and their parents for challenging developmental transitions, it is important to educate families on what they can expect and to have these conversations early and often. For example, encouraging families to consider the adolescent's abilities and willingness (versus age) to assume more treatment responsibility and recommending a gradual transition from the parent to the child or adolescent can help prevent non-adherence and subsequent declines in physical functioning [59]. Moreover, helping family's problem-solve around barriers to dietary adherence may decrease resistance and parent–child conflict associated with the process [60, 61]. In sum, all families must manage the changes and milestones characteristic of child and adolescent development, but the additional complexity of CF can complicate this process and requires considerable effort to promote optimal health and maximize quality of life among youth with CF.

Conclusion

In order to support families in achieving what can feel like lofty CF nutrition benchmarks, it is important for nutrition care to incorporate a behavioral approach that includes goal setting, caloric intake tracking, timely feedback on energy intake, and child behavioral management strategies to address child behaviors that limits intake and parent–child interactions that make mealtimes stressful. Enhancing standard nutrition care to include these components gives families a goal to work towards with the ability to know when it has been reached, engages them in problem-solving around barriers to meeting nutritional recommendations, and equips them with the necessary skills to elicit improved behavior from their child at meals. In addition, providing anticipatory guidance about developmentally normative mealtime challenges can help families know when to ask for assistance in order to address problem behaviors before they become more engrained and difficult to change. As children's energy needs increase with age, early programming for adaptive eating behavior will make it easier to reach expectations for increased energy intake. Finally, increased life expectancy for individuals with CF highlights the benefit of behavioral intervention in assisting with the transition of treatment responsibility to promote patient self-management and ease the move to adult care.

References

1. Cystic Fibrosis Foundation. Patients registry report. Bethesda, MD: Cystic Fibrosis Foundation; 2012 [November 14, 2014].
2. Ramsey BW, Farrell PM, Pencharz P. Nutritional assessment and management in cystic fibrosis: a consensus report. The Consensus Committee. Am J Clin Nutr. 1992;55(1):108–16.
3. Borowitz D, Baker RD, Stallings V. Consensus report on nutrition for pediatric patients with cystic fibrosis. J Pediatr Gastroenterol Nutr. 2002;35(3):246–59.
4. Konstan MW, Butler SM, Wohl ME, Stoddard M, Matousek R, Wagener JS, et al. Growth and nutritional indexes in early life predict pulmonary function in cystic fibrosis. J Pediatr. 2003;142(6):624–30.
5. Peterson ML, Jacobs Jr DR, Milla CE. Longitudinal changes in growth parameters are correlated with changes in pulmonary function in children with cystic fibrosis. Pediatrics. 2003;112(3 Pt 1):588–92.
6. Zemel BS, Jawad AF, FitzSimmons S, Stallings VA. Longitudinal relationship among growth, nutritional status, and pulmonary function in children with cystic fibrosis: analysis of the Cystic Fibrosis Foundation National CF Patient Registry. J Pediatr. 2000;137(3):374–80.
7. Stallings VA, Stark LJ, Robinson KA, Feranchak AP, Quinton H. Evidence-based practice recommendations for nutrition-related management of children and adults with cystic fibrosis and pancreatic insufficiency: results of a systematic review. J Am Diet Assoc. 2008;108(5):832–9.
8. Borowitz D, Robinson KA, Rosenfeld M, Davis SD, Sabadosa KA, Spear SL, et al. Cystic Fibrosis Foundation evidence-based guidelines for management of infants with cystic fibrosis. J Pediatr. 2009;155(6 Suppl):S73–93.
9. Lai HJ, Shoff SM, Farrell PM, Wisconsin Cystic Fibrosis Neonatal Screening Group. Recovery of birth weight z score within 2 years of diagnosis is positively associated with pulmonary status at 6 years of age in children with cystic fibrosis. Pediatrics. 2009;123(2):714–22.
10. Yen EH, Quinton H, Borowitz D. Better nutritional status in early childhood is associated with improved clinical outcomes and survival in patients with cystic fibrosis. J Pediatr. 2013;162(3):530–5. 3.
11. Sackett DL, Snow JC. The magnitude of compliance and non compliance. In: Haynes NRB, Taylor DW, Sackett DL, editors. Compliance in health care. Baltimore: John Hopkins University Press; 1980. p. 11–22.
12. Anthony H, Paxton S, Bines J, Phelan P. Psychosocial predictors of adherence to nutritional recommendations and growth outcomes in children with cystic fibrosis. J Psychosom Res. 1999;47(6):623–34.
13. Mackner LM, McGrath AM, Stark LJ. Dietary recommendations to prevent and manage chronic pediatric health conditions: adherence, intervention, and future directions. J Dev Behav Pediatr. 2001;22(2):130–43.
14. Passero MA, Remor B, Salomon J. Patient-reported compliance with cystic fibrosis therapy. Clin Pediatr (Phila). 1981;20(4):264–8.
15. Powers SW, Patton SR, Byars KC, Mitchell MJ, Jelalian E, Mulvihill MM, et al. Caloric intake and eating behavior in infants and toddlers with cystic fibrosis. Pediatrics. 2002;109(5):E75–5.
16. Stark LJ, Jelalian E, Mulvihill MM, Powers SW, Bowen AM, Spieth LE, et al. Eating in preschool children with cystic fibrosis and healthy peers: behavioral analysis. Pediatrics. 1995;95(2):210–5.
17. Crist W, McDonnell P, Beck M, Gillespie CT. Behavior at mealtimes and the young child with cystic fibrosis. J Dev Behav Pediatr. 1994;15(3):157–61.
18. Hammons AJ, Fiese B. Mealtime interactions in families of a child with cystic fibrosis: a meta-analysis. J Cyst Fibros. 2010;9(6):377–84.
19. Stark LJ, Jelalian E, Powers SW, Mulvihill MM, Opipari LC, Bowen A, et al. Parent and child mealtime behavior in families of children with cystic fibrosis. J Pediatr. 2000;136(2):195–200.
20. Spieth LE, Stark LJ, Mitchell MJ, Schiller M, Cohen LL, Mulvihill M, et al. Observational assessment of family functioning at mealtime in preschool children with cystic fibrosis. J Pediatr Psychol. 2001;26(4):215–24.
21. Opipari-Arrigan L, Powers SW, Quittner AL, Stark LJ. Mealtime problems predict outcome in clinical trial to improve nutrition in children with CF. Pediatr Pulmonol. 2010;45(1):78–82.

22. Mitchell MJ, Powers SW, Byars KC, Dickstein S, Stark LJ. Family functioning in young children with cystic fibrosis: observations of interactions at mealtime. J Dev Behav Pediatr. 2004;25(5):335–46.
23. Modi AC, Lim CS, Yu N, Geller D, Wagner MH, Quittner AL. A multi-method assessment of treatment adherence for children with cystic fibrosis. J Cyst Fibros. 2006;5(3):177–85.
24. Bell L, Durie P, Forstner F. What do children with cystic fibrosis eat? J Pediatr Gastroenterol Nutr. 1984;3 Suppl 1:S137–46.
25. Crist W, Napier-Phillips A. Mealtime behaviors of young children: a comparison of normative and clinical data. J Dev Behav Pediatr. 2001;22(5):279–86.
26. Piazza-Waggoner C, Modi AC, Powers SW, Williams LB, Dolan LM, Patton SR. Observational assessment of family functioning in families with children who have type 1 diabetes mellitus. J Dev Behav Pediatr. 2008;29(2):101–5.
27. Stark LJ, Bowen AM, Tyc VL, Evans S, Passero MA. A behavioral approach to increasing calorie consumption in children with cystic fibrosis. J Pediatr Psychol. 1990;15(3):309–26.
28. Stark LJ, Knapp LG, Bowen AM, Powers SW, Jelalian E, Evans S, et al. Increasing calorie consumption in children with cystic fibrosis: replication with 2-year follow-up. J Appl Behav Anal. 1993;26(4):435–50.
29. Stark LJ, Mulvihill MM, Powers SW, Jelalian E, Keating K, Creveling S, et al. Behavioral intervention to improve calorie intake of children with cystic fibrosis: treatment versus wait list control. J Pediatr Gastroenterol Nutr. 1996;22(3):240–53.
30. Stark LJ, Opipari LC, Spieth LE, Jelalian E, Quittner AL, Higgins L, et al. Contribution of behavior therapy to dietary treatment in cystic fibrosis: a randomized controlled study with 2-year follow-up. Behav Ther. 2003; 34:237–58.
31. Stark LJ, Quittner AL, Powers SW, Opipari-Arrigan L, Bean JA, Duggan C, et al. Randomized clinical trial of behavioral intervention and nutrition education to improve caloric intake and weight in children with cystic fibrosis. Arch Pediatr Adolesc Med. 2009;163(10):915–21.
32. Stark LJ, Powers SW, Jelalian E, Rape RN, Miller DL. Modifying problematic mealtime interactions of children with cystic fibrosis and their parents via behavioral parent training. J Pediatr Psychol. 1994;19(6):751–68.
33. Powers SW, Jones JS, Ferguson KS, Piazza-Waggoner C, Daines C, Acton JD. Randomized clinical trial of behavioral and nutrition treatment to improve energy intake and growth in toddlers and preschoolers with cystic fibrosis. Pediatrics. 2005;116(6):1442–50.
34. Hanley GP, Tiger JH. Differential reinforcement procedures. In: Fisher WW, Piazza CC, Roane HS, editors. Handbook of applied behavior analysis. New York, NY: Guilford Press; 2011. p. 229–49.
35. Powers SW, Mitchell MJ, Patton SR, Byars KC, Jelalian E, Mulvihill MM, et al. Mealtime behaviors in families of infants and toddlers with cystic fibrosis. J Cyst Fibros. 2005;4(3):175–82.
36. Miller DL, Stark LJ. Contingency contracting for improving adherence in pediatric populations. JAMA. 1994; 271(1):81–3.
37. Stark LJ, Opipari LC, Jelalian E, Powers SW, Janicke DM, Mulvihill MM, et al. Child behavior and parent management strategies at mealtimes in families with a school-age child with cystic fibrosis. Health Psychol. 2005;24(3):274–80.
38. Stark LJ, Miller ST, Plienes AJ, Drabman RS. Behavioral contracting to increase chest physiotherapy. A study of a young cystic fibrosis patient. Behav Modif. 1987;11(1):75–86.
39. Wahl AK, Rustoen T, Hanestad BR, Gjengedal E, Moum T. Living with cystic fibrosis: impact on global quality of life. Heart Lung. 2005;34(5):324–31.
40. Butryn ML, Phelan S, Hill JO, Wing RR. Consistent self-monitoring of weight: a key component of successful weight loss maintenance. Obesity (Silver Spring). 2007;15(12):3091–6.
41. Filigno SS, Brannon EE, Chamberlin LA, Sullivan SM, Barnett KA, Powers SW. Qualitative analysis of parent experiences with achieving cystic fibrosis nutrition recommendations. J Cyst Fibros. 2012;11(2):125–30.
42. Stark LJ, Mulvihill MM, Jelalian E, Bowen AM, Powers SW, Tao S, et al. Descriptive analysis of eating behavior in school-age children with cystic fibrosis and healthy control children. Pediatrics. 1997;99(5):665–71.
43. Wolff RP, Lierman CJ. Management of behavioral feeding problems in young children. Infants Young Child. 1994;7:14–23.
44. Kern DL, McPhee L, Fisher J, Johnson S, Birch LL. The post ingestive consequences of fat condition preferences for flavors associated with high dietary fat. Physiol Behav. 1993;54(1):71–6.
45. Birch LL, Marlin DW. I don't like it; I never tried it: effects of exposure on two-year-old children's food preferences. Appetite. 1982;3(4):353–60.
46. Cullen KW, Baranowski T, Owens E, Marsh T, Rittenberry L, de Moor C. Availability, accessibility, and preferences for fruit, 100% fruit juice, and vegetables influence children's dietary behavior. Health Educ Behav. 2003;30(5): 615–26.
47. Hearn M, Baranowski T, Baranowski J, Doyle C, Smith M, Lin LS, et al. Environmental influences on dietary behavior among children: availability and accessibility of fruits and vegetables enable consumption. J Health Educ. 1998;29(1):26–32.
48. Cystic Fibrosis Foundation. A teacher's guide to CF. Bethesda, MD: Cystic Fibrosis Foundation; 2014.

49. Ernst MM, Johnson MC, Stark LJ. Developmental and psychosocial issues in cystic fibrosis. Child Adolesc Psychiatr Clin N Am. 2010;19(2):263–83. 2.
50. Meyer TA, Gast J. The effects of peer influence on disordered eating behavior. J Sch Nurs. 2008;24(1):36–42.
51. Salvy SJ, de la Haye K, Bowker JC, Hermans RC. Influence of peers and friends on children's and adolescents' eating and activity behaviors. Physiol Behav. 2012;106(3):369–78.
52. Cullen KW, Baranowski T, Rittenberry L, Cosart C, Hebert D, de Moor C. Child-reported family and peer influences on fruit, juice and vegetable consumption: reliability and validity of measures. Health Educ Res. 2001;16(2): 187–200.
53. Segal TY. Adolescence: what the cystic fibrosis team needs to know. J R Soc Med. 2008;101 Suppl 1:S15–27.
54. Hegarty M, Macdonald J, Watter P, Wilson C. Quality of life in young people with cystic fibrosis: effects of hospitalization, age and gender, and differences in parent/child perceptions. Child Care Health Dev. 2009;35(4):462–8.
55. Dziuban EJ, Saab-Abazeed L, Chaudhry SR, Streetman DS, Nasr SZ. Identifying barriers to treatment adherence and related attitudinal patterns in adolescents with cystic fibrosis. Pediatr Pulmonol. 2010;45(5):450–8.
56. Quittner AL, Drotar D, Ievers-Landis CE, Seidner D, Slocum N, Jacobsen J. Adherence to medical treatments in adolescents with cystic fibrosis: the development and evaluation of family-based interventions. In: Drotar D, editor. Hillsdale, NJ: Erlbaum Associates Inc; 2000.
57. Johannesson M, Carlson M, Brucefors AB, Hjelte L. Cystic fibrosis through a female perspective: psychosocial issues and information concerning puberty and motherhood. Patient Educ Couns. 1998;34(2):115–23.
58. Randlesome K, Bryon M, Evangeli M. Developing a measure of eating attitudes and behaviours in cystic fibrosis. J Cyst Fibros. 2013;12(1):15–21.
59. Modi A, Marciel K, Slater S, et al. The influence of parental supervision on medical adherence in adolescents with cystic fibrosis: developmental shifts from pre to late adolescence. Child Health Care. 2008;37(1):78–92.
60. Wysocki T, Harris MA, Buckloh LM, Mertlich D, Lochrie AS, Taylor A, et al. Effects of behavioral family systems therapy for diabetes on adolescents' family relationships, treatment adherence, and metabolic control. J Pediatr Psychol. 2006;31(9):928–38.
61. DeLambo KE, Ievers-Landis CE, Drotar D, Quittner AL. Association of observed family relationship quality and problem-solving skills with treatment adherence in older children and adolescents with cystic fibrosis. J Pediatr Psychol. 2004;29(5):343–53.

Chapter 18
Nutrition and Quality Improvement in Cystic Fibrosis

Amanda Radmer Leonard

Key Points

- Quality improvement is a multidisciplinary method of understanding and improving the efficiency, effectiveness, and reliability of health processes and outcomes of care
- Patient registries are a useful tool in quality improvement work
- Benchmarking allows for the determination of best practices
- Patient and family involvement and education of care team in the techniques of quality improvement are important for success
- There are limited publications about quality improvement efforts in cystic fibrosis and nutrition
- Utilizing a standardized approach to quality improvement projects improves success

Keywords Benchmarking • Improvements • Learning and Leadership Collaborative • Nutrition • Outcomes • Patient registries • Quality improvement

Abbreviations

ACH	Arkansas Children's Hospital
CCHMC	Cincinnati Children's Hospital Medical Center
CF	Cystic fibrosis
CFF	Cystic Fibrosis Foundation
LLC	Learning and Leadership Collaborative
OGTT	Oral Glucose Tolerance Test
PDSA	Plan Do Study Act
QI	Quality improvement
REACT	Re-Education of Airway Clearance Techniques
SDSA	Standardize Do Study Act
UAB/COA	University of Alabama at Birmingham CF Center/Children's Hospital of Alabama
US	United States

A.R. Leonard, M.P.H., R.D., C.D.E. (✉)
The Johns Hopkins Children's Center, Department of Pediatrics,
Division of Gastroenterology and Nutrition, Baltimore, MD, USA
e-mail: aleonar1@jhmi.edu

E.H. Yen, A.R. Leonard (eds.), *Nutrition in Cystic Fibrosis: A Guide for Clinicians*, Nutrition and Health, DOI 10.1007/978-3-319-16387-1_18, © Springer International Publishing Switzerland 2015

Introduction

Quality improvement (QI) is a "multidisciplinary, systems-focused, data driven method of understanding and improving the efficiency, effectiveness, and reliability of health processes and outcomes of care" [1]. QI is a powerful tool that has been used in a variety of care settings to improve clinical outcomes [2–4]. With the provision of safe, patient centered, evidence-based, efficient, timely and equitable healthcare delivery chronic disease outcomes improve [5]. In cystic fibrosis (CF) QI has been utilized, along with new therapies to prolong the life expectancy of those affected with the disease [6]. These improvement techniques can be used to focus on the nutritional care of individuals with CF with the goal of improving their nutritional status and potentially their quality of life [7–11].

Quality Improvement in Cystic Fibrosis

The life expectancy of individuals with CF has increased dramatically over the last 50 years [12]. Between 2002 and 2012, median life expectancy for CF patients in the United States (US) increased from 32 to 41 years [13]. Improvements in medical outcomes for people with CF are a result of advances in basic science and therapeutic development combined with quality improvement work geared toward healthcare delivery [14]. With an increased focus on QI, the CF community has encouraged improvements in delivery of care as well as developing evidenced based and consensus based guidelines regarding standards of care [3, 15, 16]. Data transparency, as well as the refinement of patient registries to allow comparison of center processes and outcomes has also improved overall care delivery [6]. Many countries have embarked on QI projects, including the United States, Europe, Canada and Australia, but few have published their results [10, 13]. US Cystic Fibrosis Foundation (CFF) has recently documented their program so their work will be discussed in greater detail [13].

Patient Registries

One of the key tools for QI in the CF community is the use of patient registries. Patient registries are utilized in several countries including the United States, Canada, Australia, and several individual European countries [17–20]. A combined European registry, including multiple countries, was started in 2004 to allow for the inclusion of a larger population [18]. Patient registries, which capture patient data at point of care, allow for comparison both within the center and with other centers [17]. Registries allow practitioners to identify variability in care and also track progress in patient outcomes [14]. This variability can be associated with dramatic differences in outcomes [21]. Although the variability in care, and outcomes, could be used to define the "best" center, QI proponents believe that variation in outcomes data provides an opportunity for learning, not judging [22]. The US CFF patient registry, created in 1966, was initially used to track only survival [23]. Since that time it has been expanded to include more than 300 unique variables including outcomes and care processes and can be used to identify variability and measure outcomes [17]. While this variability may not always be immediately improved, identification of differences can be helpful in determining the next steps. For instance, Gutierrez and colleagues described the difference in life expectancy in Chile, in the teens, versus other countries, which are as high as 40+ years [24]. With this information, obstacles to care in Chile were identified which then increase the likelihood that inadequacies will be addressed.

Registries can be a useful tool in nutrition QI projects [7–9, 25]. Corey et al. published one of the first papers using registry data to describe nutrition related outcomes [26]. Using registry data the group compared survival data between two similar sized CF centers, one in Boston, Massachusetts and the other in Toronto, Ontario. Data showed that median survival in Toronto was better than Boston by about 7 years. One main difference identified between the two centers was their approach to nutrition. Boston prescribed a low fat diet to decrease symptoms of malabsorption, which was the generally accepted approach at that time. Toronto advocated for a high fat diet and administered more pancreatic replacement enzymes to decrease side effects from the high fat diet. Since the publication of this study a high fat diet has become the generally accepted approach for individuals with CF. In more recent years, registry data has been used to identify outcomes to improve and also to track progress [8–10].

Benchmarking

Significant variability in practice patterns and outcomes provides a great opportunity to identify clinical practices associated with the best performing centers [27]. Benchmarking, the process of using outcome data to identify high-performing centers and determine practices associated with their outstanding performance, is another aspect of QI that promotes an improvement in CF care [27, 28]. Since 2006, US CFF patient registry data (case-mix adjusted) has been shared with the public [22]. This transparency encourages center accountability and promotes QI to improve outcomes [13, 17].

Benchmarking allows the discovery, and facilitates the spread, of effective approaches to care [28]. Benchmarking assessments can be done on a small (one center) or large (multiple centers) scale [7, 27, 28] Beginning in 2006, the CFF organized two teams, one with adult caregivers and one with pediatric caregivers, to visit the top 10 performing centers in the US [27, 28]. The task of the teams was to identify best practices. Table 18.1 describes the main themes identified [27].

Spreading the Quality Improvement Message

In addition to using the registry and benchmarking to help improve outcomes, CFF also started an initiative to educate care centers on the specifics of how to implement QI work. [30]. The Learning and Leadership Collaboratives (LLC) were designed to accelerate the rate of improvement in CF care by training care teams on methods of QI [14, 30]. In 2002, after a meeting with national quality improvement leaders, CFF began to update its registry data so that it could support QI work [14, 17]. CFF also sponsored a training program on clinical improvement methods, which was launched in 2003 [21]. Standardized care, which has been shown to improve outcomes in a variety of disciplines, is an important part of the LLC training [21, 30]. The standardized care model allows for an individual approach to patient care within a standardized framework [21]. Through specific, targeted, evidenced based QI projects CF care centers were able to improve outcomes [13, 30]. James, a thought leader in healthcare QI, estimates that the medical profession could achieve as much benefit for patients if it could routinely apply and deliver current best medical knowledge, as will be achieved by the next 25 years of government funding for new biomedical research [21].

Patient and Family Involvement

Engaging patient and families in CF care has been part of many improvement efforts and is one of the goals of the CFF [9, 10, 13, 14, 22, 28, 29]. Patients and families participate on Family Advisory boards which help direct improvement work [9, 10, 22, 28, 29]. Many centers have patients and/or

Table 18.1 Key characteristics of programs with top-quintile cystic fibrosis clinical outcomes

Benchmarking themes
Systems
1. Strong leadership
2. Dedicated multidisciplinary team
3. Easy accessibility by patients and families
4. Close tracking of clinical details and outcomes
Attitudes
1. High expectations for pulmonary and nutritional status
2. Low threshold for vigorous treatment of health declines
3. Aggressive use of antibiotics for pulmonary symptoms
4. Team consensus on standard approach to care
Practices
1. Preclinic review of patients and treatment planning
2. More frequent clinic visits for identified health concerns
3. Regular patient visits with full multidisciplinary team
Patient/family engagement and empowerment
1. Patients provided with data on their clinical outcomes
2. Patients/families educated on high outcome expectations and need for early, aggressive intervention for declines
3. Patients/families encouraged to provide feedback on their clinical care experiences and concerns
Projects
1. Self-assess program outcomes and practice patterns
2. Develop projects to improve program performance of key clinical practices

Reproduced from Boyle MP, et al. Key findings of the US Cystic Fibrosis Foundation's clinical practice benchmarking project. BMJ Qual Saf. 2014;23 Suppl 1:i15-i22. with permission from BMJ Publishing Group Ltd.

family members as part of the QI, participating in meetings and working with the care team on projects [9, 10, 22]. The perspective of patients and families in QI work has motivated clinicians and provided valuable insight [14, 28].

Implementing a Quality Improvement Project

Nutrition plays an integral role in the health of individuals with CF [11, 31–33]. Nutrition assessment and interventions are important for outpatient, as well as inpatient, care [16, 34, 35]. Although CF nutrition QI projects have been reported at meetings, there are limited publications about projects specific to CF nutrition [6]. The primary approach for most centers is to focus on implementing guidelines for CF care. This section will provide an overview of the steps for implementing a nutrition related QI project. The approach described is based on the Dartmouth Microsystem Improvement Curriculum and is described in the Action Guide for Accelerating Improvement in Cystic Fibrosis Care (Action Guide) [36]. This method was used by CFF for the LLC [30]. More detailed information can be found in the Action Guide and other works devoted to QI [36].

Prior to embarking on a nutrition QI project, it is vital to assess clinic structure and function [36]. By understanding the people involved, the current state of the program, and current outcomes it will be easier to achieve desired results. The assessment should include the 5 P's: purpose, patients, professionals, processes, and patterns. Defining a purpose will guide decision making and focus improvements. Identifying your patient population and the professionals involved in their care, as well as the processes and patterns, will further describe your current system. Ideally, QI work will involve the entire care team [36, 37]. Members of a comprehensive QI team will vary depending on a variety of factors, but might include a dietitian/nutritionist, physician(s), nurse, social worker, respiratory therapist, physical therapist, behavioral psychologist, pharmacist, and a patient/parent. From this broader team, a lead team can be identified to pursue the project [36]. Once the lead team is selected a theme, global aim, and specific aims should be determined for the work. The theme and aims will help decide where the improvement efforts will focus. It is helpful to look at registry results to assist with identifying areas where improvement is warranted. Review of center outcomes can help the team choose the theme, for example nutrition care. From the broad reaching theme a global aim and smaller specific aims can be identified to define the work. For instance, with a theme of nutrition care, a global aim might be to improve the nutritional status of patients at the center. The specific aim(s) would detail the change needed to achieve this goal such as "clinic dietitian will assess all patients with a body mass index less than the 50 percentile." The actual change instituted to achieve the specific aim is referred to as a change idea. Many QI projects are not necessarily new recommendations but new approaches to applying the current recommendations or guidelines at the center [8–10]. The goal is to identify and correct inconsistencies, or to apply a new method to allow patients and families to succeed [36]. For instance, assessing BMI at every clinic visit for every patient or adopting a screening tool to assess nutrition risk. Barriers to achieving these goals can be identified and addressed as the process progresses.

In order to assess change over time improvement projects should be measurable. Metrics can be gathered from registry data or collected and organized by clinic staff. Once a measurable change idea is chosen it is often helpful to have a smaller scale pilot using a subset of patients before applying to a greater proportion of your center. This process will help identify, and correct, potential issues with the planned changes. One way to approach implementation of a change idea is a Plan Do Study Act (PDSA) Cycle (Fig. 18.1). With this approach the team plans the change, then implements the change, assesses the impact of the change, and finally takes action. Each PDSA cycle should be about a specific aspect of care. The action at the end of the cycle could be a small adjustment to the plan or moving to the next step in the improvement process. Once a PDSA cycle is complete, and the outcomes are acceptable, the process can become standardized. It may take many times through the cycle before the plan is ready to become standardized. At this point the cycles are called Standardize, Do, Study, Act (SDSA). The use of PDSA cycles allows QI work to begin on a small, manageable scale and then grow to spread throughout the care center. PDSA cycles related to the overall theme will drive improvements at your center.

Applications in CF Nutrition

Although many centers have participated in nutrition related quality improvement work, there are a limited number of publications describing these efforts [6]. This section will review the currently available published works.

The Cincinnati Children's Hospital Medical Center (CCHMC) has been working on QI for over a decade [10]. The CCHMC CF center reports a dramatic improvement in median clinic BMI (as reported in CFF patient registry) as a result of their QI work. The median clinic BMI improved from 35% in 2000 to 55% in 2010. Siracusa and colleagues report that the center focused on specific outcomes, empowering families and patients, using data effectively, standardizing the care processes,

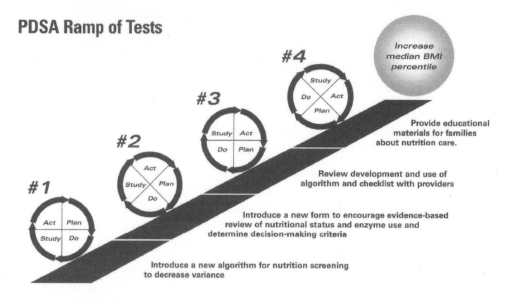

PDSA Ramp of Tests

Increase median BMI percentile

Provide educational materials for families about nutrition care.

Review development and use of algorithm and checklist with providers

Introduce a new form to encourage evidence-based review of nutritional status and enzyme use and determine decision-making criteria

Introduce a new algorithm for nutrition screening to decrease variance

Fig. 18.1 PDSA Ramp used with permission from Action Guide For Accelerating Improvement In Cystic Fibrosis Care, 2006

transformation of culture and care delivery. Benchmarking visits were conducted by the team to identify best practices. Additional dietitian staffing was added to the team in 2007 to facilitate effective and equitable care. Nutrition specific action plans, using PDSA cycles, were implemented to effect change. Although specific change ideas are not detailed in the manuscript, lessons learned at CCHMC during a decade of QI work can be found in Table 18.2.

Savant et al. describe sustained improvement in nutrition outcomes at two CF centers, the Ann and Robert Lurie Children's hospital of Chicago CF Center (Lurie Children's) and the University of Alabama at Birmingham CF Center/Children's Hospital of Alabama (UAB/COA) [9]. Both Lurie Children's and UAB/COA improved and sustained nutrition outcomes through implementation of CFF practice guidelines for CF nutrition management. Improvement was achieved through changes in the care delivery processes, nutrition interventions, team engagement, and data display. Specific nutrition interventions included a standardized clinic worksheet to assess patient data and a nutrition algorithm. The nutrition algorithm included increased visit frequency for patients who were determined to be at nutritional risk and individualized action plans for patients with inadequate nutritional status. Action plans focused on the specific needs of the patient included enzyme adjustment, increased caloric intake, and mealtime behaviors. Both centers also offered "dietitian only" visits to those patients with suboptimal nutritional status. With these changes significant improvements were made in mean clinic BMI at both centers. Lurie Children's mean BMI increased from 42.2% in 2002 to 54.4% in 2004. The mean clinic BMI has continued to be above the 50th percentile for 10 years. Similar improvements were seen at UAB/COA. In 2002 the mean BMI at UAB/COA was 37.2% and it increased to 44.2% by 2005. A mean BMI above 50th percentile has been maintained for 9 years at UAB/COA.

Leonard and colleagues implemented a standardized nutrition risk assessment and treatment protocol to improve nutrition outcomes [8]. A nutrition risk category, optimal, acceptable, concerning, risk or failure, was assigned at each clinic visit based on BMI, weight change, and linear growth (Fig. 18.2). The concerning category was developed to catch small changes in nutritional status before they developed into nutrition risk or failure. Patients in this category had a BMI above the 50th

Table 18.2 Lessons learned during a decade of quality improvement process

Lesson learned
1. Start with a project with an established baseline that is easy to measure and trend over time
2. Choose a project that is meaningful to both care team members and patients
3. Bring members to the team who are committed to the success of the project, including patients and families
4. Include formal training in QI, a QI coach and team members with dedicated time for QI work
5. Have regular meetings to review results and plan next steps

Reproduced Siracusa CM, et al. The impact of transforming healthcare delivery on cystic fibrosis outcomes: a decade of quality improvement at Cincinnati Children's Hospital. BMJ Qual Saf. 2014;23 Suppl 1:i56-i63. with permission from BMJ Publishing Group Ltd.

percentile but did not gain weight between clinic visits. The goal of this approach was to provide early intervention and more frequent follow-up in the hope of preventing a decline in nutritional status. Patients identified as "concerning," "nutrition risk," or "nutrition failure" were assessed using the treatment protocol. The protocol included assessment of caloric intake, nutrient absorption, and risk for cystic fibrosis related diabetes (CFRD). Based on the treatment protocol an individualized treatment plan, including more frequent follow-up, was developed with the patient and family. During the 15-month study period the median BMI percentile of the subjects improved from 37.8 (2006) to 42 (2007). Since the report the protocol has been adopted for the entire pediatric clinic (unpublished data). Median clinic BMI percentile has improved from 43 in 2006 to 50.7 in 2012 [12].

Some groups report improvements in nutritional outcomes as a result of QI work targeting the entire treatment plan [7, 38]. For example, Kraynack reports that as part of their QI initiative they identified and treated patients with and at risk for nutrition failure but did not elaborate on techniques or outcomes [7]. Arkansas Children's Hospital (ACH), as part of an LLC project, aimed to increase the percentage of patients with four or more outpatient visits, as recommended by CFF [38]. With this initiative they also noted an increase in BMI. It is possible that the more frequent visits led to better access to nutrition care. The group later developed a nutrition pathway to provide consistent nutrition support. The nutrition pathway included screening weight, length, and BMI to determine nutrition risk category and an individualized nutrition plan for at risk patients.

Although the majority of CF nutrition QI work is geared toward improving weight and BMI, some centers focus on other aspects of care that impact nutrition, such as screening for CFRD [8, 39]. The CHRISTUS Santa Rosa Children's Hospital CF Center focused improvement efforts on screening for CFRD [39]. They implemented a clinic based algorithm to improve compliance with oral glucose tolerance test (OGTT). The goal of the algorithm was to provide consistent parameters for ordering and interpreting OGTT results. During the 6-month study period there was a statistically significant improvement in screening with OGTT from 65 to 89%. However, in the year following the implementation of the algorithm, the completed OGTT rate fell to 79%, despite a high (97%) rate of physician ordering. The group suggests that barriers to compliance with OGTT need to be explored.

**The Johns Hopkins Cystic Fibrosis Center
Nutrition Algorithm: Nutrition Classification**

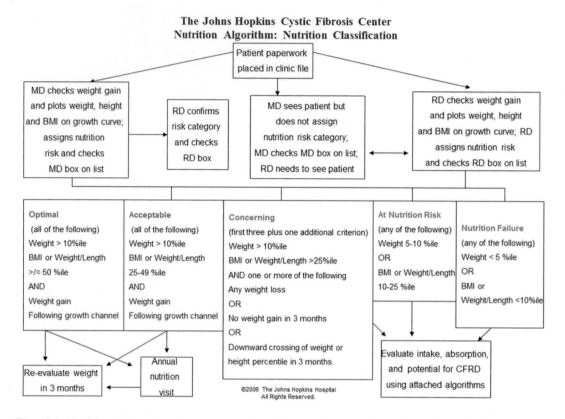

Fig. 18.2 Nutrition classification algorithm used from Leonard A, et al. Description of a standardized nutrition classification plan and its relation to nutritional outcomes in children with cystic fibrosis. J Pediatr Psychol. 2010;35: 6–13. by permission of Oxford University Press

Applying these concepts, as well as those from other QI projects has the potential to improve outcomes in CF. Although screening for nutritional status is a common first step in nutrition QI work, there is little published data about screening [40]. McDonald validated a nutrition risk screening tool for children and adolescents with CF ages 2–20 years. The tool assigns points based on weight gain, height velocity, and BMI and stratifies the patient into low, moderate, or high risk. The purpose of the quick screening is to standardize nutrition risk categorization and provide clinical direction for determining those individuals at nutrition risk who would benefit from more extensive medical nutrition therapy. Modifying currently available tools to fit your center population is also a useful approach.

There are concepts from QI work in other aspects of CF that can be applied to the nutrition arena as well. For example, the CF Center at Monmouth Medical Center had improvements in clinic pulmonary function outcomes with the Re-Education of Airway Clearance Techniques (REACT) program [41]. REACT focused on re-educating patients and families about the importance of, and approach to, airway clearance. Knowledge about airway clearance and barriers to adherence were also assessed. A similar education program could be used with nutrition topics including a knowledge assessment, identification of barriers to success, and re-education.

Conclusion

CF is a complex disease and care requires the interdependent cooperative work of patients, parents, families, and the health care professionals [22]. Quality improvement is a means to provide the best possible care and improve outcomes. There are a variety of quality improvement factors that have influenced CF care including patient registries, benchmarking, patient and family involvement, collaborative learning, effective data management, and a culture of improvement [3]. Although there is little published data about nutrition QI projects, many centers have worked in this area [6]. As QI work in this area continues, it will ideally lead to a culture of quality, with expectations of ongoing improvements in CF care and life expectancy.

References

1. McPheeters ML, Kripalani S, Peterson NB, Idowu RT, Jerome RN, Potter SA, Andrews JC. Closing the quality gap: revisiting the state of the science (vol. 3: quality improvement interventions to address health disparities). Evid Rep Technol Assess. 2012;208(3):1–475.
2. Berwick DM. The science of improvement. JAMA. 2008;12(299):1182–4.
3. Stevens DP, Marshall BC. A decade of healthcare improvement in cystic fibrosis: lessons for other chronic diseases. BMJ Qual Saf. 2014;23 Suppl 1:i1–2.
4. Kaplan HC, Brady PW, Dritz MC, et al. The influence of context on quality improvement success in healthcare: a systematic review of the literature. Milbank Q. 2010;88:500–59.
5. Crossing the quality chasm: a new health system for the 21st century: Institute of Medicine of the National Academies. National Academy Press: Washington, DC; 2001.
6. Schechter MS, Gutierrez HH. Improving the quality of care for patients with cystic fibrosis. Curr Opin Pediatr. 2010;22:296–301.
7. Kraynack NC, McBride JT. Improving care at cystic fibrosis centers through quality improvement. Semin Respir Crit Care Med. 2009;30:547–58.
8. Leonard A, Davis E, Rosenstein BJ, Zeitlin PL, et al. Description of a standardized nutrition classification plan and its relation to nutritional outcomes in children with cystic fibrosis. J Pediatr Psychol. 2010;35:6–13.
9. Savant AP, Britton LJ, Petren K, et al. Sustained improvement in nutritional outcomes at two paediatric cystic fibrosis centres after quality improvement collaboratives. BMJ Qual Saf. 2014;23 Suppl 1:i81–9.
10. Siracusa CM, Weiland JL, Acton JD, et al. The impact of transforming healthcare delivery on cystic fibrosis outcomes: a decade of quality improvement at Cincinnati Children's Hospital. BMJ Qual Saf. 2014;23 Suppl 1:i56–63.
11. Yen EH, Quinton H, Borowitz D. Better nutritional status in early childhood is associated with improved clinical outcomes and survival in patients with cystic fibrosis. J Pediatr. 2013;162:530–5.
12. Cystic Fibrosis Foundation Patient Registry. 2012 annual data report. Bethesda, MD: Cystic Fibrosis Foundation; 2012.
13. Marshall BC, Nelson EC. Accelerating implementation of biomedical research advances: critical elements of a successful 10 year Cystic Fibrosis Foundation healthcare delivery improvement initiative. BMJ Qual Saf. 2014;23 Suppl 1:i95–103.
14. Marshall BC, Penland CM, Hazle L, Ashlock M, Wetmore D, Campbell 3rd PW, Beall RJ. Cystic fibrosis foundation: achieving the mission. Respir Care. 2009;54:788–95. discussion 795.
15. Borowitz D, Baker RD, Stallings V. Consensus report on nutrition for pediatric patients with cystic fibrosis. J Pediatr Gastroenterol Nutr. 2002;35:246–59.
16. Stallings VA, Stark LJ, Robinson KA, et al. Clinical practice guidelines on growth and nutrition subcommittee. evidence-based practice recommendations for nutrition-related management of children and adults with cystic fibrosis and pancreatic insufficiency: results of a systematic review. J Am Diet Assoc. 2008;108:832–9.
17. Schechter MS, Fink AK, Homa K, et al. The cystic fibrosis foundation patient registry as a tool for use in quality improvement. BMJ Qual Saf. 2014;23 Suppl 1:i9–14.
18. Stern M, Bertrand DP, Bignamini E, et al. European cystic fibrosis society standards of care: quality management in cystic fibrosis. J Cyst Fibros. 2014;13 Suppl 1:S43–59.
19. Stern M. The use of a cystic fibrosis patient registry to assess outcomes and improve cystic fibrosis care in Germany. Curr Opin Pulm Med. 2011;17:473–7.

20. Wiedemann B, Steinkamp G, Sens B, et al. German cystic fibrosis quality assurance group. The German cystic fibrosis quality assurance project: clinical features in children and adults. Eur Respir J. 2001;17:1187–94.

21. James BC. The cystic fibrosis improvement story: we count our successes in lives. BMJ Qual Saf. 2014;23: 268–71.

22. Sabadosa KA, Batalden PB. The interdependent roles of patients, families and professionals in cystic fibrosis: a system for the coproduction of healthcare and its improvement. BMJ Qual Saf. 2014;23 Suppl 1:i90–4.

23. Warwick WJ, Pogue RE. Cystic fibrosis. An expanding challenge for internal medicine. JAMA. 1977;238: 2159–62.

24. Gutierrez HH, Sanchez I, Schidlow DV. Cystic fibrosis care in Chile. Curr Opin Pulm Med. 2009;15:632–7.

25. Antos NJ, Quintero DR, Walsh-Kelly CM, et al. Improving inpatient cystic fibrosis pulmonary exacerbation care: two success stories. BMJ Qual Saf. 2014;23 Suppl 1:i33–41.

26. Corey M, McLaughlin FJ, Williams M, et al. A comparison of survival, growth, and pulmonary function in patients with cystic fibrosis in Boston and Toronto. J Clin Epidemiol. 1998;41:583–91.

27. Boyle MP, Sabadosa KA, Quinton HB, et al. Key findings of the US cystic fibrosis foundation's clinical practice benchmarking project. BMJ Qual Saf. 2014;23 Suppl 1:i15–22.

28. Schechter MS. Benchmarking to improve the quality of cystic fibrosis care. Curr Opin Pulm Med. 2012;18: 596–601.

29. Britton LJ, Thrasher S, Gutierrez H. Creating a culture of improvement: experience of a pediatric cystic fibrosis center. J Nurs Care Qual. 2008;23:115–20.

30. Godfrey MM, Oliver BJ. Accelerating the rate of improvement in cystic fibrosis care: contributions and insights of the learning and leadership collaborative. BMJ Qual Saf. 2014;23 Suppl 1:i23–32.

31. Konstan MW, Butler SM, Wohl ME, et al. Investigators and coordinators of the epidemiologic study of cystic fibrosis. Growth and nutritional indexes in early life predict pulmonary function in cystic fibrosis. J Pediatr. 2003;142: 624–30.

32. McPhail GL, Acton JD, Fenchel MC, et al. Improvements in lung function outcomes in children with cystic fibrosis are associated with better nutrition, fewer chronic pseudomonas aeruginosa infections, and dornase alfa use. J Pediatr. 2008;153:752–7.

33. Steinkamp G, Wiedemann B. Relationship between nutritional status and lung function in cystic fibrosis: cross sectional and longitudinal analyses from the German CF quality assurance (CFQA) project. Thorax. 2002;57: 596–601.

34. Ferkol T, Rosenfeld M, Milla CE. Cystic fibrosis pulmonary exacerbations. J Pediatr. 2006;148:259–64.

35. Flume PA, Mogayzel Jr PJ, Robinson KA, et al. Clinical practice guidelines for pulmonary therapies committee. Cystic fibrosis pulmonary guidelines: treatment of pulmonary exacerbations. Am J Respir Crit Care Med. 2009;180: 802–8.

36. Action guide for accelerating improvement in cystic fibrosis. Cystic Fibrosis Foundation version 1. 2006.

37. Tiddens HA. Quality improvement in your CF centre: taking care of care. J Cyst Fibros. 2009;8 Suppl 1:S2–5.

38. Berlinski A, Chambers MJ, Willis L, et al. Redesigning care to meet national recommendation of four or more yearly clinic visits in patients with cystic fibrosis. BMJ Qual Saf. 2014;23 Suppl 1:i42–9.

39. Rayas MS, Willey-Courand DB, Lynch JL, et al. Improved screening for cystic fibrosis-related diabetes by an integrated care team using an algorithm. Pediatr Pulmonol. 2014;49:971–7.

40. McDonald CM. Validation of a nutrition risk screening tool for children and adolescents with cystic fibrosis ages 2–20 years. J Pediatr Gastroenterol Nutr. 2008;46:438–46.

41. Zanni RL, Sembrano EU, Du DT, et al. The impact of re-education of airway clearance techniques (REACT) on adherence and pulmonary function in patients with cystic fibrosis. BMJ Qual Saf. 2014;23 Suppl 1:i50–5.

Index

E.H. Yen, A.R. Leonard (eds.), *Nutrition in Cystic Fibrosis: A Guide for Clinicians*, Nutrition and Health, 265
DOI 10.1007/978-3-319-16387-1, © Springer International Publishing Switzerland 2015